ASHWORTH, P. M. 1973.
Cardiovascular disorders.

Cardiovascular Disorders

patient care

Cardiovascular Disorders

patient care

Pat M. Ashworth SRN SCM
Department Sister, Intensive Therapy Unit, Regional Cardiothoracic Centre, Broadgreen Hospital, Liverpool

Harry Rose SRN RFN RNT BTA
Principal Tutor, Broadgreen Hospital, Liverpool; Examiner, General Nursing Council for England and Wales

Foreword by

F. Ronald Edwards, MD FRCS
Consultant Cardiologist, United Liverpool Hospitals

Baillière Tindall · London

First published 1973

ISBN 0 7020 0420 0

Published in the United States of America by
the Williams and Wilkins Company, Baltimore.

Printed in Great Britain by
Cox & Wyman Ltd
London, Fakenham and Reading

Foreword

There has been a change in the pattern of nursing over recent years and the introduction of progressive patient care in various forms has resulted in the nurse being exposed in some part of her training to a high concentration of seriously ill patients. This varies particularly in cardiac disease where many patients, as a result of cardiac failure, coronary artery disease or surgery, require a standard of nursing care and surveillance that must be related to the fact that cardiac arrest may occur at any time. A doctor may not be immediately available, and the life of the patient will for a time depend upon the nurse's knowledge of the underlying condition and her ability to undertake the correct emergency treatment until help arrives. Apart from the management of the acutely ill cardiac patient, the realization that convalescence from severe cardiac disease is a prolonged process which is much helped by the attitude of the attending staff cannot be overemphasized.

Miss Ashworth and Mr Rose have combined in this book a valuable guide to those engaged in treating heart disease, in which very clear indications are given as to what should be done, how it is done and why it is done. All aspects of cardiac disease are covered with a full discussion on acquired and congenital conditions and disease of the coronary arteries. Miss Ashworth has drawn on her many years of practical experience in charge of a large intensive care ward and Mr Rose has contributed the more academic sections from his long experience as Senior Nursing Tutor.

One of the most valuable chapters is on the impact of heart disease, not only on the individual, but on the family. The social consequences of chronic illness can be immense and the handling of the various problems is succinctly presented.

This book has the advantage that it can be opened anywhere and the reader will receive composite information on the subject which he or she requires. This has resulted in a certain amount of repetition, but has enabled the requisite knowledge to be obtained rapidly.

The overall result is a volume which will be of great value to the reader, both for primary instruction, and also as a constant reference manual.

F. RONALD EDWARDS

Preface

This book is intended to help nurses understand and enjoy their work with patients suffering from cardiovascular diseases, be it in special units, in general wards or in the patient's own home, since this will encourage even better nursing care for the patient. It is designed for trained nurses working with these patients in all situations and for the more senior nurses working towards their final examinations and subsequent registration. With the advance of medical science and technology, medicine has become more and more specialized, and it is not surprising that nursing, too, tends to resolve into specialities; the specialist in cardiovascular nursing should also find this book helpful.

No doubt some nurses will wish to find information on a particular topic without needing to read through the whole book; each section has been written to facilitate this, although doing so has inevitably resulted in some repetition. In order that there should be a minimum of interruption while reading, descriptions of investigations, of the chemistry and haemodynamics in cardiovascular conditions and of the drugs used in treatment, are placed towards the end of the book; the reader can refer to them when necessary.

The incidence of cardiovascular disorders and their impact on the patient, the family and the community as a whole are examined in the first chapter, together with the response which each makes in its turn. These responses are common to all conditions and should be borne in mind as each condition is considered. Nursing is sometimes defined as 'attending to the physical, emotional and social needs of the patient'. The manner in which these needs may be attended to is discussed in relation to the pathology of the condition and the medical and surgical treatment. Where the cause can be identified, stress is placed on the part the nurse can play in its prevention.

Heart failure is probably the form in which most nurses first meet cardiovascular disease, so the chronic form is described early.

Next, considerable attention has been paid to the emergency care and treatment of a patient who has suffered cardiac arrest, with the subsequent care and attention required. Nursing the patient with coronary artery disease is then described, and it was felt appropriate to include here some notes on ECG monitoring with an oscilloscope.

Congenital heart conditions are then described, with the relevant treatment and care. This is followed by consideration of those conditions acquired after birth or which develop as the individual grows older; the possible medical and surgical treatments are indicated.

The preparations for an operation on the heart, the postoperative care and the recognition and treatment of the possible complications are described in some detail. Vascular conditions and operations are considered in a separate chapter.

Anatomy and physiology are used to introduce particular topics, to increase understanding or to clarify detail of the abnormality or treatment under discussion. It is assumed that the reader has a basic knowledge of these subjects.

Since specialized nursing is usually carried out in a special unit, the last chapter has been devoted to the cardiovascular unit in the hospital, with suggestions for in-service training and for the organization of a ward. The coronary care unit is described, as well as the principles of care in an intensive therapy unit. This chapter also includes a consideration of the ethics of performing those life-saving measures which the nurse in the unit may frequently encounter.

An increased understanding of any subject often stimulates the appetite for further related reading. Appended is a list of current books which may be found helpful. No one textbook can contain all the knowledge required by the 'cardiovascular nurse'.

We have received much help and inspiration from others. In particular we would like to thank Miss V. Jenkinson, with whom it all began; Dr C. Evans was most helpful with haemodynamics and electrolytes; Mr P. J. Molloy, now in Belfast, read and made useful comments on the chapters relating to cardiac and vascular surgery. We must also express our appreciation to the many other medical and nursing staff at Broadgreen Hospital, Liverpool, for the assistance they have so kindly given. We would also like to thank Mr F. Ronald Edwards for reading the script and writing a foreword; and we cannot forget Miss M. E. Williams, who typed and retyped the manuscript. Finally, our thanks to our publishers, Baillière Tindall, for their suggestions and help, and for their permission to reproduce illustrations from the following books: Figs 11 and 12A from *Anaesthetics for Nurses* (*Nurses' Aids Series*) by Joan Hobkirk; Figs 1, 2, 19, 54, 105 and 106 from *Anatomy and Physiology for Nurses* (*Nurses' Aids Series*) by K. F. Armstrong and S. Jackson; Figs 18, 26–37, 59, 60C and 65 from *Cardiology* (*Concise Medical Textbooks*) by D. G. Julian; Fig 4 from *Hutchison's Clinical Methods* by D. Hunter, R. R. Bomford and D. G. Pennington; Figs 21, 23, 25, 60A, B and 94 from *Nurses' Guide to Cardiac Monitoring* by Peter Hubner; and Figs 42, 47 and 72 from *Paediatric Nursing* (*Nurses' Aids Series*) by M. A. Duncombe and B. E. Weller.

Liverpool
September 1972

Pat M. Ashworth
Harry Rose

Contents

1
The impact of heart disease

Folk-lore and everyday colloquial expressions are an indication of the importance we attach to the heart and the blood. 'The heart of the matter' is the centre or hub of the topic under discussion around which everything else revolves; people are described as being stout-hearted, faint-hearted, hard-hearted, soft-hearted, and even big-hearted; emotions are registered in such expressions as 'my heart was in my mouth' and 'my heart stood still'; situations can 'pull on the heart strings', and of course most of us have come across the term 'broken-hearted'.

Throughout the ages blood has been regarded as an essential of life, and has sometimes been invested with magic or mysterious properties, as in the shedding of blood to appease the gods and the drinking of blood, especially of a valiant enemy, to increase physical or supernatural strength.

It can be easily understood how any disease of the heart and any loss or disorder of the blood is felt to be a threat to the existence of the individual. But individuals are members of larger groups—be it family, township, nation or the world as a whole — so cardiovascular disease affects not only the individual but also the community of which he is a member. We will look first at the extent of cardiovascular disease as shown by some national and international statistics.

The extent of heart disease

The total number of deaths in England and Wales during 1969 was 579 378. Of these diseases of the heart and blood vessels caused 214 029 deaths (37% of the total), with ischaemic heart disease causing 139 428 (23%) and cerebrovascular disease 79 728 (14%). In that year male deaths from coronary heart disease rose to

80 728, an increase of 1139 compared with 1968; female deaths from this cause (58 554) were marginally fewer. That deaths from cardiovascular disease in England and Wales are increasing can be seen from the annual report of the Chief Medical Officer of the Department of Health and Social Security, who gives the following figures under the heading 'deaths from arteriosclerotic heart disease including coronary thrombosis':

1946	32 847 deaths
1954	66 901 deaths
1964	106 290 deaths
1965	113 451 deaths

In 1968 the introduction of the International Classification of Disease made it possible to examine specifically the trends of morbidity by cause, and the following statistics are given:

	1966	*1967*	*1968*	*1969*
Ischaemic heart disease	130 113	129 204	138 617	139 428
Cerebrovascular disease	77 540	76 988	80 352	79 728

From the statistics quoted by the Chief Medical Officer there is undoubtedly an increase in deaths due to cardiovascular disease. At this point it is perhaps worth while to note that he stresses cigarette-smoking as a predisposing factor in cardiovascular disease.

The table issued by the World Health Organization listing death rates from arteriosclerotic and degenerative heart disease in the age group 45–54 years shows that between 1955 and 1967 there was a general increase in these rates, with the exception of the U.S.A., Japan and Switzerland.

In different countries there are different methods of diagnosis and classification, therefore it is wise to be cautious in making any comparison between countries; nevertheless, throughout the world an increase can be seen.

Not only is there an increase in the number of deaths, but there is a change in the age at which these deaths occur. Although the WHO figures cover the middle age groups, there is also an increase

Table 1. Death rates from arteriosclerotic and degenerative heart disease in the 45–54 age group

Country		*Death rate (per 100 000 inhabitants)* 1955	1960	1966	1967	*Changes (%)* 1967/55
Australia	Total	159·8	182·4	203·9	204·6	+28
	Male	247·0	287·0	324·4	325·0	+32
	Female	65·2	71·9	81·3	82·1	+26
Austria	Total	72·4	83·3	80·8	88·6	+22
	Male	113·9	144·7	147·1	165·7	+45
	Female	37·1	34·7	31·9	32·2	−13
Canada	Total	171·6	191·5	185·9	187·4	+ 9
	Male	277·0	307·6	312·0	314·7	+14
	Female	59·0	69·0	59·3	6·50	+ 3
		(1956)				
Czecho-slovakia	Total	74·1	76·8	93·9	101·3	+37
	Male	114·1	127·2	159·7	178·1	+56
	Female	36·5	29·3	32·3	29·7	−19
Federal Republic of Germany	Total	90·0	97·3	107·6	102·3	+14
	Male	134·2	159·5	186·5	179·7	+34
	Female	51·9	48·5	49·7	46·0	−11
Finland	Total	173·8	186·1	226·1	244·7	+41
	Male	305·8	340·1	436·7	468·6	+53
	Female	59·2	53·4	51·4	60·1	+ 2
France	Total	30·3	40·2	42·1	41·7	+38
	Male	49·2	67·8	73·3	72·4	+47
	Female	12·0	13·5	12·2	12·2	+ 2
Hungary	Total	84·5	91·7	104·1	111·2	+32
	Male	109·2	119·2	148·5	160·7	+47
	Female	61·9	67·2	65·3	67·9	+10
Italy	Total	69·7	75·7	78·0	78·9	+13
	Male	97·2	114·7	125·1	127·5	+31
	Female	43·6	38·8	34·2	34·0	−22

Table 1. *continued*

Country		*Death rate (per 100 000 inhabitants)* 1955	1960	1966	1967	*Changes (%)* 1967/55
Japan	Total	53·6	45·7	39·2	39·1	−27
	Male	58·3	52·9	51·5	50·4	−14
	Female	49·0	39·1	28·9	29·9	−39
Netherlands	Total	69·9	73·3	98·0	106·9	+53
	Male	115·1	128·7	173·7	191·2	+66
	Female	27·2	20·9	25·6	26·2	− 4
Sweden	Total	69·5	69·4	76·5	79·7	+15
	Male	106·9	108·3	125·7	133·7	+25
	Female	32·5	30·1	26·8	25·4	−22
Switzerland	Total	78·0	79·3	85·7	75·9	− 3
	Male	117·1	124·7	135·8	126·2	+ 8
	Female	41·8	33·9	37·1	27·3	−35
England and Wales	Total	109·1	121·2	144·5	140·9	+29
	Male	181·3	208·3	248·0	244·0	+35
	Female	40·1	37·6	44·6	41·6	+ 4
United States of America	Total	210·6	216·0	215·7	211·8	+ 1
	Male	342·2	358·5	357·7	351·8	+ 3
	Female	82·2	78·2	81·9	80·3	− 2
Venezuela	Total	97·5	118·6	96·7	102·1	+ 5
	Male	127·3	158·1	126·8	139·6	+10
	Female	65·1	75·1	65·2	61·7	− 5

Figures issued by the World Health Organization (1969).

in the number of those under 40 years who are falling victim to fatal heart disease. This means that many of the people at risk are the fathers and breadwinners in families where there are young children, and they are also those whose contribution to the nation's economy, both as worker and taxpayer, is important. Cardiovascular degenerative disease tends to occur 10–15 years earlier in men than it does in women; it is thought that in some way women are protected by their female hormones.

The effects of heart disease

The effect of heart disease can be seen in the individual, both physically and psychologically, in the family and in society as a whole.

The individual

The individual will experience the symptoms associated with his particular condition, and he will need to curtail his activities, both physical and mental, so that his way of life and enjoyment of it will not be quite the same as that of a healthy person. Each age group will have its own special problems and must make its own adjustments both in individual activities and in relationships with others.

Any infant is dependent upon its parents, but an infant with a heart condition will be even more so, and will need more protection. The doctor will discuss with the parents the child's incapacity and the limits of activity within which an attempt should be made to keep him. Some children are self-limiting, in that they find their level of tolerance and do not go beyond it, but there is always the possibility that other children may entice them on to further and possibly harmful activity. The feelings and reactions of the parents may vary: some can accept the situation with equanimity, others may become somewhat despondent. They may be impatient for a cure and not accept the explanations of the doctor, but rather seek an alternate medical opinion in order to have the child treated earlier than advised. Some may pretend that the child is not really incapacitated and force it beyond endurance.

On the other hand, there may be a tendency for the parents to do too much for the child, preventing him from taking part in those activities that are within his capacity. They may never allow him to play with other children, or even to walk and run about, for fear he should become excited. Occasionally parents may confine a child to rest in a room, not allowing other members of the family to disturb him. Sometimes special foods and toys may be bought, which the family can ill afford. Too much attention is paid to him and every whim is attended to. The child grows up overdependent on its parents, afraid to leave them or be separated from them, and also unable to make contact and happy relationships with other children or even with adults. Any tendency for underprotection or overprotection should be guarded against. Problems are not always easy to detect, but if suspected the doctor, health visitor, children's welfare officer or nurse should explain the child's condition to the parents and advise on the best ways of helping him.

The school child needs intellectual and emotional stimulus and contact with other children, and will often be involved in the rough and tumble of play. While children may sometimes appear cruel and oppressive in the play group, they can also be understanding and assign a more passive role to companions with heart disorders. Parents should inform the teachers of the limits of the child's activity, so that the teacher can take special care and foster his growth without appearing to show any special favour. The school nurse and the school medical officer should be informed of the child's condition, and the school welfare officer may visit the parents and the home in order to help where possible. In some areas special arrangements are made to transport handicapped children to school, and the child whose physical activities are curtailed by a heart condition may be able to take advantage of them. Liaison between parent, school nurse, teacher and welfare officer is most important.

Adolescence is a period with its own special difficulties, the child gradually awakening to the wider aspects of life as well as undergoing the normal changes of puberty; he begins to adjust to the reality of the world and to leave the shelter of parental protection. As he grows up he should be guided by the doctor, nurse, parent and any other person from whom advice will be taken, about the effects of exercise, growth and the metabolic changes through which his body is going, so that he may be able to regulate his activities in relation to his illness. This may be difficult for him for it is a time when his friends, colleagues and peers are often joining in more and harder physical group projects away from home. The adolescent with a heart condition is tempted to participate but risks overtaxing his strength; but there is also the opposite danger, that he may shun the company of his own age group and become a lonely and unfulfilled youth. This may lead to an overdependence on his parents. Life may be further complicated by the need to find work—work which will not only fulfil his aspirations, but also be suited to his limited physical abilities. There will indeed be a great need for understanding on the part of his parents and of his peers, and guidance at this time will need to be positive yet acceptable as well as wise.

The young adult will no doubt desire to marry and bring up children, but before doing so he would be wise to discuss the situation with his future wife (or a girl with her husband) so that they can prepare together for the future, and, of course, they would be wise to discuss this with their family doctor.

When a heart condition develops during adult life, the reaction may be great. The patient may not be able to enjoy life as he had previously and thus will need to seek other, probably quieter, forms of activity. A man may not be able to work and support his family, or even himself. A mother may not be able to care for her children and needs to lean heavily upon the husband. Either may experience a feeling of inadequacy and become depressed; there may be anxiety too, and fear for the future of both self and family. There may be a tendency to overcompensate by an exaggerated independence, doing even more physical activity and refusing help, an unwarrantable euphoria pervading all; on the other hand there may be a tendency for the patient to do less than he is capable of and thus to develop an overdependence upon others which, in turn, may put a strain upon the family and upon family relationships.

Relationships with children may need to be physically more passive but, although the parent may not be able to romp and run, he will still be able to encourage the children's play and guide their growth and general development.

The doctor will explain the condition to the patient and to his wife (or in the case of a woman, her husband), indicating the extent of activity permissible. The health visitor and social worker can advise about the social assistance available. The patient is encouraged to do as much as he can, seeking ways which, while within his limitations, will help to maintain his personal dignity and prevent him from feeling too much of a responsibility to his family.

During middle age, when there is a greater risk of heart disease, especially among men, the onset of heart disease is an even greater blow. Often sudden and unexpected, it interferes with the pattern of life. Although most patients are able to make the appropriate changes in the manner of living, and are able to arrange adjustments in their work, accepting the 'warning' of the sudden attack, there are others who tend to resist this need. The family, the nurses and the advisors may feel their efforts are in vain, but they must patiently seek every opportunity to encourage the patient to rest and to take things easy.

The elderly often accept a diagnosis of heart disease with greater calm than do the young. Perhaps it is because they develop a philosophical outlook often expressed as 'one has to die of something'. Nevertheless, by taking all the appropriate precautions and following medical advice, they can, and do, live to an old age. Patients and those caring for them must all remember the patient's need to take part in physical and mental activity to the fullest extent possible and to retain a feeling of independence.

The family

The effect on the family of having someone with heart disease will vary. Some families tend to make great efforts to help; brothers, sisters, older parents and children usually give some assistance. Having in the family a patient who suffers from heart disease is often a cohesive force, binding together members of the family who might otherwise fail to contribute to the family well-being. There may be a fear that the condition is familial, in which case each member should seek medical advice about his own condition. Other families may tend to reject the unfortunate sufferer or regard him as a burden, and every effort must be made to bring about a change in this attitude; unfortunately in some cases it does become necessary to find an alternative place for the patient to live. There may be a tendency for the family to overprotect the patient, insisting upon doing for him those things which he could really do for himself, fussing over him and getting unduly anxious when he does not appear as well as usual. Those visiting, such as the doctor, health visitor, community nurse and welfare workers, will be aware of these possibilities and will look out for them.

Each patient presents individual problems and these may vary with the severity and the stage of the condition. Advice and guidance need to be adapted to the individual's condition as well as to the total situation.

The community

The effect of heart disease on the community is less readily seen. For every day away from work there is a corresponding loss of production of work. An indication of the amount of time lost through cardiovascular disease can be gained from a study of the causes of incapacity shown on certificates for National Insurance sickness benefits. In 1968 the total number of days lost through arteriosclerotic and degenerative heart disease was 17 million; for men, this was a 50% increase since 1958. Under the heading of other diseases of the circulatory system there was also an increase, albeit less dramatic: but from these statistics, there is undoubtedly a considerable loss of time from cardiovascular disease, and this time and type of disease is increasing.

One important effect of the presence of cardiovascular disease and the suffering it causes is that the community has taken steps to treat it, to alleviate the suffering it causes and to prevent it.

With modern advances in drug therapy, anaesthesia, surgery, resuscitation techniques and special facilities such as coronary or intensive therapy units, it is now possible to restore to a full and useful life not only children born with abnormal hearts, but also many of those who acquire cardiovascular disease later in life. Nurses have a vital part to play in the cardiac team, and they are taking on new and greater responsibilities as they fulfil, in the modern age, their traditional role to 'heal sometimes, to relieve often and to comfort always'.

Since the development of closed cardiac massage by Kouwenhoven and his colleagues in the United States in 1960, it has been possible for nurses to restore both circulation and respiration and so to keep the patient alive until the arrival of medical help. Thus a nurse is often the first person to start the modern miracle of bringing back to life someone whose vital functions have ceased.

Services for the cardiac patient

Heart disease causes physical suffering which is alleviated to a very great extent by the doctors and nurses who care for the patient. It also has other effects which, to the patient, may be a greater source of worry than is his physical condition—worries about his work, his family and his life in society as a whole. Quite often his physical condition prevents his solving by himself the problems which arise, so he may turn to the doctor or to the nurse for guidance. The nurse must be familiar with the resources available in the community, and in view of her knowledge of his condition and her insight into his needs and by using her ingenuity she may be able to assist in creating conditions which the patient might find helpful in the fulfilment of his needs.

Communities differ, be they countries, towns or neighbourhoods, but there are usually some means by which assistance can be obtained. These may have arisen from governmental action and legislation, as are provided by the Department of Health and Social Security in England through the hospital boards or the health and social services of the Local Authorities. They may be organizations to which the patient belongs as a form of insurance, or as a voluntary body on a national or local scale whose aim is to assist those in need of help.

Social workers are trained to help individuals and families with personal and social problems and to make full use of the range of social services available. The medical social worker assists with problems connected with illness, and which, being a source of anxiety to the patient, may hinder his recovery. She makes a careful study of the patient's illness and his personal and social background, and discusses with the doctor and nurse those factors which may be relevant to treatment and after-care. The problems may be of work, income or housing, all of which play an important part in the care of the patient. The medical social worker knows the statutory as well as the voluntary agencies available to assist the patient. Her professional skill and understanding are used to help the patient deal with any difficulty in his personal life, or to make necessary social changes in order that he may benefit from treatment.

The patient's condition may necessitate a reduction in physical activity and a consequent reduction in the amount of work he can do, with a change of job to one of a lighter nature or even one involving no physical work at all. In some types of employment it may be possible for someone suffering from heart disease to work shorter hours or to change his type of work, and as soon as there is an indication that the patient may later be able to work again, even in a different capacity, the employer should be approached. Some employers run their own retraining schemes for sick and handicapped employees. Alternatively, if the patient must leave his job, he may be able to benefit from rehabilitation services or from the Disablement Resettlement Service of the Department of Employment. The medical social worker will explore these avenues quite early; the sooner the patient can be given some reassurance as to his future work and income, the sooner he will be able to relax and obtain full benefit from his treatment and care.

When the patient is unable to work he may have no means of earning enough money to provide for himself and for his family. He will most probably qualify for some financial assistance from national insurance schemes such as the Social Security sickness benefits, or from other insurance schemes either at work or as a private arrangement, or from organizations such as 'penny in the pound' or sickness funds which provide money in time of illness and incapacity to work. Some employers pay a part or even the whole of a patient's salary for a period of time. Charitable institutions may donate financial grants in individual circumstances. All these sources should be tapped in order to alleviate financial hardship.

The occupational therapist might be able to teach the patient light crafts, such as needlework, leatherwork or basketry, which would relieve the patient of the boredom and frustration of enforced idleness, and which might at the same time bring in a little in the way of finance.

There is the possibility that the house in which the patient lives may be so built that he cannot easily move from one part to another because of long corridors or stairs. It might be ideal for the patient to find another house, or alternatively it might be possible to make changes such as removing walls, installing lifts and putting bathroom, bedroom and living-room all on the same floor. However, provision of alternative housing, or alteration to existing accommodation for those suffering from heart disease, is not always easy. There may not be an alternative house, or even if there is the patient may not find it convenient to move because of family ties or other limiting circumstances. Changes in the structure of a house may be expensive, and indeed, if the patient is only the tenant, such changes may not meet with the approval of the landlord. The social worker should be asked to make enquiries into the circumstances before such advice is given.

For the patient who is ill at home, assistance from the Community Nursing Services should be sought; the District (Home) Nurse comes to give nursing care, and the Health Visitor to give advice and to act as liaison with the other social workers and social services.

The housewife may require assistance in caring for the house and family. Sometimes some members of the immediate family may be able to provide this. Otherwise the social worker may be able to arrange for a home help to assist with the housework and the shopping. She may be able to arrange for children to attend a nursery, and for assistance with the laundry. Sometimes a period of convalescence or holiday can be arranged. Special services may be provided as part of the arrangements for the care of the disabled and handicapped and for which the patient with heart disease may qualify. In Great Britain a register of handicapped people is maintained by each Local Authority.

Voluntary bodies such as the Red Cross Society, the Fellowship of the Chest and Heart Association and the Women's Royal Voluntary Service usually have means of helping those who are ill or handicapped, and much worth while help is given by youth organizations in sitting with helpless patients, decorating rooms and taking for an outing those who find it difficult to leave the house. The Health Visitor and the Social Worker will know how to put the patient in contact with them.

While the patient suffering from heart disease is in hospital it is essential for the nurse caring for him to remember the social facilities available. The patient may be worried about his or her immediate condition, but one can be certain that there will be considerable anxiety as to what the future holds, the man thinking of the financial support for his wife and family and the woman of her possible inability to care for her husband, children and home. At the earliest opportunity the nurse should introduce the medical social worker to the patient and to the wife or husband as well. She can then look into the patient's and the family's needs during the period of hospitalization. If they can be attended to, the patient will feel reassured and be able to settle down. Similarly, before discharge, the medical social worker, acting as liaison with the community services, can make arrangements for the return home, and set in motion the arrangements for rehabilitation and re-adjustment to life outside the hospital. The nurse should contact the Community Nursing Services regarding the need for further nursing and advice after the patient goes home. The doctor from the hospital will inform the patient's doctor at home of his condition, the treatment carried out, the prognosis and any special recommendations for the continuation of treatment. He will most probably discuss some aspects of these with the patient and his family. If all these arrangements are made before the patient goes home the future will not look so bleak. With assurance that preparations have been made and that assistance is available, the patient can be discharged with that self-confidence and calmness so necessary for those with cardiovascular disease.

Causes and prevention

Heart disease does indeed cause considerable upset to the patient, his family and the community in general. It is not surprising therefore that steps are being taken to ascertain the causes of this disease and, where possible, prevent its occurrence.

Causes

A considerable amount of research is being carried out into the actual causes of cardiovascular conditions and how they might be prevented, in hospital, research units and other institutions. The cost of this may be met out of government funds, but it is often carried out as a result of donations from private individuals, companies or foundations. Particular mention might be made of the British Heart Foundation and the Chest and Heart Association, both voluntary bodies in the United Kingdom. Not only do they sponsor research, but they also publish pamphlets and hold meetings for those suffering, for nurses, doctors and social workers and for the families who are caring for them.

It is worth while remembering that the main factors aggravating cardiovascular disease are our social habits and that much of the suffering and the financial burden need not happen if there were a change in the way of life currently considered normal by many people.

A working group set up by the WHO on Epidemiological Studies in Ischaemic Heart Disease (report number Euro 5011, London, December 1968) gave smoking habits as the main cause. Cigarette-smoking causes harm directly by its vasoconstrictor effect and indirectly by the damage it does to the lungs. A more recent publication (*Nature, London,* June 1971) suggests that expectant mothers who smoke cigarettes are likely to have children suffering from heart disease. Obesity is also believed to be a major contributory factor, and obesity follows overeating and lack of exercise. Thus two of the most common social habits in western society, cigarette-smoking and overeating, are seen to be the two most common factors contributing to cardiovascular disease.

Hypertension also predisposes to cardiovascular disease. It is suggested that hypertension may result from environmental stress and from dietary factors. In western society, where cardiovascular disease is most commonly seen, it is often considered normal that the blood pressure should rise with advancing age, yet this is not so in people who live a less sophisticated life. It has been shown (for example, WHO November 1969) that among the nomads of Northern Kenya the blood pressure does not rise with age, but, when young men from these tribes join the Kenya Army, it rises within the first two years.

Infections such as rubella in women during the first 8–12 weeks of pregnancy may result in congenital heart disease. There is the possibility of a similar effect from taking some drugs during the same period, although as soon as such drugs are suspected they are withdrawn from circulation.

Prevention

Prevention of cardiovascular disease, so widespread and so serious, is equally as important as treatment. A considerable amount of time, effort and money is being spent on health education and the removal of those factors predisposing to these diseases, by governments, health educationists and by voluntary bodies. Again, the work of the British Heart Foundation and of the Chest and Heart Association is worthy of mention, through the meetings they sponsor, and the pamphlets they publish. Doctors participate both in their private capacity and as members of the associations. The British Medical Association publishes useful booklets in the *Family Doctor* series.

Nurses are health teachers and as such are able to make a considerable contribution. All over the world nurses come into contact with people with whom they can talk informally, be it in the hospital, the clinic, the works surgery or the home. Each occasion is an opportunity to point out the dangers of cigarette-smoking and obesity, and the value of a balanced health-giving diet and adequate exercise. The avoidance of emotional stress can be a more difficult subject, but in this the nurse helps by her calm manner, her undisturbed appearance and her fine grasp of essentials. Another opportunity to extol the need and the means of preventing heart disease is when the nurse is invited to speak on health matters in schools, institutes or other public meetings. Many nurses are parents and can give good advice and example to their children. In some way or other, all nurses come into contact with young people, who often need to be brought to understand that cigarette-smoking and overeating over a long period can be dangerous, just as dangerous as drug addiction, and that once acquired the habit can be just as difficult to break. Each nurse is an individual with her own sphere of influence; people take notice not only of what she says but also of what she does. Her deeds as well as her words will be taken as an example of healthy living.

2
Heart failure

The heart

The heart is a pump. A pump is a mechanism which takes fluid from one point and delivers it to another. As blood arrives in the great veins it is transferred through the heart to the arteries. By means of this transfer, the great veins are prevented from getting over-full and a supply of blood is ensured through the arteries to the tissues and organs of the body.

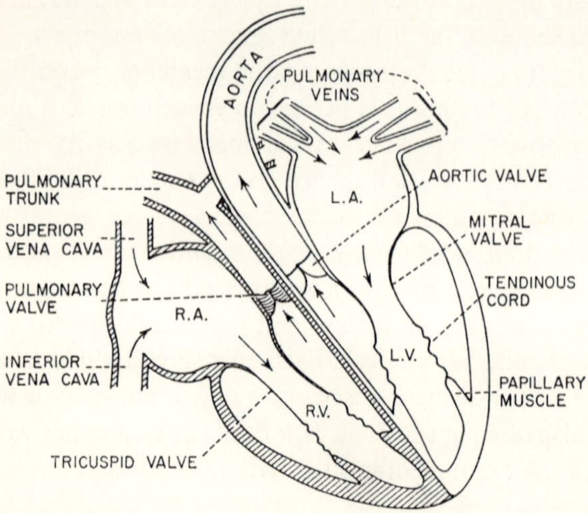

Fig 1. The structure of the heart.
L.A., Left atrium. L.V., Left ventricle. R.A., Right atrium. R.V., Right ventricle.

Having a left and right side, the heart is a double pump. Each side consists of an atrium or receiving chamber, through which the blood passes or waits until it can pass into the ventricle or discharging/pumping chamber (Fig. 1). Between the atria and the ventricles lie the atrioventricular valves (the mitral on the left and the tricuspid on the right), the purpose of which is to prevent blood passing back from the ventricle into the atrium, and between the ventricles and the great arteries lie valves consisting of three semilunar cusps (the aortic on the left and the pulmonary on the right), the purpose of which is to prevent blood from returning to the ventricle once it has been ejected into the artery. In this way the flow of blood is maintained in one direction only.

The muscle in the walls of the atria is thinner than that in the walls of the ventricles. This is understandable when it is remembered that the contraction of the atria is only to propel blood into the ventricles when the latter are already almost full, and thus to cause a small increase in the volume and pressure of the blood in the ventricle prior to the beginning of ventricular contraction. The muscle of the left ventricle is thicker than that of the right; whereas the left ventricle has to pump blood under great pressure into the arteries supplying the whole of the body, the right ventricle has to pump it only into the pulmonary arteries and lungs at a relatively lower pressure, as the pulmonary artery soon divides into short thin-walled arterioles, which offer only limited resistance to the flow of blood.

The failing heart

A pump loses its efficiency when its active force is insufficient to overcome the resistance set up either by a narrow outlet or by the pressure of the fluid on the other side. It is not completely efficient if the valve leaks, allowing fluid to flow back into the vessel from which it was intended to move it. Similarly, the heart becomes inefficient if the muscle loses its power to move blood onward or when the valves are incompetent and some of the blood flows back into the chamber which it has just left.

Acute heart failure

In some patients the onset of heart failure may be acute, the heart suddenly being unable to deliver sufficient quantities of blood to the tissues. This happens when there is death of myocardium due to an infarct; when there is interference with its activity, as in tamponade, and the compression within the pericardial sac prevents the ventricle from filling; in injury to the heart, when blood is ejected through a hole in the heart wall rather than through the appropriate valve; when the muscle is being poisoned, as in the toxaemia of diphtheria; when there is mechanical obstruction to the flow of blood, as in the presence of a blood clot too big to pass through the valve and in pulmonary oedema; and when the lungs are too congested to allow the entry of more blood. The patient

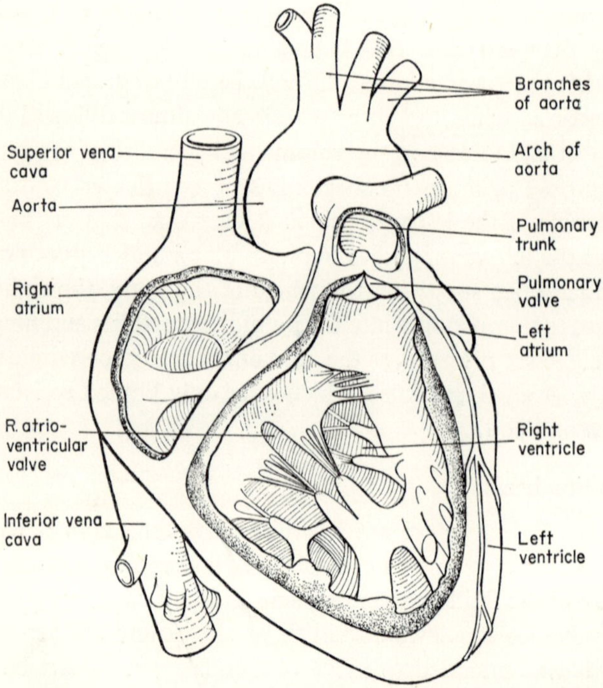

FIG 2. **The structures of the right side of the heart.**

may die suddenly or show the signs and symptoms of acute circulatory failure, due to cardiogenic shock, such as pallor, tachycardia, low blood pressure, cool clammy skin, weakness, oliguria, peripheral cyanosis and mental confusion. Treatment is urgent; an account of the emergency measures required will be found in Chapter 3.

Chronic heart failure

In other patients the onset of heart failure is more insidious. When some condition prevents the heart from performing its function of transferring blood from the veins to the arteries, the heart itself attempts to overcome the deficiency. Whilst it is able to make good the deficiency it is said to be 'compensating'. When the tissues are receiving insufficient blood a series of reflexes take place (described in Chapter 11) in order to bring about a better distribution of blood.

One such reflex is an increase in the rate at which the heart beats (tachycardia), which thus increases the cardiac output. However, the more frequent contraction will necessitate a greater consumption of oxygen. In tachycardia the time required for systole is the same as when at rest, but the time for diastole is reduced, thus the time for replenishment of the energy sources in the heart is reduced. The myocardium will become fatigued and unable to compensate, and eventually may even stop beating.

When the heart or one of its chambers cannot pass on its contents, some blood remains inside. Blood continues to come in from the venous side, but, as the chamber is never emptied it gradually distends due to the excess quantity of blood inside. At first this stretching of the muscle fibres brings a more forceful systole. After sometime it is unable to contract so forcefully and may become so weak as to allow permanent dilatation of the chamber, or even of the whole heart. However, as the chamber increases in size it tends to become chronically distended during diastole and requires an increased effort and increased amount of oxygen to bring about contraction in an attempt to empty it.

As a result of the stronger contractions made in order to empty the chamber and to push the blood onwards, the heart muscle enlarges (hypertrophy). Sometimes the wall of one chamber hypertrophies, or it may be that the whole heart does so. The size of the enlarged heart may be seen on X-ray of the chest, and also there may result a displacement from its normal anatomical position, e.g. the apex may be located more laterally than usual. The normal apex beat can be found by feeling with the finger or listening through a stethoscope placed near the left nipple or under the left breast in the fifth intercostal space about 7 cm from midline, and within the mid-clavicular line (Fig. 3). No additional fibres grow, but the existing ones become thicker. At first the thickening strengthens the contraction of the fibre and the total effect is to enable the heart to compensate. Unfortunately the fibres become so thickened that they press on the blood vessels supplying the myocardium, eventually interfering with its oxygen supply, the contractions become weaker and the heart is then said to be failing. There is also a tendency for the hypertrophied fibres to be

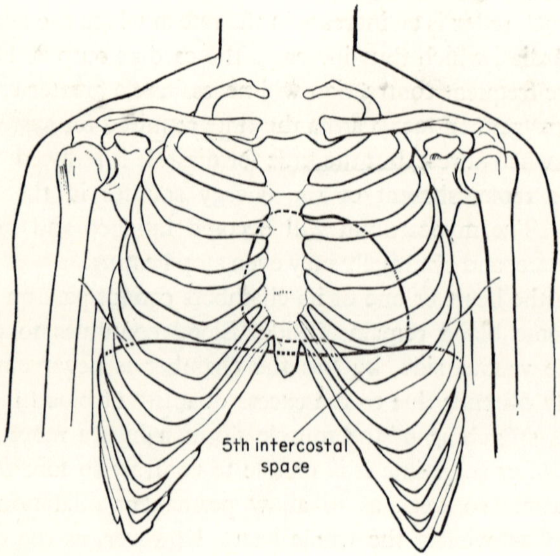

FIG 3. The position of the apex of the heart in the fifth intercostal space, about 7 cm left of the midline.

replaced by fatty infiltration and fibrous tissue, thus reducing the amount of muscle available for contraction.

Congestive heart failure

Blood entering the heart from the great veins is transferred through to the arteries leaving it. Sometimes the amount of incoming venous blood is too great for the heart to pass on. As more and more blood arrives it accumulates in the veins, and pressure within the veins rises. The high venous pressure causes a rise in pressure at the venous end of the capillary and oedema occurs in the tissues (see Chapter 10); the tissues or organs are then said to be congested. When the left side of the heart fails, the pressure rises in the pulmonary veins, and in right-sided failure the pressure rises in the systemic veins. The high venous pressure and congestion and oedema in the tissues and organs are often the cause of the features of chronic heart failure. When congestion occurs as a result of heart failure, the term congestive heart failure is often used.

The congestion in the veins due to heart failure is further aggravated by an increase in the total blood volume due to the retention of sodium and water by the kidney. The reason for this retention is not fully known; one theory is that, owing to a poor supply of blood to the kidney resulting from the heart failing, there is a diminished filtration in the glomerulus of the nephron. There seems to be little doubt that a greater part is due to increase in the reabsorption of sodium and water in the uriniferous tubule. In patients with advanced heart failure there is an increase in the secretion of aldosterone which, by its action on the distal part of the tubule, promotes further reabsorption of sodium. It is also suggested that a poor supply of blood to the brain causes an increased secretion of antidiuretic hormone which in turn brings about reabsorption of yet more water by the tubules. It is as if the body attempts to make adjustments for a low cardiac output by increasing the blood volume, not realizing that when the blood volume is really sufficient, an increase only leads to congestion.

Although both sides of the heart may fail together, either side alone may fail, and it is possible to consider right- and left-sided heart failure separately. It should be remembered that failure on one side of the heart may entail more vigorous attempts to compensate by the other side, and that this in turn may lead to failure of both sides.

For example, let us examine the process of heart failure following mitral stenosis. The narrowed mitral valve interferes with the easy flow of blood from the left atrium to the left ventricle. The left atrium does not completely empty, and the residual blood in addition to the incoming blood leads to a rise in pressure. The wall of the atrium hypertrophies and tends to distend. Blood from the pulmonary veins cannot easily enter the atrium, so the pressure in these veins rises and congestion in the lungs ensues, producing the symptoms of left-sided heart failure. As the lungs are congested the right ventricle needs to pump more forcefully to push the blood through them. It in turn hypertrophies, becomes distended with blood and fails. The blood in the right atrium, unable to enter the right ventricle, impedes the flow of blood from the venae cavae. Congestion occurs in the large veins from the head and from other organs and tissues of the body, producing the symptoms of right-sided heart failure. In this example, right-sided failure followed left-sided failure.

Left-sided heart failure

Left-sided heart failure may occur as a result of damaged heart muscle, when the heart muscle has been replaced by fibrous tissue or when the muscle is necrosed, as in coronary artery disease. It also occurs in hypertension, especially when due to arteriosclerotic disease, and in aortic valve disease such as aortic stenosis.

Right-sided heart failure

Right-sided heart failure also occurs as a result of damaged heart muscle. It follows pulmonary valve stenosis. As already described, it may follow left-sided failure, e.g. due to mitral stenosis. It can also occur as a result of lung conditions such as pulmonary embolism and chronic bronchitis. A particular form of heart failure following upon lung disease is known as cor pulmonale.

When a patient's heart is failing, it is failing not only to provide an adequate supply of blood to the tissues and organs, but also to transfer blood from the veins to the arteries, thus allowing the pressure of the blood in the veins to rise. It is worth remembering this because, clinically, the symptoms which arise are more often than not caused by the rise in venous pressure and the congestion of the tissues and organs, rather than by their not receiving an adequate blood supply.

Symptoms

As the symptoms occur they are usually indicative of whichever side of the heart is failing. At first they may be few, and at rest there may be none, although the patient may notice that at the end of the day he feels more tired than he used to. In left-sided heart failure he may notice that he gets short of breath on exertion but that it passes when he rests for a while. The dyspnoea may increase and may occur more frequently; eventually it is present when the patient lies flat, the use of more pillows making breathing easier. At this stage he may be coughing, especially at night, producing a sticky frothy sputum; there may be some blood in the sputum or it may look pink. Some patients experience attacks of dyspnoea at night; such attacks require urgent treatment. The condition is often referred to as paroxysmal nocturnal dyspnoea or cardiac asthma and will be considered later in this chapter.

In right-sided heart failure the patient may notice that towards the end of the day his feet and ankles swell, but that this disappears when he has been lying down for a short time. Actually the oedema does not really disappear, but the fluid is distributed to a more central part of the circulation. As the condition progresses the amount of fluid retained in the tissues increases and he notices that he is putting on weight. The oedema affects the legs and thighs and, when he sits for a long time, occurs round the sacrum; it becomes noticeable in any dependent part of the body. The abdomen begins to distend due to the presence of ascites, and the patient may also attribute this to putting on weight. The liver becomes congested and enlarged, so he may complain of pain over the right hypochondrium and find it tender to touch. Liver function may be intefered with and sometimes mild jaundice may be present. Other abdominal organs become congested, leading to nausea, anorexia, indigestion and flatulence. Pleural effusion (hydrothorax) may compress the lungs, making breathing somewhat difficult. There may be insomnia and in later stages the patient may become confused.

Signs

On examining the patient, note should be taken of the degree of dyspnoea, of whether the patient obtained relief by sitting up, of any tendency to cough and, if productive, of the nature and amount of sputum, including any signs of haemoptysis.

The presence and distribution of cyanosis would be observed, whether peripheral, central or both. In peripheral cyanosis the congestion in the veins causes the blood to flow slowly through the tissues, there is excessive reduction in oxyhaemglobin, the extremities become cyanosed and cold, but the mucous membranes of the tongue remain unaffected. It is usually indicative of right-sided failure. Central cyanosis characteristically affects the tongue. It results from inadequate oxygenation in the lungs due to left heart failure and lung disease and intracardiac shunts. The cyanosis may be generalized, in which case the cyanosed extremities are warm. In heart failure the cyanosis is often mixed, due to peripheral and to central causes.

Any oedema of the ankles, legs and thighs, buttocks and sacrum should be noted, together with any tautness of the skin and the

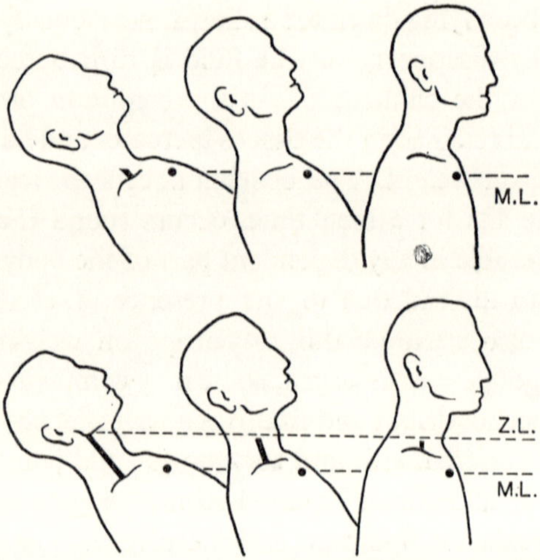

FIG 4. Visible pulsation of the jugular veins.
In health the vertical height of the column of blood in the jugular veins is about level with the manubrium sterni (M.L.), whatever the position of the patient. In heart failure, when right atrial pressure is increased, the vertical height of the column is increased and is above the manubrial level (M.L.), whatever the position of the patient.

extent to which pitting of the oedema takes place. The presence of abdominal distension and of ascites should be noted.

In right-sided failure blood cannot enter the right atrium and the superior vena cava and jugular veins in the neck become congested (engorged) with blood, the column of which moves (pulsates) at each atrial contraction (Fig. 4). Usually pulsation of the jugular veins may be seen only when the patient lies flat; at an angle of 45° it will be barely perceptible at a point horizontal with the manubrium sterni, and as he becomes more erect it completely disappears. When the central venous pressure is raised, the jugular vein can easily be seen to pulsate at an angle of 45°, and it will be present as the patient moves higher. Doubt as to whether the pulsation is in an artery can be removed by pressure: a vein collapses easily and an artery needs much firmer pressure. An estimation of the rise in venous pressure can be made by measuring the distance between the uppermost level of the pulsation in the jugular vein and an imaginary line drawn horizontal with the sternal angle (manubrium sterni): the greater this measurement, the greater the central venous pressure. A more accurate estimation can be made by inserting an intravenous catheter attached to a manometer.

On listening to the heart sounds through a stethoscope a third heart sound may be heard due to distension of the ventricle. Usually only two sounds are heard, the first due to closing of the atrioventricular valves, the second due to closing of the semilunar valves. Following these the third heart sound makes the whole sequence seem like a galloping horse and is termed 'gallop rhythm'. It is heard particularly in right-sided heart failure.

The rate of the pulse will most probably increase. Its rhythm may be regular or irregular, depending upon the cause of the failure. The volume may be small due to low cardiac output. In left-sided failure there may be a rhythm of alternate weak and strong pulse beats called 'pulsus alternans', which is best detected using a sphygmomanometer. It is sometimes desirable to compare the pulse rate with the heart rate. One nurse counts the apex beat whilst the other counts the pulse rate. Any difference in rate is known as the 'pulse deficit'. It is useful to assess any pulse deficit when there is irregularity of the pulse, as in atrial fibrillation, or when there is a slow pulse, as in digitalis poisoning. The blood pressure may be low or at the lower end of the range of normal limits.

Management of the patient

In managing a patient suffering from heart failure the objectives are threefold: first to alleviate the symptoms, secondly to bring the patient out of heart failure to a state where the heart can compensate for additional strains and thirdly to treat the cause of the heart failure if possible.

Rest in bed

Physical activity adds to the work of the heart by increasing the oxygen needs of the tissues, and the venous return of blood to the heart. To keep this at a minimum the patient must rest. He should be put to bed and encouraged to rest in the position he finds most comfortable; very often this is with the head and shoulders supported on pillows. When there is dyspnoea it may be essential for him to sit upright in order to breathe (orthopnoea). In this position the diaphragm can move more freely, being less hindered by the abdominal contents than in recumbency. The arms should be supported on pillows and not allowed to drag by the side from the shoulders. When dyspnoea is very severe, or when a change of position would be more comfortable, some patients find it helpful to lean forward with the arms resting on a bedtable on which has been placed a pillow. By raising the arms slightly the size of the thorax is increased, thus allowing the entry of more air into the lungs and resultant better oxygenation of the blood. To prevent the patient slipping down the bed a footboard or foam rubber pillow can be placed against the feet.

When the congestion is severe some patients are best nursed sitting in an armchair, head, shoulders and arms supported by pillows, with the feet on a small stool. Alternately, special 'cardiac' beds are sometimes available, in which the springs and mattress can be folded so that the resultant position is similar to that of a chair.

Bedclothes should be light in weight, so that when the patient feels like moving he can do so with a minimum of hindrance and effort. The weight of the bedclothes can be removed from the feet and legs by the careful placing of a bed-cradle. Anything which the patient may need should be placed within easy reach–such things as sputum carton, tissues for wiping the mouth and a drink.

Physical rest can be further enhanced if the patient is emotionally calm. A bunch of flowers or photograph placed so that they can easily be seen will help relaxation, as also will the view from a window, or even a television. The room should be well ventilated and kept at a comfortable temperature.

Movement of limbs

Although the patient is being encouraged to rest, that rest should not mean immobility. As the heart is failing to pump the circulation is poor, and thrombophlebitis (deep vein thrombosis) tends to occur especially in the legs. Movement of the legs should take place at intervals. If the patient can do it himself he should be asked to move the toes and ankles and to bend his knees each hour whilst he is awake, but should he be too weak, the nurse should passively carry out these exercises and gently massage the calf of each leg for him.

Relief of pressure

The areas of skin subject to pressure should receive care and attention. Every two hours the position of the patient should be changed so that one area is relieved of the weight of the body and another takes it. This can be achieved by positioning the patient inclined to one side or the other. Not only is the supply of the blood to the skin poor as a result of the heart failure, but the weight of the patient occludes the blood vessels, reducing even further the supply of blood to the tissues, so that there is danger of the skin deteriorating and pressure sores occurring. Damage to the skin over the pressure areas also predisposes to pressure sores, so any movement of the patient should be achieved by lifting him clear of the bedclothes and thus preventing friction between them and the patient's skin. The bottom sheets and the patient's nightwear should be free from folds and creases, which may act as a small but relatively intense area of pressure.

General cleanliness

In the early stages of heart failure, the nurse may be able to wash and dry only the face and hands without undue disturbance of the patient, but as soon as possible a daily bath should be given. In addition to cleaning the skin and providing a measure of comfort and ease, bathing the patient gives the nurse the chance to talk to him and to assess his condition, and also an opportunity to observe the extent of the oedema and the general condition of this skin.

Special attention should be paid to the mouth, especially when the patient is breathing through it, is producing sputum or is restricted in the amount of fluid he may drink.

Emptying the bowels

The bowels should be emptied as the need arises; failure to do so causes vague discomfort. The longer the act of defaecation is put off the harder the faeces become and even more difficult to pass later. Some patients find it difficult to use a bedpan for defaecation; straining should be avoided as it increases the work load of the heart. Most physicians would give permission for the patient to use a commode or sanichair brought to the bedside, the nurses taking great care to lift him out of and back into bed. Patients who are having difficulty in opening the bowels often get rather worried about it. The insertion of a glycerine suppository is often sufficient to alleviate the constipation.

Calmness

The patient may know or suspect that he has something wrong with his heart, or he may be somewhat concerned about his health and physical condition. Moreover, he may be worried about the effect of his illness and/or hospitalization on his family, his work or his social life. All this anxiety and emotional upset is not conducive to physical rest, often being the cause of the patient tossing and turning about in bed rather than lying still. In addition the sympathetic nervous system will have a stimulating rather than a relaxing ing effect on the heart. The nurse's role is to encourage the patient to rest with the aim of improving his health so that he can soon return to his normal way of life. A pleasant manner, clear and soft speech, graceful movements and efficient performance of nursing skills will instill in the patient a feeling of confidence in her ability. She should talk to him without tiring him, tactfully giving information and answering questions. By her conscientious observation she will know when to approach for the fulfillment of a need and when to retire, allowing him to rest. She will advise his visitors and relatives about his condition, and as to what they can do to help. The medical social worker may be able to resolve some of his problems and her services should be sought at the earliest opportunity.

The nurse observes

In observing the patient, the nurse will assess his general condition, comparing it with previous observations, and noting any progress or deterioration. She will note anything which tends to disturb him and also those things which help him to relax. She will look for and note the extent of any cyanosis, whether it is of the face and fingers (peripheral), of the mucous membranes of the mouth and tongue (central) or perhaps both. She will also note whether the extremities feel cold or, on the contrary, feel warm. Any dyspnoea will be noticed, as will the rate and depth of breathing and the use of accessory respiratory muscles, and also those factors which aggravate or relieve dyspnoea. Any tendency to cough will be observed and, should any sputum be produced, whether it is mucoid, frothy or contains blood. The pulse should be taken and recorded at least four-hourly or more often in the early stages, the rate, volume and rhythm being recorded. The apex beat may be taken at the same time to ascertain any discrepancy between them. If a cardiac monitor has been attached to the patient, or if a central venous pressure line has been set up, these will be recorded as the doctor instructs. The amount and distribution of oedema will be noted, and whether it is decreasing or becoming more marked. The amount of urine passed will be recorded, its colour, specific gravity and any abnormalities, such as the presence of protein which may indicate renal damage. When his condition warrants, the patient should be weighed each day; together with the observation on his urinary output and the amount of oedema, this will give an indication as to the decrease or increase in the amount of fluid being retained in the body.

The doctor examines

The doctor examines the patient, assesses his condition and orders the appropriate treatment. In doing so he will carry out a general examination for which the nurse will prepare the patient, and at which she will assist both the patient and the doctor by loosening his clothing, helping the patient to move and physically supporting him.

Tests and investigations

More detailed tests and investigations may be ordered, such as a radiograph of the chest, electrocardiogram, cardiac monitoring, central venous pressure, blood urea, blood gases and electrolyte content of the blood. Sometimes the results of these clinical investigations may be needed before the doctor can prescribe treatment. The nurse assists the doctor and/or the technicians when the investigations are being carried out, ensuring the maximum comfort and minimum distress for the patient. Some of the clinical investigations will probably be repeated as the days go by to estimate the improvement and progress made, and to ascertain the effects of the treatment prescribed.

Drugs

The drugs which may be ordered by the doctor as part of the treatment vary with the severity of the condition, and also according to whether there is predominantly right-sided failure (generalized congestion) or left-sided failure (pulmonary failure). For present purposes, right-sided failure will be considered first; a patient in acute left-sided failure will be discussed later.

Digitalis, or one of its derivatives, e.g. digoxin, is given to improve the efficiency of the heart beat. It increases the force of the heart contraction by directly stimulating the myocardium; the ventricles are emptied, the cardiac output is increased and the central venous pressure lowered. By improving the blood supply to the kidneys it assists in the elimination of excess fluid with a consequent increase in urinary output. Digitalis slows down the rate at which the ventricles contract, thus allowing a longer rest between beats, and allowing an increase in coronary circulation. In view of this the nurse will count the pulse before administering the drug; if below 60/min, it would be advisable to take the apex beat and if that is below 60 to withhold the drug and inform the doctor. More details about the dosage, modes of administration and side-effects can be found in Chapter 11.

Diuretics, i.e. frusemide or one of the thiazide group of compounds, are given to improve the efficiency of the kidneys. Details of their mode of action can be found in Chapter 11. The patient passes more urine, the amount and frequency of which should be recorded, and the fluid lost decreases the congestion and oedema. Large quantities of urine can be passed in the early stages, so it is wise to have a urinal close at hand. Diuretics tend to cause a loss of potassium, so potassium supplements will most probably be ordered to be given at the same time. Estimation of the electrolyte content of the blood and of potassium in particular are requested. When digitalis is also being given, the potassium deficiency increases the tendency for digitalis poisoning to occur.

Spironolactone may be ordered when oedema persists in spite of the administration of frusemide and thiazide diuretics. For its mode of action see Chapter 11.

Sedatives may be ordered to ensure maximum rest for the patient. In the early stages, and especially if dyspnoea is present, 10–30 mg morphine may be prescribed, unless respiratory failure makes respiratory depression dangerous. Should there be any tendency to vomit, it may be given as a preparation incorporating cyclizine (e.g. Cyclimorph) or it can be controlled by 25 mg chlorpromazine. Tranquillizers may be ordered if the patient is anxious. At night, sleep is important; the nurse should make the patient as comfortable as possible and the doctor may order a hypnotic drug such as 1·0 g chloral hydrate with perhaps 0·6 ml tincture of opium. Barbiturates, such as butobarbitone, may be ordered if necessary, but in elderly patients these tend to cause confusion, hence the use of chloral hydrate as first choice.

Oxygen will probably be given if the patient has dyspnoea and obtains relief by its administration. However, when the heart failure follows upon respiratory disease, such as cor pulmonale, oxygen must be given cautiously, as it may depress still further the respiratory centre, which has already become insensitive to the excess carbon dioxide, and which is being stimulated only by the deficiency in oxygen (hypoxia, hypoxaemia). Some patients benefit from oxygen when it is given through small polythene tubes shaped to resemble spectacles with a small extension into each nostril. Others prefer or benefit from a light-weight face mask, e.g. of the Venturi pattern, the flow being adjusted to 4–6 litres/min.

Diet

The diet should consist of foods which are to the patient's liking, but which are easily digested. Meals should be small in amount, given at frequent intervals rather than in large quantities. As the patient is relatively inactive he will not require a diet of high calorie value. In view of sodium and fluid retention, the doctor may order a diet low in sodium, e.g. 500 mg in contrast to the average daily 2 g. On the other hand it may be sufficient to give the patient the foods which he likes but to withhold additional salt. Some doctors set limits to the intake of fluid, but with low sodium diets and/or modern diuretics this is not always considered necessary, the patient being permitted to drink in order to assuage his thirst. In those patients with kidney dysfunction and urine retention, the doctor may order restriction of protein in the diet, but if there is proteinuria, additional protein will be required. It is wise to measure and record the fluid intake so as to be able to compare it with the urine output and with the loss in weight as the congestion and oedema subside.

Procedures

When pleural effusion persists and interferes with breathing, aspiration of the fluid may be necessary. Similarly, ascites in the abdominal cavity may be relieved by paracenteses. Gross oedema of the subcutanous tissues of the legs may be relieved by the insertion of Southey's tubes, the patient sitting at rest in an armchair and the legs supported on a stool.

Acute pulmonary oedema

The attack

In left-sided heart failure the heart is unable to transfer blood from the pulmonary veins into the aorta, and consequently the pressure in these veins rises. The pressure in the capillaries of the lungs also rises until it is higher than the osmotic pressure of the blood, and this allows a transudation into the alveoli of the lung, at first of fluid, and later perhaps of blood, and the condition of pulmonary oedema occurs. It occurs in patients with mitral stenosis and when there is left ventricular failure due to hypertension, aortic valve disease and damage or death of myocardium as in arteriosclerosis and coronary infarct.

Usually there are early signs of heart disease, but patients sometimes suffer attacks of sudden onset with no preceding clinical history.

A typical attacks occurs at night when the patient has been resting, probably asleep for a few hours, and perhaps has slipped into the recumbent position. In this position blood tends to leave the legs and increases the venous return to the heart. The extra blood passing through the right atrium to the right ventricle brings about a more rapid heart beat and corresponding increase in output by the right ventricle into the lungs. However, the left ventricle fails to keep up with the additional strain, or the blood cannot pass through the mitral valve if it is stenosed, and the blood congests in the lungs. The vessels become engorged and acute pulmonary oedema ensues.

The patient wakes up breathless and feels as if he is suffocating. He sits up breathing fast and deep, but the sensation gets worse; he panics and may rush to open a window in search of the air he so badly needs. He starts coughing; at first the sputum is mucoid and frothy, but later it becomes pink with blood, a sight which terrifies him even more. The pink frothy sputum increases and he feels as if he is choking—he is literally drowning in his own secretions. He continues his breathless struggling until he is exhausted and confused and he sinks on the floor, into a chair or back into the pillows, depending on where he happens to be at the time (Fig. 5). The attack in some ways resembles an attack of asthma, and is sometimes referred to as 'cardiac asthma'. It is also frequently called 'paroxysmal nocturnal dyspnoea'.

The nurse acts

When such an attack occurs at night in a ward of patients, the nurse will be badly frightened until she realizes what is happening and what can be done about it. She will have noticed the patient's dyspnoea or orthopnea, the cough, the sputum and the anxiety. She will also notice that he is grey in colour, his skin cold and moist and his mucous membranes and fingernails becoming

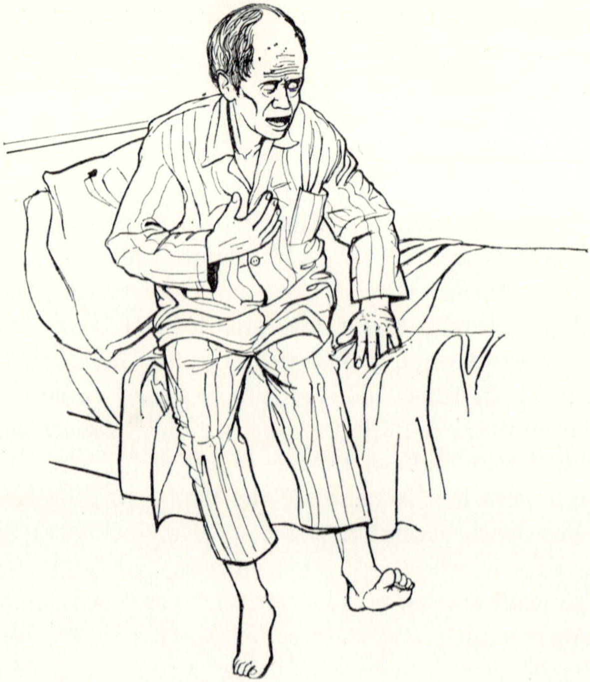

FIG 5. **A patient suffering from an acute attack of paroxysmal dyspnoea (cardiac asthma).**

cyanosed. She will try to get him to sit up in bed or in a chair, maintaining her own calm and efficient manner and encouraging the patient to entrust himself to her care. She will summon the doctor at the earliest opportunity, as the need for medical treatment is urgent.

The patient is kept upright supported with pillows and, if he finds it helpful, leaning forward on to a pillow or a pillow placed on a bed table. Sitting in a chair is sometimes easiest for the patient, but it may make examination and nursing care a little more difficult. The object of keeping the patient in this position is to allow pooling of the blood in the sacral area and lower limbs, so that correspondingly less blood flows back to the heart. Allowing the heart to rest in this way will be one way in which it is helped to recover. The skin is allowed to remain cool, no attempt is made to warm or wrap up the patient.

Oxygen can be administered to increase its proportion in the air in those alveoli not filled with oedematous fluid. As this is taken up by the blood, the patient may feel a certain amount of relief.

The doctor acts

The doctor will most probably order 10–30 mg morphine by injection. This will relieve the acute anxiety of the patient and any pain he may be feeling. It tends to decrease the need for oxygen in the tissues. Its action depresses the respiratory centre mildly, rapid forced but shallow respirations become slower, quieter and deeper and the patient is better able to rest.

An injection of 250–300 mg aminophylline, perhaps slowly by the intravenous route, relieves bronchospasm and, by its effect of dilating the bronchi, relieves dyspnoea. It also has a strengthening effect on the heart beat.

Following this a diuretic, e.g. 20 mg frusemide or 50 mg ethacrynic acid, may be given by injection so as to reduce the congestion as quickly as possible.

All these actions are taken to allay the breathlessness and reduce the pulmonary oedema as much as possible. As his condition improves, digitalis or one of its derivatives will be given to both strengthen and rest the heart.

Venesection is an older method of treatment of the emergency. About 500–700 ml of blood are rapidly withdrawn from a vein, there is a resulting decrease in venous return and, as less blood is pumped by the right ventricle to the lungs, pulmonary congestion decreases as the lungs reabsorb the fluid which has escaped. Although the heart gains temporary relief, the patient loses a considerable amount of blood, which takes time to replace; thus he gains little in the long run.

Another method of delaying the venous return and giving a little relief to the heart is to apply tourniquets to the four limbs, tight enough to prevent venous return, but not tight enough to interfere with arterial supply. The tourniquets on a limb are loosened one at a time, and then re-tightened, so that at any one time the venous return from three limbs is being slowed down.

The patient's progress

Until the patient's anxiety is relieved, and there is an improvement in his condition, the nurse stays with him, trying to anticipate all his needs so that he moves as little as possible, and explaining the procedures. Her very presence is reassuring to him, she is someone with whom to share his distress. She should give an air of confidence in her approach to him. Should she need to leave the bedside or to fetch help, her absence must be as brief as possible.

It may take from two hours to two weeks or even longer to bring the heart out of failure. As a result of measures taken, the congestion gradually decreases and the urgent symptoms subside. The patient will feel better and will want to move about and to do things for himself, even whilst lying in bed. This is usually permitted for it is encouraging to the patient and lessens any anxiety he may have been feeling. Movement in bed also reduces the tendency for hypostatic pneumonia and thrombophlebitis to occur. The patient may be allowed to sit up supported by pillows but with his legs dangling from the bed. Eventually he will be permitted to sit up in a chair for a few hours. The move from bed to chair should be made gradually, the nurse first preparing the chair, then dressing the patient appropriately and finally assisting him out of bed on to his feet and from there lowering him gently into the chair. It is useful to count the pulse before and after this movement to ensure that it was not too much for the patient. If all goes well, another day he will be allowed to take a few steps around the room, eventually to take a bath or shower and gradually to perform all the activities of everyday life. During this period of increasing ambulation the nurse will continue to make the observations mentioned earlier, so as to detect quite early any deterioration in his condition or any return of the congestion. The medication ordered by the doctor may be continued, often in smaller maintenance doses.

In the meantime the doctor will have assessed the cause of the heart failure and, where possible, e.g. in hypertension, hyperthyroidism, etc., will institute the appropriate treatment.

Returning home

The future pattern of life will be discussed with both the patient and his family. He will be advised to exercise with moderation but never to the point of breathlessness or fatigue. He will be advised to rest at intervals during the day, perhaps putting up his feet on a stool or couch, and to spend at least 10 or even 12 hours in bed at night—preferably asleep. If he is to continue taking any medication, e.g. digitalis, he will be advised about the importance of doing so. Similarly, if there are any adjustments to his diet, they will be explained to both patient and his family. He will be advised not to smoke. He should visit his doctor regularly, and especially if there should be any recurrence of breathlessness or swelling. The medical social worker will be asked to see him, to assist with any domestic difficulties and to advise where she is able.

The ultimate

Unless the cause of heart failure can be removed, e.g. in mitral valve disease, a patient who has recovered from congestive heart failure or acute left ventricular failure is likely to suffer further attacks. They may be precipitated by chest infections, extra exertion, a worsening of the causal condition or degeneration of the heart muscle. Successive attacks may be overcome, but the measures become less and less successful, each attack leaving the patient in a worse general condition than before. He may become a semi-invalid, requiring much care and attention whilst at home. The attacks become more severe and eventually he dies. With this in mind, the nurse should be calm, gentle and attentive to his needs, filled with the knowledge that if she cannot help him to recover, she can at least ensure that he suffers a minimum of discomfort when he dies.

3 Emergency care

Wherever patients with cardiac disease are nursed dramatic situations are liable to occur. These include the occurrence of acute conditions such as acute left heart failure and pulmonary oedema, or cardiac tamponade, or absolute emergencies such as cardiac arrest. Such an occasion can be very frightening for all concerned. If the nurse knows that she is well prepared for it she will be able to take the necessary action quickly and efficiently, organize others to help and at the same time provide support for the patient concerned (if he is conscious), the other patients in the ward and less experienced staff, so that psychological trauma is minimized. With proper preparations a nurse can accept such conditions as demanding all her skill and efficiency, but nevertheless regard them as being almost routine, since she knows what is expected of her and is aware that resuscitation may well be successful.

Cardiac arrest may happen unexpectedly, but it is often possible to identify patients at risk, i.e. in whom it is most likely to occur. Some of the important precipitating factors are recent myocardial infarction, major cardiac operations, hypoxia, metabolic acidosis and disturbance of the intracellular and extracellular potassium balance. An oscilloscope attached to a patient at risk may show early indications of approaching dangers and allow successful preventive measures to be taken. It will also make possible the detection of asystole or ventricular fibrillation immediately it occurs.

Cardiac arrest

If the heart has ceased to beat at all (asystole) or the ventricles are quivering but not contracting effectively (ventricular fibrillation) circulation ceases. In consequence the tissues no longer receive the oxygen supply vital to their life and work, waste products accumulate and, unless circulation is rapidly restored, the tissues will die. The organs most dependent on a plentiful supply of oxygen will suffer first. The brain, kidneys and liver all use up oxygen rapidly in performing their various functions and are most susceptible to damage.

After *three minutes* without circulation brain damage may be irreversible.

Resuscitation

Since speed is essential the necessities for resuscitation (Fig. 6) must be readily available in any acute hospital. For convenience and mobility they are usually stored together on a trolley. In many hospitals it is the practice to have a cardiac massage board and Waters' bag or Brook airway on each ward, and the other requirements strategically placed for easy access by several wards.

Oxygen supply to the body must be restored to the body within three minutes. This means re-establishing circulation and ventilation of the lungs. The immediate steps taken are:

1. Confirm cardiac arrest.
2. Clear the airway.
3. Restore circulation by giving the patient a sharp blow over the sternum with the side of a clenched fist, followed, if the heart does not start beating, by closed cardiac massage.
4. Re-establish respiration.

This can all be done by one person, each 10 beats of closed massage being followed by ventilation of the lungs twice. However, help should be summoned as soon as possible and the resuscitation trolley sent for. One person then maintains circulation, pausing only to ascertain that the chest moves with artificial ventilation, while the other maintains ventilation, pausing to palpate the carotid or femoral pulse to see that cardiac massage is effective.

If resuscitation is being performed effectively, the patient's colour will usually improve, the pupils will become smaller if they were dilated, spontaneous heart beat and respiration may commence and the patient may become conscious. In any case, permanent tissue damage can usually be held at bay until medical help arrives and further treatment can be instituted.

Throughout all the emergency procedures the nurse must

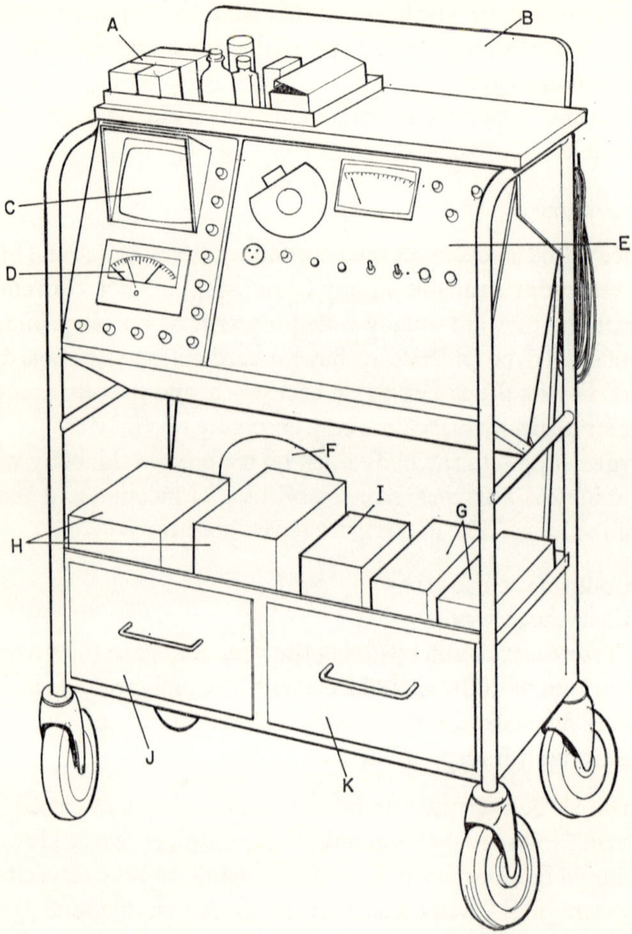

FIG 6. A cardiac massage trolley.
A, Drug tray, including medicated swabs and ampoule files. B, Cardiac massage board. C, Oscilloscope and leads. D, Heart rate meter. E, Defibrillator. F, Self-inflating bag. G, Intravenous equipment and fluids. H, Syringes and needles of various sizes. I, Zinc oxide plaster, spare laryngoscope batteries and bulbs, Doyen's mouth gag, tongue forceps and metal spatula. J, Ventilation equipment: airways, masks, Waters' bag, catheter mount and connections, laryngoscope, endotracheal tubes in various sizes and artery forceps. K, Defibrillator electrodes and electrode jelly.

remember that the patient may be conscious and may need constant reassurance, explanation and comfort by voice or physical contact. Fortunately many patients do not remember this terrifying experience afterwards, but a few are able to describe their feelings. This is particularly true if at any point the patient is intubated and curarized, which abolishes normal signs of consciousness.

A more detailed description of resuscitation procedures follows.

1. *To confirm cardiac arrest* the carotid or femoral pulses are palpated. If these pulses are absent, the patient is, or rapidly becomes, unconscious and respiration ceases, which in itself is sufficient confirmation.

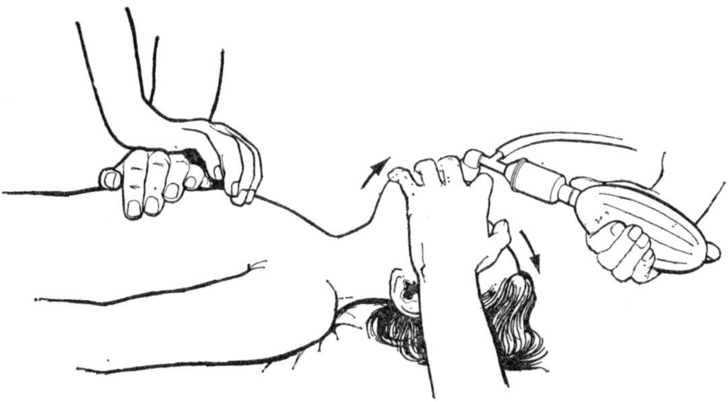

FIG 7. **External cardiac compression and ventilation with a Waters bag and mask.**
Note the position of the hands. Pressure is exerted only over the lower third of the sternum, with the heels of the hands. Note also the position of the head. The chin is held well up to keep the airway clear. The mask must fit the face well to maintain the gas pressure inside during ventilation.

Resuscitation should not be delayed until the pupils dilate since this may take 45 seconds and vital time may be wasted.

2. *To clear the airway* the chin is lifted up and the jaw pulled forwards. Secretions or vomit are removed from the mouth by wiping them out, or by aspiration if a suction machine is at hand. A clear airway is essential; without it the lungs cannot be ventilated, and indeed respiratory obstruction may be the cause of the arrest.

3. *To perform closed cardiac massage* (Fig. 7), the patient should be laid flat. The heel of the operator's hand is placed over the lower

third of the patient's sternum, the other hand placed over it and pressure exerted to compress the heart between the sternum and the spine 70–80 times/min. The sternum should move about 4 cm, the amount of pressure needed varying according to the size of the patient and the rigidity of the chest wall. (Pressure must be much less than this in the young; it is performed with one hand on a child and with two fingers over the middle third of the sternum on a baby.) Since closed massage is only really effective if there is a rigid surface under the chest a cardiac massage board should be put in place as soon as possible, unless the bed is rigid and the mattress firm. A pillow should be put under the patient's head, because a subdural haemorrhage can be caused by bouncing the head on a rigid surface during massage. Accidental injuries caused during resuscitation, such as fractured ribs or ruptured liver or spleen, are usually due to excessive or misplaced force. Pressure must only be applied over the sternum, not over the ribs.

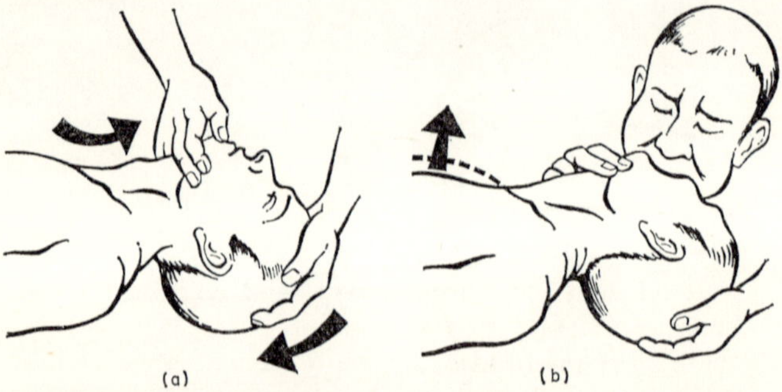

Fig 8. **Mouth-to-mouth-and-nose respiration.**
A, The correct position of the head. B, Inflation of the lungs is shown by an upward movement of the chest. In mouth-to-mouth respiration the operator's left hand or cheek would be used to occlude the nose.

4. *Ventilation of the lungs* can be performed in emergency by the mouth-to-mouth expired air method (Fig. 8). The operator lifts the patient's chin to clear the airway, takes a deep breath, places her lips to form a seal round the patient's mouth and breathes air into the lungs. The patient's nose must be nipped to prevent the escape of air or, in the case of a child, both nose and mouth would be covered by the operator's mouth. This is the oldest and simplest method, but it has the disadvantages that it is aesthetically unde-

sirable and that the expired air does not have a high oxygen content. There is also the question of infection, particularly in units where a nurse may perform resuscitation several times in one day, possibly on infected patients.

Apparatus such as the Brook airway (Fig. 9) solves some of these problems, and is easily stored and relatively inexpensive. However,

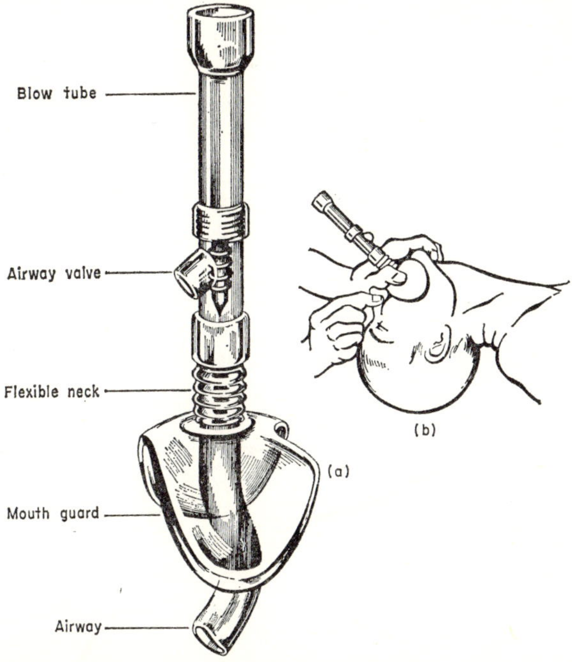

FIG **9. The Brook airway for insufflation of the lungs.**
A, The Brook airway. B, The airway in position. The mouthguard is pressed against the face and the nostrils are pinched to prevent leakage of air.

in hospital it is usually possible to ventilate the patient with oxygen. This improves the chances of successful resuscitation, especially if the patient was hypoxic before the emergency.

Artificial ventilation may be performed with a self-inflating bag with oxygen inlet, or with a Waters' bag (Figs 10, 11). In either case, the airway must be clear, the mask should be a good airtight fit over the face and the chest must be seen to rise and fall with ventilation.

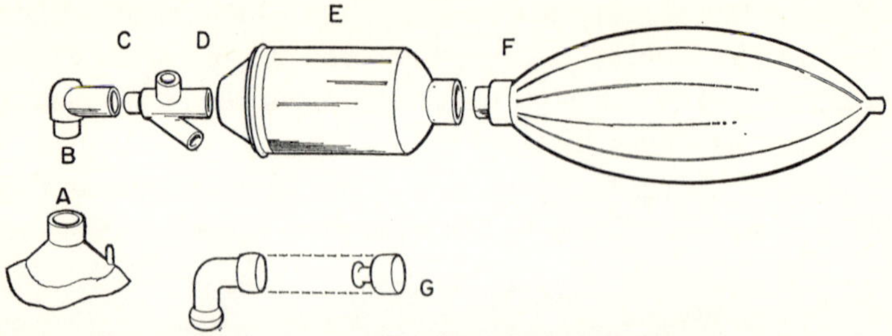

FIG **10. The Waters' circuit for manual ventilation.**
A, Face mask. B, Mask angle mount. C-D, Expiratory valve. E, Waters' canister. F, Waters' bag and adaptor. G, Catheter mount.

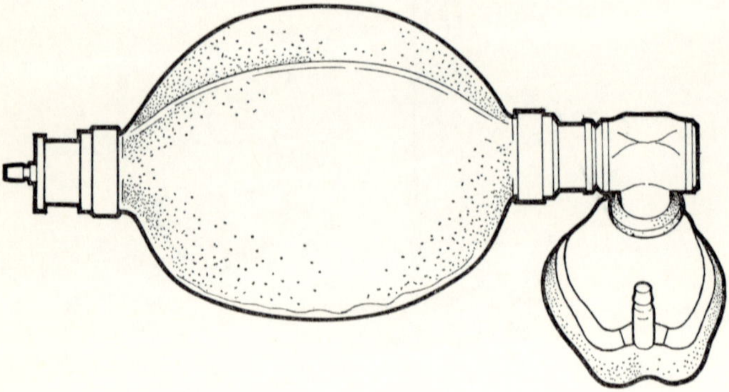

FIG **11. The Ambu Ruben resuscitator.**
The mask is placed over the patient's mouth and nose, the jaw being kept well forward. When the bag is compressed, air is forced into the patient's lungs. The expired air escapes through the non-return valve (1); the bag refills through the air inlet valve (2). Some types of bag have an inlet for oxygen.

When a doctor arrives he will usually pass an endotracheal tube (Fig. 12). In some units nurses are specially trained to do this. The requirements are a cuffed endotracheal tube, a laryngoscope, a syringe to inflate the cuff, artery forceps to clamp the cuff tube and a catheter mount to attach the endotracheal tube to the expiratory valve. If manual ventilation is continued for long a Waters' canister filled with soda lime is required to absorb carbon dioxide.

Once circulation and ventilation of the lungs have been re-established, more specific measures can be taken.

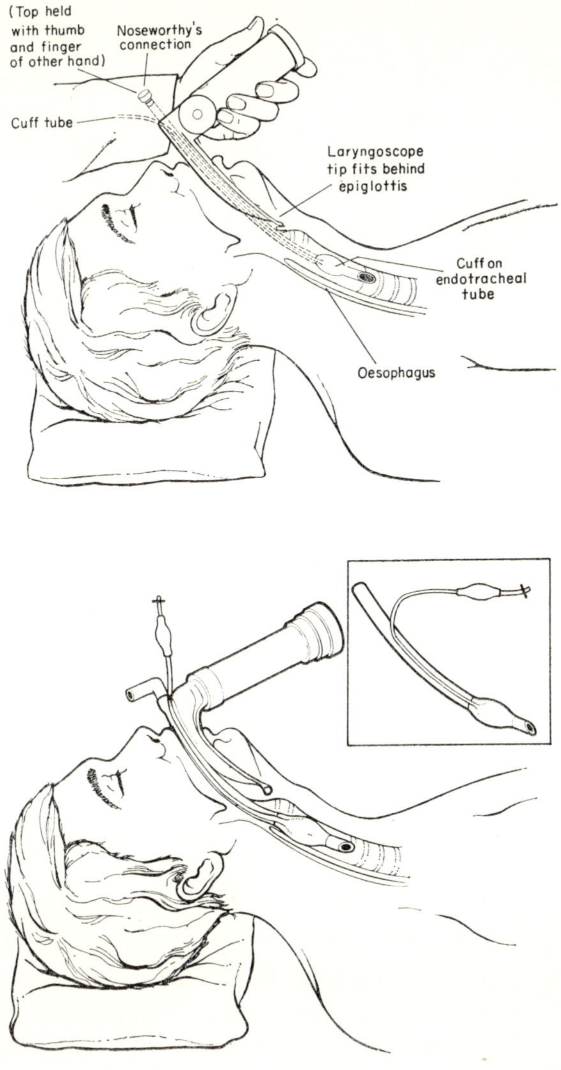

FIG **12. Intubation.**
A, Insertion of the MacIntosh laryngoscope. The top of the Nosworthy's connection is held with the finger of the other hand, and the tip of the laryngoscope fits behind the epiglottis. B, The laryngoscope and endotracheal tube in position. The cuff has been inflated. The inset shows details of the tube. In practice the laryngoscope is removed immediately after intubation and before the cuff is inflated.

The electrocardiogram

An oscilloscope is attached to show the electrocardiogram. If this shows ventricular fibrillation electrical defibrillation may be performed. The machine is connected to an electrical supply; the electrodes are covered with saline pads or conductive jelly to protect the patient's skin and placed on the patient's chest (Fig. 13).

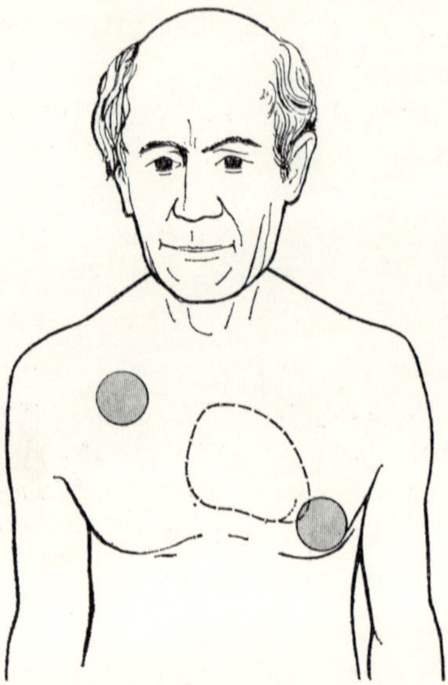

FIG 13. **Usual sites for application of the defibrillation electrodes.**

An electrical shock of pre-set intensity is then passed through the heart. This abolishes electrical activity in the heart for a brief period and may allow the sino-atrial node to take over again as pace-maker. *No person must be in contact with the patient or bed while defibrillation takes place, otherwise that person will also receive the shock and may need resuscitation.*

Intravenous infusion

An intravenous infusion is needed as soon as possible for the administration of fluids and drugs. These may include:

1. *Sodium bicarbonate* 8·4%. The longer the patient has been hypoxic due to cardiac arrest or other causes the greater will be the

degree of metabolic acidosis. At least 100 ml sodium bicarbonate 8·4% or the equivalent is usually given, and further requirements calculated from the results of blood gas and acid–base balance estimation. A sample of blood should be taken into a heparinized syringe from an artery as soon as possible so this investigation can be done. Uncorrected acidosis may prevent successful resuscitation.

2. *Adrenaline* 1 in 1 000 to 1 in 10 000; the nurse must always check which strength is required. This circulates as the heart is massaged and may stimulate coarse ventricular fibrillation in an asystolic heart. Defibrillation can then be performed.

3. *Calcium chloride* 1%. This may be used to stimulate contraction of the heart.

4. *Isoprenaline* 2 mg in 500 ml, or even stronger solutions, may be given to stimulate the heart, increase the heart rate and raise arterial pressure. The number of drops per minute is specified by the doctor and this rate must be strictly maintained. Too rapid infusion of this solution may precipitate cardiac dysrhythmias. The infusion bottle should, of course, be marked with the amounts of drugs added, but it is wise to mark the infusion set also, near the control clamp, so that the rate is not altered without thought, for example when giving other drugs. The oscilloscope must be observed carefully, especially when the infusion rate has just been altered.

5. *Lignocaine* 50 mg immediately followed by a continuous infusion may be used to control cardiac dysrhythmias by decreasing the irritability of the heart muscle.

6. *Potassium chloride* may be given if it is suspected that a low intracellular potassium is a contributory cause of dysrhythmias. It may be added to the infusion or 0·5–1 g may be given directly intravenously by a doctor. Insulin and glucose may be ordered at the same time, because they increase the rate at which potassium passes into the cells.

7. *Mannitol* 12·5% 100 ml may be ordered to increase the urine output. This both dehydrates the patient, so that cerebral oedema due to cerebral hypoxia is less likely, and encourages the function of the kidneys which may have suffered from hypoxia. Frusemide (Lasix) may be given intravenously for the same purpose. It is

wise to put a urinal in place as soon as possible to catch the expected flow of urine, or to insert a urethral catheter.

8. *Hydrocortisone* 100–200 mg may be ordered to increase the arterial pressure.

9. Infusion of *plasma-expanding solutions* such as the various kinds of dextran solutions may be ordered to increase tissue perfusion and prevent 'sludging' in the peripheral vessels.

10. Occasionally *phenoxybenzamine* (Dibenyline) may be ordered to dilate the peripheral vessels and reduce resistance to circulation. If this is used extra infusion of fluid will be needed immediately to increase the circulatory volume and fill the peripheral vessels without decreasing the arterial pressure.

Drugs which raise the arterial pressure by constricting peripheral vessels are not used, since these may diminish blood supply to the kidneys.

Artificial pacemakers

Artificial pacemaking may be necessary. A small electrical current is passed through the heart intermittently to stimulate contractions at a pre-set rate. This may be performed with external electrodes but this method is relatively inefficient and may be painful to the patient. Usually a catheter is inserted via a peripheral arm vein or the jugular vein as an emergency procedure and connected to an external pacemaker.

The responsibilities of the nurse

It is now acknowledged that if patients are to have the best possible chance of recovery, nurses must be competent and willing to perform basic resuscitation measures, i.e. closed cardiac massage and artificial ventilation. Although this sounds a heavy responsibility, it is obviously a worthwhile and satisfying one if it enables a patient to live when he would otherwise have died. The nurse is the person most frequently present when a cardiac arrest occurs.

Nurses are now sometimes asked to take on further responsibilities, such as tracheal intubation and electrical defibrillation. For example, in coronary care units it may be the policy for a nurse to defibrillate immediately she diagnoses ventricular fibrillation, without any preliminary measures. Both for the good of the patient

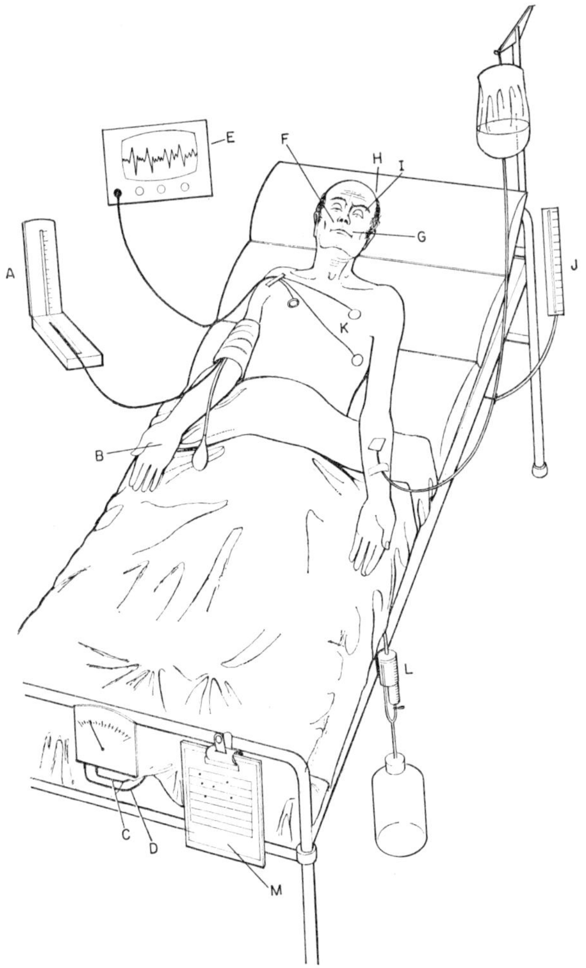

FIG **14. Observations to be made after cardiac arrest.**
A, Arterial pressure. B, Is normal movement present on command? C, Peripheral temperature (the foot might be felt). D, Core (rectal) temperature. E, Heart rate and rhythm shown on the oscilloscope. F, Oxygen (equipment omitted for clarity). G, Is the patient capable of normal speech? H, Colour. I, Pupil reaction. J, Venous pressure (might be measured). K, Type and rate of respiration. L, Urine output. M, Chart for all observations.

and for the legal protection of the nurse it is important that she should not take on such responsibilities even at the request of a doctor unless certain criteria are fulfilled. These are:

1. That the nurse is confident that she has been properly taught and is competent to perform the procedure.
2. That it is in accordance with the policy of the hospital nursing administration, and the employing authority that she should do so. Even so, she is still liable for her own error or incompetence.

Once the immediate crisis is over the patient may be conscious and breathing spontaneously, or he may still be in a critical state. In any case he requires careful observation (Fig. 14) and possibly drug therapy, and good nursing care. Special points to be observed are:

1. The heart rate, rhythm and arterial pressure, and respiration. Any marked variation in these should be reported immediately.

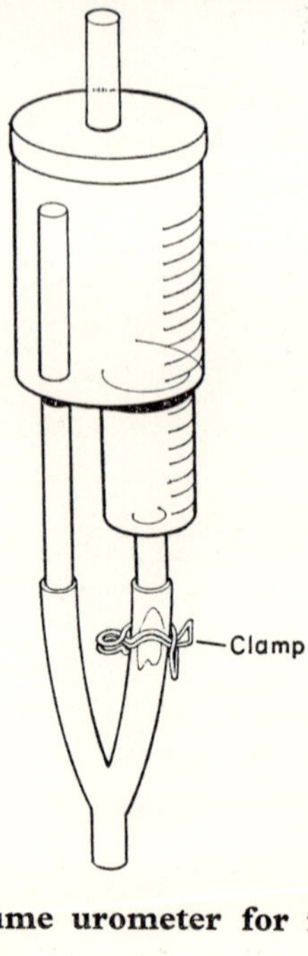

FIG **15. Precision volume urometer for measurement of small amounts of urine.**

An oscilloscope is usually used to allow the cardiac rhythm to be observed.

2. The colour and peripheral tissue perfusion. It should be noted whether the extremities are pink and warm or cold and pale due to vascoconstriction.

3. The urine output should be observed carefully (Fig. 15), oliguria being reported if it occurs. Kidney function may be impaired due to the anoxic period resulting from cardiac arrest.

4. The state of consciousness, orientation, ability to obey commands and move all limbs. Temporary or permanent cerebral damage may result from cerebral hypoxia.

Sometimes the patient may fail to regain spontaneous respiration or it may be felt that the effort and oxygen consumption involved in respiration is undesirable. In this case ventilation of the lungs is maintained artificially by a respirator. This involves considerable responsibility for the nurse.

CARDIOPULMONARY RESUSCITATION CHART

Name John BROWN

Date 8·12·72

Ward

Time	12·35AM	12·40	12·45	12·50	1am						
External cardiac massage	✓	✓	✓	✓							
Internal cardiac massage											
Artifical ventilation	✓	✓	✓	✓							
Intubation		✓									
Defibrillation		X2	✓	✓							
I.V. Sodium bicarbonate		100ml 8·4%			50ml 8·4%						
I.V. calcium chloride											
I.V. adrenaline			10 ml 1–10 000								
I.V. lignocaine					50mg	1mg/min					

FIG 16. A chart such as this is a useful and quick method of recording the management of a case of cardiac arrest. Other drugs or intravenous solutions can be recorded in the spare lines.

Intermittent positive pressure respiration

Early respirators consisted of a large box or shell which fitted over the whole patient up to the neck, or just from neck to waist. A bellows connected to this box produced a negative pressure inside it, intermittently. This pulled the chest wall outwards, and air entered through the mouth and nose into the lungs because the atmospheric pressure was higher than the box pressure.

More recent intermittent positive pressure respirators work the opposite way, by intermittently blowing air under pressure into the lungs through a cuffed endotracheal or tracheostomy tube. These respirators are smaller and do not impede access to the patient for treatment or nursing care; and many are much more adaptable to the patient's respiratory needs. Their uses now include prolonged artificial ventilation in cardiac or respiratory failure, to maintain adequate respiration and reduce the work involved in this.

Respirators may be powered by electricity, e.g. the East-Radcliffe respirator which consists basically of bellows operated by an electrically powered machine. Alternatively they may be gas-powered, when a controlled amount of gas under pressure is supplied intermittently. The Bennett and Bird respirators are examples of this.

The most important adjustments permitted by most respirators are:

1. *Rate of respiration.* This may be altered by a direct control or by altering the rate of inspiration and expiration. Alteration of the inspiration/expiration ratio may also be possible.

2. *Positive pressure.* The force with which the air is blown into the chest. Change in pressure usually goes with change in

3. *Volume.* This may be measured as the amount of air inspired in one breath (tidal volume) or over one minute (minute volume). In practice the volume of expired air should be measured to reduce the chances of a false reading. Since the pressure and volume are interdependent on some machines, the pressure is set (i.e. pressure controlled) while on others the volume is set (volume controlled). This volume will be delivered regardless of the resulting pressure, though on most machines there is a pressure limit.

4. *Gas composition control.* Some machines allow administration

of anything from room air up to 100% oxygen, and possibly added anaesthetic gases. In the latter case a closed-circuit system with soda lime canister to absorb the carbon dioxide is used to economize on expensive gases. With a closed circuit system oxygen *must* be added. Other machines have less variable oxygen–air dilution controls.

5. *Humidification* of inspired air is essential. Dry gas administered over several hours or days will cause drying of the secretions and obstruction to efficient respiration. Air may be moistened by passing over hot water in a thermostatically controlled container, or by a fine mist of spray from a humidifier or nebulizer.

6. *Hand operation* is usually available for emergency use, but may depend on the gas supply if the machine is gas-powered.

7. *Negative pressure* to assist expiration and help to maintain venous return and cardiac output.

8. *Patient-triggering*, which allows the machine to give a full inspiration in response to the patient's inspiratory effort. The amount of effort needed from the patient to operate the machine is regulated by the sensitivity control.

The machine controls are usually set by an anaesthetist according to the patient's size, volume needs and lung compliance (the ease with which the lungs can be inflated), among other considerations. Negative pressure may be needed to prevent hypotension. During spontaneous respiration the negative pressure in the chest aids venous return. If the respirator supplies constant positive pressure this may reduce venous return of blood to the heart, and hence the cardiac output falls.

However, in controlling pulmonary oedema constant positive pressure is maintained to prevent exudation of fluid into the alveoli from the circulation. Bronchospasm may make it necessary to prolong expiration and so allow time for the air to pass out through the narrowed bronchi.

Although it is not usually a nurse's function to set the respirator controls, she should know the levels set for any patient under her care in case they should change. She should also know whether she may alter the controls, under what circumstances, and what to do if the respirator fails. This knowledge is vital for the patient's safety.

Care of the patient

A nurse must accept the responsibility for the constant observation on any patient with a respirator. She must stay with the patient, that is she must be within sight and earshot in case the respirator fails or becomes disconnected or the endotracheal tube kinks. This nearness to the patient is essential to safeguard the patient's life. Loss of voluntary respiration and of speech is very frightening to a conscious patient, and the proceedings must be explained by the nurse as often as necessary. Any patient will be much easier to care for if confident that the nurse knows how to manage both patient and machine. Communication may be difficult and a word indicator or writing materials should be used when possible, but patience is essential.

Spontaneous respiratory efforts will interfere with mechanical ventilation. Hyperventilation may be used initially to remove more carbon dioxide and so reduce the stimulus to respiration. This may be followed by respiratory depressant drugs, e.g. 1–4 mg phenoperidine (Operidine) intravenously hourly or as necessary, or 10 mg morphine when necessary. A paralysing drug such as tubocurarine (Tubarine), 5–30 mg intravenously, may be given, preferably with a sedative to reduce the patient's awareness. A fully curarized patient is quite unable to move, but may be fully conscious, able to see, hear and feel. The nurse must remember this at all times and explain the situation to visitors.

Change of position two-hourly improves lung expansion, relieves pressure areas and often improves the patient's comfort. At least 2 nurses are usually necessary; one should be responsible for seeing that the endotracheal tube is not pulled out, and that ventilation is maintained. Good positioning and passive exercises are important. Tracheobronchial secretions should be aspirated before and after turning the patient, and whenever they can be heard or felt through the chest wall. This must be done quickly and efficiently without introducing infection or causing hypoxia or unnecessary trauma. Excessive or unduly frequent suction may increase tracheobronchial secretions, trauma and the risk of infection. Viscid secretions may be loosened by increased humidification or by putting 5 ml of sterile saline down the tube hourly. 'Artificial sighing' to maintain good lung expansion may be performed intermittently by increasing the respirator pressure for a few breaths, or by manual ventilation with a Waters' bag.

Prolonged pressure from the inflated endotracheal tube cuff will cause necrosis of the trachea, with the risk of fistula formation or later tracheal stenosis. To avoid this, either a small air leak is allowed round the cuff or the cuff is deflated at least 4–6-hourly, after tipping the patient's head downwards (unless this is contra-indicated) and aspirating secretions from the pharynx and trachea. Aspiration from the trachea is performed as the cuff is released. Oronasal secretions or regurgitated fluid may cause pneumonia if allowed to run down the trachea. With the cuff deflated air will usually leak up through the larynx or round the tracheostomy, and the patient should be warned of this. After five minutes the cuff should be reinflated with the minimum of air necessary to stop the air leak. Tracheal necrosis may also occur if the respirator tubing is allowed to pull on the tracheostomy tube, so causing the distal end of the tracheostomy tube to press on the side or rear wall of the trachea.

The paralysed or unconscious patient will develop corneal ulceration if the eyes are allowed to remain open and the cornea dry. This may be prevented by instilling sterile paraffin or methyl cellulose drops two-hourly and keeping the eyes closed and possibly covered or 'blinking' them artificially. If they are kept padded the eyes should be opened at regular intervals to see if there is any inflammation and to allow visual contact if the patient is conscious. With some patients a piece of zinc oxide adhesive tape stuck horizontally across the upper part of the eyelids (over the tarsal plate) may suffice to keep the eyes closed but allow them to be opened for observation or visual contact. It may be necessary to close the lids with non-allergic adhesive tape placed vertically.

Nutrition and fluid intake must be maintained. Gastric feeding is the natural and best method, orally or by tube if necessary. Calorie, protein, electrolyte and fluid intake can be adjusted to the patient's needs. Usually a high-calorie, high-protein diet is required. If gastric feeding is contra-indicated, for example, if peristalis is absent, intravenous feeding will be necessary.

Bladder and bowel function should be regulated as necessary, since a distended abdomen may raise the diaphragm and interfere with ventilation of the lungs, apart from causing discomfort to the patient.

When continuous artificial ventilation is no longer necessary the patient is usually allowed to breathe spontaneously for increasing periods of time, until the respirator is no longer used at all.

Observations and records

The best indication of efficient ventilation is a pink, restful patient, with the chest moving well in time with the respirator. However, certain records are necessary. Blood pressure and heart rate are recorded half-hourly at first, later hourly, or occasionally even two-hourly if the records have been steady and the patient's condition is good. Hypertension and tachycardia may indicate hypoventilation, particularly if the patient is flushed, restless and sweating. These are all signs of carbon dioxide retention. Hypotension may be due to hyperventilation.

The respirator pressures and minute or tidal volume are recorded hourly, though observed more frequently. A rising pressure or falling volume (according to which is pre-set) may indicate retention of secretions, a collapsed area of lung, a pneumothorax or decreasing lung compliance.

The respirator rate is recorded hourly, alterations will usually affect the volume.

If a closed-circuit system of ventilation is used with a soda lime canister, the canister must be changed at regular intervals, and the change recorded. A dye indicator in the soda lime changes colour when it no longer absorbs carbon dioxide efficiently. This will show whether the soda lime needs changing more or less often.

Records of drugs administered, oxygen flow-rate, nursing treatment, change of position, and the patient's condition and state of consciousness are important. Medical records should include orders for drugs, respirator settings, oxygen requirements and fluid and dietary needs.

Care of the respirator

No respirator should be transferred from one patient to another without adequate cleaning and sterilization. Humidifers should be

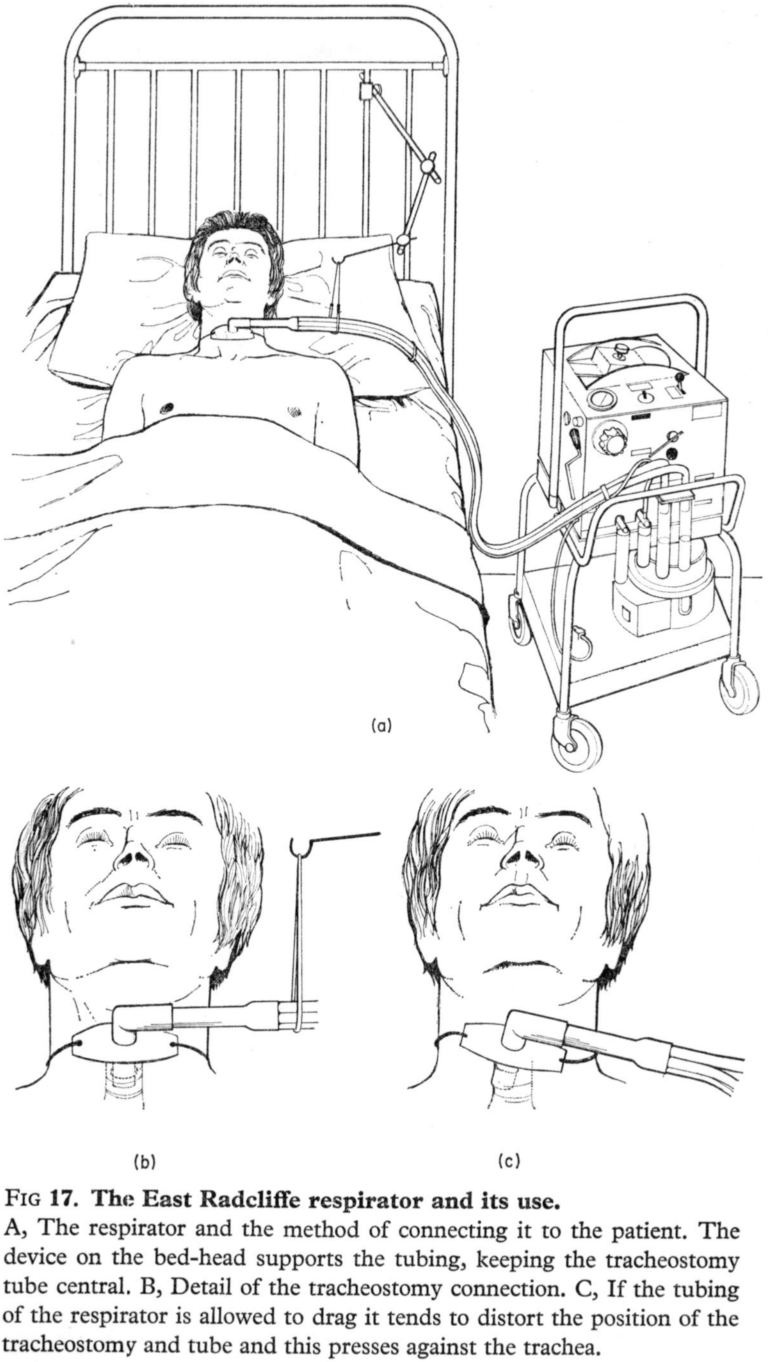

FIG 17. The East Radcliffe respirator and its use.
A, The respirator and the method of connecting it to the patient. The device on the bed-head supports the tubing, keeping the tracheostomy tube central. B, Detail of the tracheostomy connection. C, If the tubing of the respirator is allowed to drag it tends to distort the position of the tracheostomy and tube and this presses against the trachea.

refilled as necessary without stopping ventilation, and if heated should be checked at intervals to detect excessive or inadequate heating. The minimum temperature should be 60–65° C to avoid the growth of organisms in the humidifer.

All tubing and connections must be kept firmly attached, and the tubing supported so that it does not pull on the patient's tracheal tube, and excess condensation drains downwards. Water traps and tubes must be emptied when water accumulates in them.

The nurse caring for a patient with a respirator needs an observant eye, a listening ear, trained hand and great patience and sympathy. Her patient's well-being and even life depend on these.

4

Coronary artery disease

The heart, like any other organ of the body, depends on its blood supply to bring oxygen and other metabolic requirements and to carry away waste products. Just distal to the aortic valve are the two coronary orifices through which blood enters the right and left coronary arteries (Fig. 18). These split into branches supplying mainly the right and left sides of the heart respectively; and blood

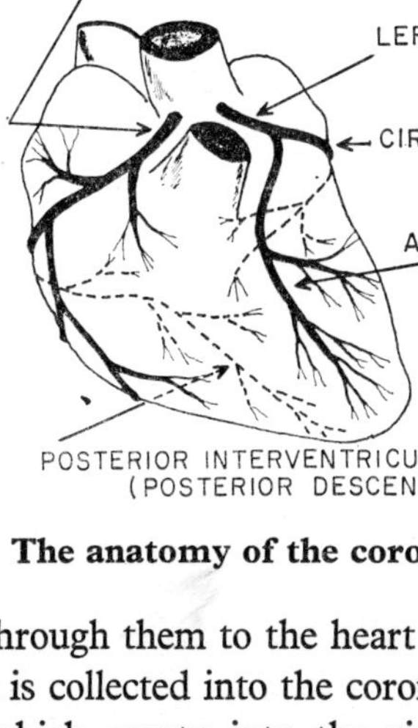

FIG 18. **The anatomy of the coronary arteries.**

flows through them to the heart for the greater part during diastole. It is collected into the coronary sinus and two other smaller veins which empty into the right atrium. Several small veins empty directly into the right atrium and ventricle. When a coronary artery becomes narrowed, usually due to atherosclerosis, the blood supply may still be adequate during rest, particularly if a collateral circulation has developed. During exercise, however, as the heart works harder to increase its output, its own blood supply may become inadequate to meet the increased needs, and angina pectoris occurs. The pain of angina pectoris is retrosternal, may spread up into the jaw or through the shoulder and down one or both arms (more often the left) and there is a gripping sense of oppression in the chest. It may be provoked by a big meal, exercise, anxiety or excitement, but is usually relieved by a few min-

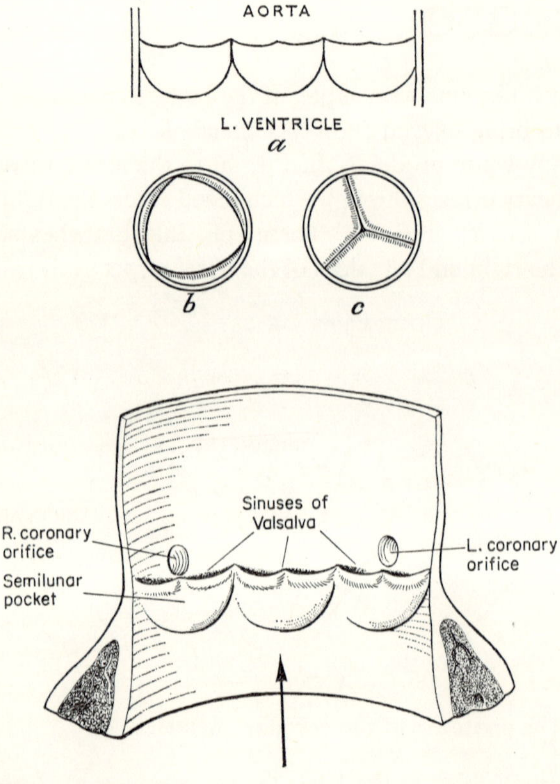

FIG **19. The aortic valve.**
a, Laid open. *b*, Seen from above open. *c*, Seen from above closed.

utes rest, by inhaling the contents of an amyl nitrite capsule or by 0·5–1 mg glyceryl trinitrate sublingually. At first the angina may occur infrequently, but as the lumen of the coronary artery decreases it may occur more frequently, provoked by less and less exercise until the patient is completely incapacitated. This is sometimes knnow as coronary insufficiency.

When angina has occurred it may be possible for the patient to continue a fairly normal life by recognizing his limitations, avoiding excessive exercise or excitement and taking long-acting coronary dilators such as pentaerythritol tetranitrate (Mycardol) regularly and, if necessary, glyceryl trinitrate before extra exertion or when angina begins. It is sometimes possible to improve the blood supply to the heart by surgical procedures, described later in this chapter.

Coronary occlusion

The typical patient admitted to hospital with coronary occlusion is an overweight man of 40 or more, with a responsible but sedentary job, who gives a history of waking in the night with severe chest pains, tachycardia, nausea, a feeling of weakness and a cold sweating pale appearance. What has happened is that a narrowed coronary vessel has become blocked by an atheromatous plaque, or by clotting on the roughened intima of the artery. This immediately cuts off the blood supply to a small or large area of myocardium which is thus damaged and may die (infarction). There may be no history of angina, and because of the site of pain and the nausea the patient may consider that he had indigestion. Unless the pain is severe or continues for a long time he may not seek medical aid.

Myocardial infarction is usually the result of atherosclerosis. The predisposing factors are therefore the same and include obesity, increasing age, lack of exercise, anxiety and overwork, hypertension, diabetes and a high blood cholesterol or uric acid level (even without signs of gout). It is rarer in women before the menopause, owing to hormonal effects, but it is becoming more common in relatively young men. However, since age is a factor and there are an increasing number of old people, many of the patients seen with myocardial infarction are elderly.

Probably the most important treatment after a coronary occlusion is rest, so that demands on the heart are reduced until collateral circulation is established, electrical instability decreased and cardiac efficiency improved. If home circumstances are good and quiet and help adequate, it may be considered best to nurse the patient in his own home rather than risk moving him. Often admission to hospital is thought best because of the possibility of complications, which may prove fatal unless promptly treated, and because it may be difficult at home to ensure rest for the patient without his worrying about relatives caring for him.

Ideally the patient should be transported to hospital in a specially equipped and staffed 'Coronary Flying Squad' ambulance, but as yet this service is available in very few places. On reaching the hospital admission procedure must be quietly and efficiently carried out, giving the patient confidence that he is among people who are friendly and competent to give him the best possible care. He is lifted gently into a comfortably warm bed, preferably in a quiet part of the ward, and put in a semirecumbent position to reduce cardiac work, allow the patient to see round him and relieve any dyspnoea. Oxygen is given at once, because with myocardial infarction both the arterial oxygen tension and the cardiac output may be reduced, and hypoxia will increase myocardial damage. (If there is a history of cough and sputum it is essential to give only 25–30% oxygen, and watch for any signs of respiratory failure and carbon dioxide retention.) Many patients find nasal cannulae more comfortable than a mask, and communication and feeding are easier with these, as it is not necessary to keep removing the source of oxygen.

The heart rate rhythm and the blood pressure are recorded and an electrocardiograph is taken as soon as possible. An oscilloscope or monitor may be attached so that the cardiac rhythm can be observed easily. The patient is examined by a doctor, a history obtained and any necessary treatment ordered and carried out, Drugs ordered usually include 10–15 mg morphine intramuscularly to relieve pain and anxiety, and possibly a sedative such as 30 mg phenobarbitone three times a day. Digoxin and a diuretic such as frusemide may be ordered if there are signs of heart failure.

If a relative has accompanied the patient to hospital she should be interviewed as soon as possible. Some of the patient's medical history and details for the case-sheet may be obtained from the relative to save the patient effort. Information should be given regarding the diagnosis, likely progress and condition, and also visiting arrangements and what gifts may be brought for the patient. It is wise to explain that too many visitors may be tiring at this stage, and it is best if only those very well known to the patient visit at this time. The sudden severe illness of a previously healthy member of the family, particularly in the middle of the night, is a traumatic experience and the visitor, like the patient, may be in need of all the help and reassurance which can be provided. As soon as possible the visitor should be allowed to see the patient, but may be advised to stay only a short time to avoid tiring him.

As has been said, rest and observation are a vital part of early treatment, and ideally the patient spends the first 48–72 hours, the period of greatest risk, in a coronary care unit designed to be quiet and peaceful, as well as having all the facilities to deal with complications. The heart rate and blood pressure are recorded half-hourly at first, and the rhythm checked by palpation, auscultation, or by observing the oscilloscope.

The need for information must always be weighed against the inevitable disturbance to the patient, and the frequency of blood pressure recordings is reduced as soon as possible. Rest must be mental as well as physical, and when necessary the nurse must provide information about what is going on and reassurance. She must learn to judge when the patient wants to talk, when he is frightened and needs her presence at the bedside even for a brief moment intermittently, when he is worried about death or his family and may be helped by a visit from the Chaplain or medical social worker and when he has pain and needs an analgesic. She must note and report any cardiac dysrhythmias, cyanosis, pain, dyspnoea or other signs and symptoms.

Usually fluids and light diet are all the nutrition required at this stage, and it may be less effort to drink through a straw or from a cup and eat from a plate within easy reach than to be fed by a nurse. All fluid intake and output must be carefully recorded. Some people feel that fluids should not be given iced or very hot in case this stimulates the vagus and provokes cardiac dysrhythmias. Fresh fruit juice freshens the mouth, helps to supply extra potassium and may help to regulate the bowels. As the patient improves the diet may be increased, but should be well balanced and easily digested. A low-calorie diet may be necessary if obesity is a problem, or a low-cholesterol or low-sodium diet may be ordered.

Many physicians now allow these patients to be helped out of bed on to a commode for defaecation, as this is usually less effort than using a bedpan in bed. Straining must be avoided and a mild aperient may be included in the medicines ordered by the doctor.

After myocardial infarction almost all patients can and should be moved gently at regular intervals, and their pressure area care and personal hygiene maintained. This makes them more comfortable, helps them to rest and prevents pressure area necrosis, a particular risk when the circulation is poor or the patient sweating. However, in the period shortly after coronary occlusion, and while the patient has pain, dyspnoea, cyanosis or cardiac dysrhythmias, close observation is necessary during nursing care, and it may be necessary to omit the full bed-bath routine and change the position as little as possible during pressure care. Gentle passive movements of the feet and legs should be carried out and the calves massaged intermittently to prevent the deep vein thrombosis which is a very real risk. Chest complications are also a risk and short periods of deep breathing should be encouraged.

Medical staff usually examine the patient at intervals to detect any signs of complications, and order any changes in treatment.

Apart from the routine urine examination and haemoglobin estimation, investigations ordered usually include serum enzyme estimations, e.g. serum glutamic oxaloacetic transaminase (SGOT), serum glutamic pyruvic transaminase (SGPT) and lactic dehydrogenase (LDH) daily for the first 3 days, and serum cholesterol and uric acid; also serum electrolytes. Any sputum should be sent for culture, and if there is any glycosuria the blood sugar should be estimated. Some physicians prescribe anticoagulant therapy using the longer-acting drugs such as warfarin or phenindione, in which case it is necessary to estimate the prothrombin index at regular intervals so that drug dosage can be adjusted as is appropriate. If heparin intravenously or intramuscularly is used, a regular dose of 5000–10 000 units is given and the prothrombin index is not helpful. Estimation of the acid–base balance and blood gases may be necessary, particularly if the patient is hypotensive, cyanosed or tissue perfusion is poor. Either hypoxia or acidosis may depress cardiac action and increase damage.

Intravenous sodium bicarbonate, the dose calculated according to the base deficit, may be ordered and may produce immediate obvious improvement in the patient's condition (Fig. 20).

If there are no complications and the patient's condition improves he may be allowed to increase his activities, helping to wash himself, and eventually getting out of bed and starting to walk round the ward. At one time patients were kept in bed for 4–6 weeks with this condition, but many physicians now allow them to get up after 7 days and to walk freely around the ward by the end of 2–3 weeks, on the principle that the heart will more quickly

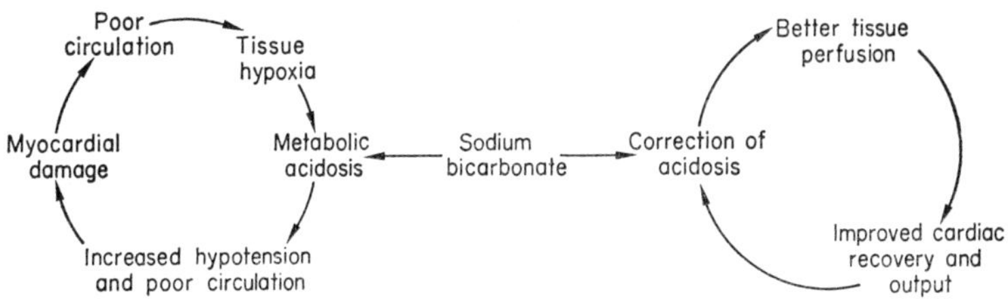

FIG **20. The effect of sodium bicarbonate.**

develop a collateral circulation if exercise is progressively increased. The important thing is that any recurrence or onset of signs and symptoms must be observed and reported early, so that treatment can be changed and activity limited as necessary. At the same time, nurses must not give the patient the impression that they are waiting for something to happen, so observation must be unobtrusive.

The period of rehabilitation both in hospital and after discharge is very important. Both patients and relatives must realize that 'having a heart attack' does not necessarily mean the life of a complete invalid. Activities must be introduced gradually, and sudden violent physical exertion must always be avoided. Many people live a full and quite active life for many years after a coronary occlusion, though recurrence is fairly common. The important thing is that the patient should learn to take warning and slow down or reduce his exertions if he is unduly breathless, excessively tired or has chest pain. Yet he should take adequate exercise within his limitations. The medical social worker may be able to help by arranging for his employer to have a lighter job ready for the patient when he is fit to return to work.

The future support of his family may be a source of considerable anxiety to a breadwinner, and the knowledge that he will be able to return to work may assist his recovery. It may be necessary to arrange a brief period of convalescence away from home after discharge, particularly if home circumstances are unsuitable and there are a lot of stairs. Help from the medical social worker may be needed to find suitable permanent accommodation, for example, by contact with the local housing authority.

On discharge, full instructions must be given regarding diet, other restrictions and the 'follow-up' appointment. Usually only a moderate intake of alcohol is allowed. An adequate supply of any necessary drugs should be given, making sure that the patient understands how and when to take them, and the dangers of not taking them and of allowing anyone else to take them. If anticoagulants are given, he should also be warned of any side-effects to look for, e.g. dark or blood-stained stool or urine, or other bleeding. Helpful printed cards are available for distribution to patients having such drugs. The letter to the patient's family doctor should reach him as soon as possible after discharge.

Complications

The commonest complications of coronary occlusion are cardiogenic shock, cardiac failure (see Chapter 2), cardiac dysrhythmias and, less commonly, deep vein thrombosis (see Chapter 8), arterial embolism, ventricular aneurysm, ruptured ventricle or occasionally a ventricular septal defect.

Cardiogenic shock

In this condition the cardiac output is low, the peripheral tissues cold and pale or cyanosed, and the patient is hypotensive, sweating and lethargic and mentally detached from his surroundings or confused and restless. The urine output is low. The heart rate is usually rapid, but may be abnormally slow, particularly if there is any degree of heart block. The pulse pressure, i.e. the difference between the systolic and diastolic pressure, is decreased. The prognosis for these patients is poor unless the condition can be reversed fairly quickly. A high concentration of humified oxygen should be given, 6–10 litres by mask or nasal cannulae. The patient is kept at rest lying flat unless dyspnoea makes it imperative to sit him up a little. Passive foot movements and leg massage may be performed to decrease the risk of venous thrombosis, but otherwise disturbance should be reduced to a minimum. Blood gas estimation will reveal a low Po_2 and metabolic acidosis. Correction of this by intravenous infusion of 100–200 ml, as sodium bicarbonate 8·4%, as calculated from the base deficit, often produces marked clinical improvement. The patient becomes pinker, warmer and the urine output may improve. Low molecular weight dextran infusion may be ordered to reduce 'sludging' and improve peripheral tissue perfusion.

Drugs which may be used include isoprenaline infusion to stimulate the heart and improve tissue perfusion, phenoxybenzamine to dilate peripheral vessels, reduce peripheral resistance and improve perfusion and diuretics such as mannitol or frusemide intravenously to stimulate urine output. Digitalis in some form may be indicated. If the heart rate is abnormally slow, 60/min or less, 0·6 mg atropine or isoprenaline infusion may be ordered to increase the heart rate, or a transvenous pacemaker catheter may be introduced and attached to an electrical pacemaker set at the desired rate. Where possible a demand pacemaker is used for safety, since this will cease to function if the patient's spontaneous rate overtakes the rate set.

At one time vasoconstrictor drugs such as metaraminol were used in an effort to raise blood pressure. This is now rarely done because they reduce still further the blood supply to the kidneys and peripheral tissues, so that renal function is decreased still further and metabolic acidosis increased. Hypotension, e.g. blood pressure 90/60, may be accepted without too much concern if the tissue perfusion is good, i.e. the patient pink and warm and the urine output good. Venous pressure may be measured to assess how much fluid should be given and detect fluid retension and heart failure.

Nursing these patients involves careful observation, recording of the various parameters such as heart rate, arterial pressure, urine output and possibly venous pressure, and reporting any adverse changes, accurate administration of the treatment ordered, and maintenance of the best basic nursing care compatible with the patient's condition. For example, it may not be possible for some hours to turn the patient for full sacral pressure area care, but the heels are often even more at risk and are accessible to treatment without disturbing the patient. In the acute stage catheterization is often necessary to allow accurate hourly measurement of urine output.

Inexperienced nurses may wonder why one patient receives much more intensive treatment and observation than another in an apparently similar condition. It must be realized that measures justifiable for a patient who has a real if slim chance of return to a worthwhile life may be unjustified for a patient with no such expectation because of age or condition.

Cardiac failure

This has already been described in Chapter 2.

Cardiac dysrhythmias

Many of the deaths which occur after coronary occlusion are due to dysrhythmias, which can be treated successfully if detected early enough. It is often for this reason that an oscilloscope is used to display cardiac rhythm for the first 48–72 hours, the period of greatest risk, or longer if dysrhythmias are observed; these will be discussed in a separate section later in this chapter.

Arterial embolism

Clot formation in the left atrium may take place when the atrium fibrillates instead of contracting forcibly. When ischaemia or infarction of ventricular muscle involves the endocardium clot may form over the damaged area. In either case at any time the clot may become dislodged and be swept through the arterial system until it reaches an artery small enough to obstruct its passage.

The principles of treatment of arterial embolism are the same whatever the cause, but may have to be modified when it is associated with ischaemic heart disease because of the cardiac condition. For example, a patient with a saddle embolus obstructing circulation to the legs and a tachycardia of 200/min cannot be subjected to surgical removal of the embolus until the cardiac dysrhythmias has been controlled and the general circulation restored to as near normal as possible. During and after operation adequate oxygenation and maintenance of circulatory volume without overloading are particularly important.

Ventricular aneurysm

This may form as a result of necrosis and subsequent fibrosis of an infarcted area of the ventricular wall, most commonly in the left. There is a danger that it may enlarge and rupture.

The aneurysm may be seen on X-ray screening as a pulsating dilatation attached to the ventricular wall. The ECG shows the typical infarction pattern even more than 6 months after the original episode of coronary occlusion. Sometimes the aneurysm can be removed surgically and the healthy muscle sutured, or a reinforcing patch of synthetic material sewn over the area. Cardio-pulmonary bypass technique is necessary.

Cardiac dysrythmias and electrocardiograph abnormalities

As already stated, cardiac dysrhythmias may be one of the complications of coronary occlusion. They may also occur owing to conditions of metabolic origin, e.g. acidosis, drugs, hypoxia, trauma, and cardiac disease, or postoperatively.

Any persistent tachycardia may increase myocardial damage, since it decreases the period of diastole during which coronary blood flow is at its maximum. Hypotension due to low cardiac output also decreases myocardial circulation. This may occur with a rapid or abnormally slow rate. Normally the various parts of the heart contract in regular sequence in response to impulses passing through the conduction system from the sinu-atrial node, through the atrial muscle, the atrioventricular node, down to the bundle of His, the right and left bundle branches, and out through the fibres of Purkinje to the ventricular muscle. When heart muscle is damaged by ischaemia or subjected to abnormal conditions, such as hypoxia, acidosis, hypothermia or too much or too little of certain electrolytes such as potassium in the circulation, transmission of normal impulses may be altered, or impulses may be fired off from abnormal sites in the heart muscle. The shape of the complexes seen on the electrocardiogram varies according to the direction in which the impulses travel and the speed of conduction. Impulses taking an abnormal pathway are said to be aberrant.

Electrocardiogram monitoring with an oscilloscope

Many of the deaths which occur after coronary occlusion or in certain other conditions of metabolic origin, postoperatively or due to drugs, hypoxia, trauma or other cardiac disease, are due to cardiac dysrhythmias which can be successfully treated if they are detected early enough. For this reason patients known to be particularly at risk may be attached to an oscilloscope (Fig. 21) so that the electrical impulses passing through the heart and the

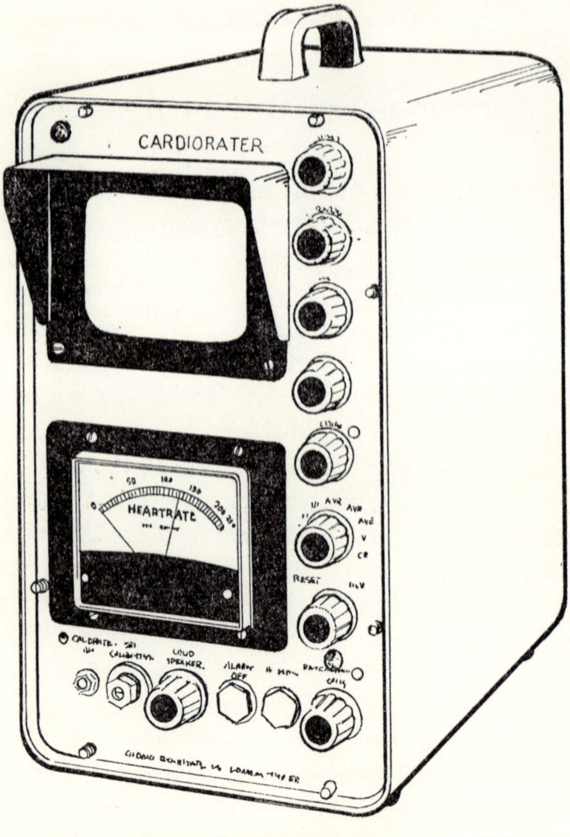

FIG 21. Cardiac oscilloscope (Cardiac Recorders Ltd).

cardiac rhythm can be observed frequently without disturbing the patient.

To do this metal electrodes (Fig. 22) are attached to the wires leading to the oscilloscope and to the patient's skin, preferably to the chest wall. Electrodes attached to the limbs are less successful as

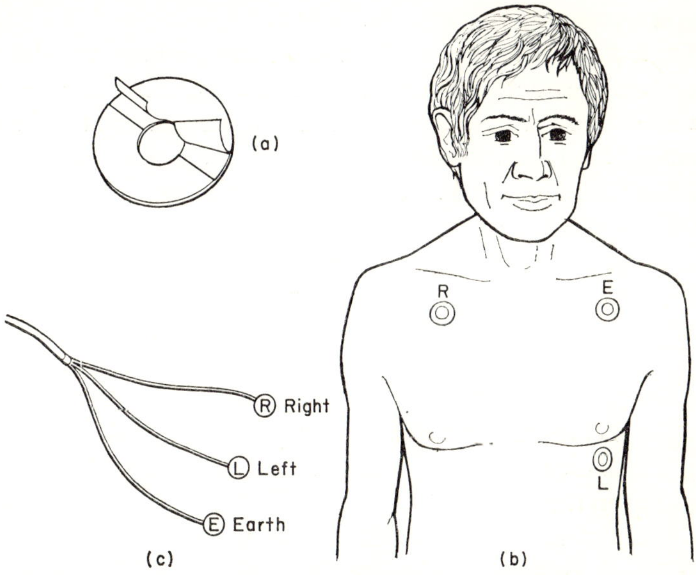

FIG 22. **A type of chest electrode for ECG monitoring.**
A, The double-sided adhesive ring is stuck to the plastic disc and the protective paper is peeled off the second side. B, The disc is then attached to an area of clean dry skin on the chest wall. Electrode jelly is applied to the skin within the plastic ring. Various positions can be used for the electrodes but after a sternal incision those shown are usually convenient. C, The metal electrodes are then snapped on to the appropriate discs.

any muscle movement causes interference with the tracing on the screen. Rubber straps to attach to limb electrodes are particularly undesirable as they impede circulation in patients already at risk of venous thrombosis.

Metal needle electrodes may be used, but to avoid repeated punctures of the skin plastic rings secured by double-sided adhesive rings are often used to secure the metal electrodes.

The procedure for attaching the patient to the oscilloscope is as follows. First, if the patient is conscious, it is explained to him that the machine will provide the staff with information about how his heart is beating, so that they need not disturb him too much, but can adjust his treatment as necessary. It will cause him no sensation and plays no part in keeping his heart beating, it merely records. As the electrodes are attached each step is explained in simple terms.

The machine is plugged in to the electricity supply and switched on. A fine line of light should soon start to run continuously across the screen. On most machines there are controls to adjust the focus and brightness as necessary. The area to which the electrodes are to be attached must be clean, dry and not hairy. The skin is rubbed lightly to achieve good contact and the electrodes applied with a layer of electrode jelly to provide good contact with the skin. The jelly used routinely for recording electrocardiographs is not usually suitable for long-term monitoring, because it is rather rough and has a high sodium content and causes soreness of the skin if left on too long. If the skin does become sore the area used should be changed at regular intervals. The cable, which is next attached to the oscilloscope, is secured so that it does not continually drag on the electrodes.

On most machines it is necessary to adjust a knob to select the lead which best displays the cardiac rhythm. The size of the pattern displayed and the speed at which it crosses the screen can be adjusted by the appropriate knobs, usually labelled 'gain' or 'sensitivity' and 'velocity' or 'speed', respectively.

A heart rate meter may be part of the machine. The upper and lower desirable limits for the heart rate can be set, so that an alarm sounds when these are passed. There may be a flashing light or audible signal to indicate each systole. If an audible signal is used it should be set as low as possible while still audible. Even so, it should be remembered that such a sound can be very disturbing to a patient, especially if it becomes irregular.

The patient should not be able to watch his own monitor, because this tends to increase anxiety.

Monitoring problems and how they might be solved

1. A straight line on the monitor.

...rmly attached and switched on?
...tly?
...appropriate lead?

...n (Fig. 23A, B).
...ned and is there enough elec-

...ratus in use which is inadequately ...plug broken? It may help to try using a ...cal socket, to avoid cables lying across each other or against the metal bed frame.

3. An irregular wavy line, without formed pattern.
   Has the patient had a cardiac arrest?
   Are all plug and electrode contacts good?
   Is a wire broken?

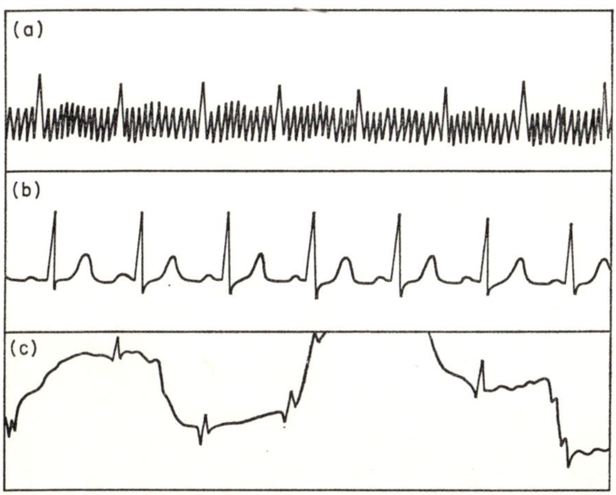

FIG **23. Faults in monitoring.**
A, The 'fuzzy' trace. B, The 'fuzzy' trace after correction. C, Wandering base-line.

4. Wandering baseline, i.e. the whole pattern is moving up and down the screen (Fig. 23C) This is usually due to movement of the electrodes, or of the area to which they are attached.

These technical faults can usually be corrected quite easily if the apparatus is good, but the nurse must report any other abnormalities noted, e.g. tachycardia, bradycardia or change in rhythm (see cardiac dysrhythmias, pp. 76–82).

When cardiac monitoring is discontinued the patient must be assured that he no longer needs it and that he is now recovering. Many patients feel insecure at this stage, and fear either that their heart is more likely to stop when the monitoring has been discontinued, or that no-one will notice if their heart does fail. Because of this they may at first need a little extra attention from the staff until confidence returns.

Patterns displayed

The pattern displayed on an oscilloscope is similar to that seen on an electrocardiograph, a description of which will be found in Chapter 9 (see Fig. 96, p. 212.) When abnormalities are observed on an oscilloscope it is often necessary to take an electrocardiograph strip for more detailed perusal and for record.

Typical myocardial infarction pattern

This shows on leads which have the positive electrode 'facing' the injured surface, e.g. Lead I and AVL if the infarction is anterior, Leads II, III and AVF if it is inferior. It has three main features:

1. The pathological Q wave is broad and deep in leads other than AVR (which normally has a broad, deep Q). This is due to an electrical 'hole' where there is completely dead tissue which allows

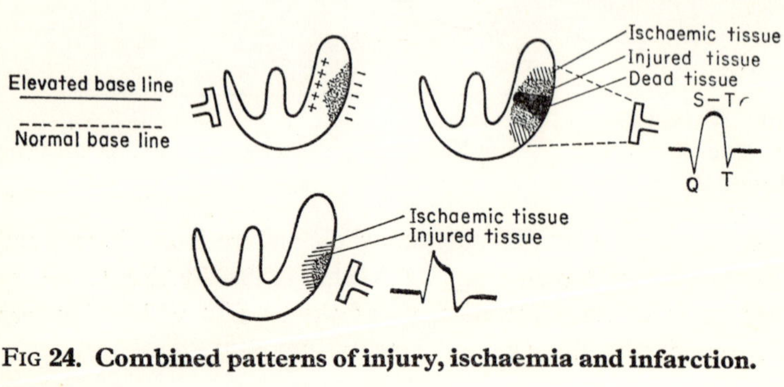

FIG **24. Combined patterns of injury, ischaemia and infarction.**

the electrode to record the activity of healthy muscle in the opposite ventricle through it.

2. Raised S–T segment. Injured muscle emits a continuous negative current which results in a depressed baseline. When the healthy muscle is stimulated it changes from electrically positive to negative. There is then no flow of current and the baseline rises to its normal level, which makes the S–T segment appear raised. This segment is also coved, i.e. convex upwards.

3. A symmetrical inverted T wave which is due to myocardial ischaemia. Within a few weeks the S–T segment returns to normal, the T wave becomes very tall and returns to normal, and only the pathological Q waves remain. It is therefore possible to estimate the age of the infarct from the electrocardiograph.

Sinus rhythm

This is the normal rhythm of the heart (Fig. 25), with a normal ECG complex. In sinus tachycardia and sinus bradycardia the rate

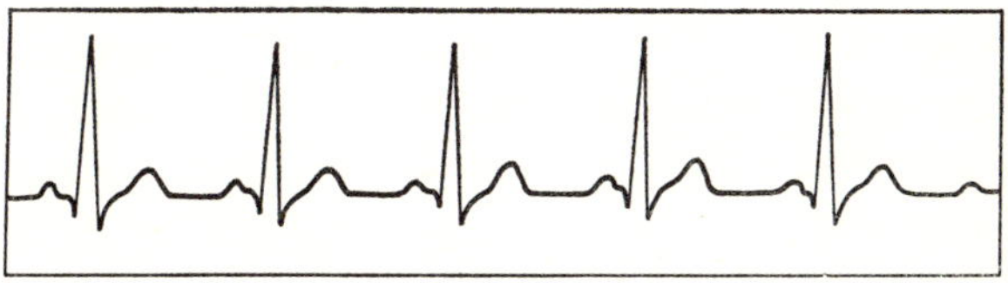

FIG **25. Sinus rhythms.**

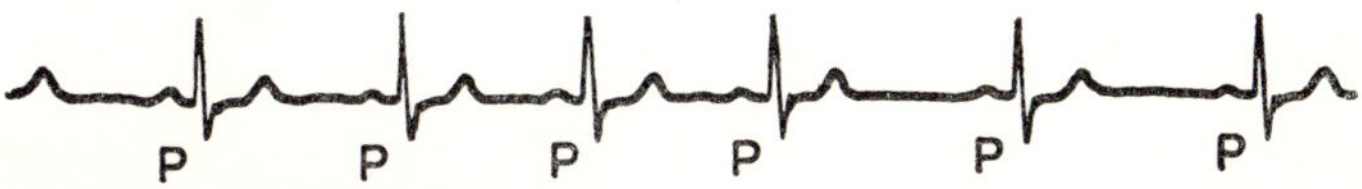

FIG **26. Sinus dysrhythmia.**

Note the gradual change in RR interval, with each QRS complex being preceded by a similar P wave.

is abnormally fast or slow respectively, but the rhythm otherwise normal.

Tachycardia is normally associated with emotion, exercise, pyrexia, heart or circulatory failure, or drugs such as atropine. Bradycardia commonly occurs during sleep, in athletes or in association with raised intracranial pressure or obstructive jaundice (direct effect of bile salts on the sinu-atrial node).

Sinus dysrhythmia

The complexes are normal, but the rate increases with inspiration and decreases during expiration. This is a normal physiological phenomenon seen most commonly in young people.

Premature atrial contraction or atrial extrasystole

The complex occurs earlier than expected, and has an abnormally shaped (bizarre) P wave. This is due to an impulse fired from an abnormal site in the atrial muscle. The impulse may reach the

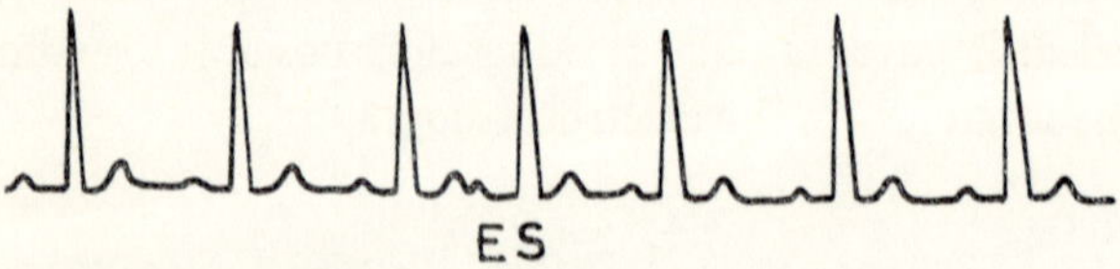

FIG **27. Atrial ectopic beat.**
Note at ES a premature P wave followed by a QRST of normal appearance.

atrioventricular node while it is refractory, i.e. not yet recovered from the previous impulse, in which case conduction to the ventricle does not take place. The P wave may be lost in the previous complex, so that there is no visible complex, but a prolonged interval before the next one.

The P–R interval may be normal or short, depending on the distance from the ectopic focus to the AV node, or prolonged due to an incompletely recovered AV node.

Ventricular conduction may be normal (normal QRS) or aberrant, due to an impulse arriving when only one bundle branch is sufficiently recovered for normal conduction. The QRS will then be bizarre. The compensatory pause is incomplete, i.e. the complex following the extrasystole occurs before it would have done had the sinus rhythm not been disturbed.

Occasionally atrial extrasystoles are not significant, but if they occur frequently, may herald atrial fibrillation.

Paroxysmal atrial tachycardia

The atria contract rapidly and regularly at up to 240 beats/min in response to stimuli from an ectopic focus (Fig. 28). The distorted P wave may be lost in the previous complex and the QRS may be normal, or distorted due to aberrant conduction. Therefore it may be impossible to determine whether the tachycardia is

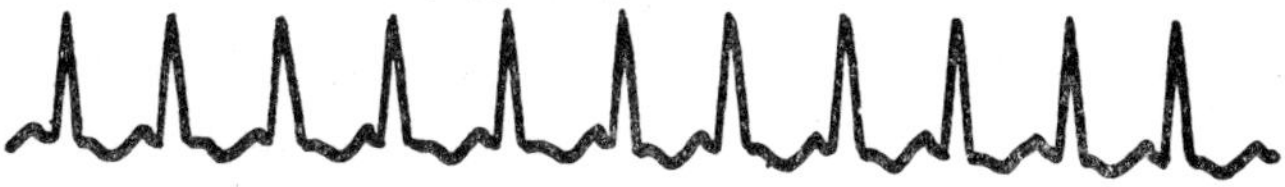

FIG 28. **Atrial tachycardia.**
Showing QRS complexes of normal width, at a rapid rate and with regular RR intervals.

Atrioventricular nodal rhythm

atrial or nodal (AV node) and either may be referred to as a paroxysmal supraventricular tachycardia.

This rhythm is dangerous where there is already myocardial damage or if it persists for long periods.

Atrial fibrillation

P waves are replaced by an irregular wavy line, with ventricular complexes (QRS) occurring at irregular intervals (Fig. 29).

Instead of contracting forcibly in response to stimuli from the sinu-atrial node the atria twitch and quiver, with small areas of the

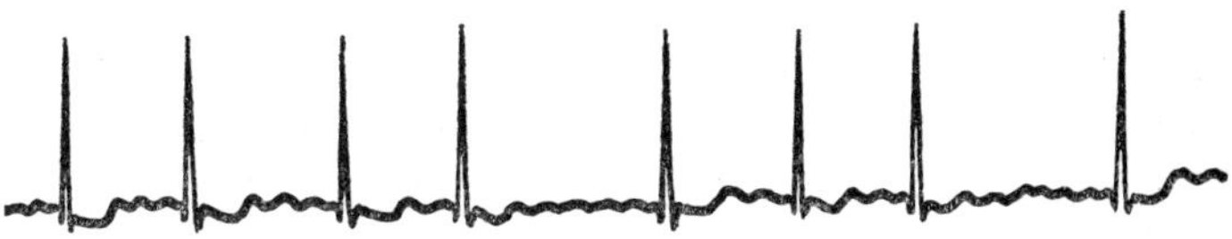

FIG 29. **Atrial fibrillation, with complete irregularity of atrial and ventricular rhythms.**

atrial muscle contracting and relaxing independently in a completely disorganized manner. The AV node is quite unable to conduct all the 400–600 impulses/min which reach it irregularly. The rate of ventricular contraction, the degree of ventricular filling and the force of contraction are all irregular. The peripheral pulses are therefore irregular in rate, rhythm and volume, and the rate felt may be less than the apex rate.

The ventricular rate may be 120–150, in which case the cardiac output and consequently the blood pressure and peripheral perfusion are decreased. Digitalis in some form is the appropriate treatment for this condition. It increases the refractory period of the AV node so that the ventricular rate slows, ventricular filling and contraction increase and consequently cardiac output rises. This also improves coronary circulation.

Atrial fibrillation occurs in association with mitral and tricuspid valve disease, coronary disease, thyrotoxicosis and constrictive pericarditis, and is not an uncommon complication of cardiothoracic surgery in older people.

Atrial flutter

This appears on the oscilloscope as a characteristic regular 'sawtoothed' pattern, often with 2, 4, 6 or even more P waves to each QRS (Fig. 30). Sometimes the ratio of P waves to QRS complexes

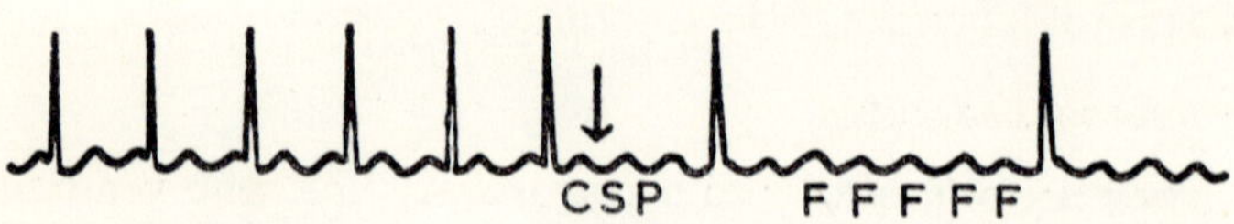

FIG 30. **Atrial flutter.**
Note that the flutter waves are difficult to discern until carotid sinus pressure is applied.

varies according to the degree of AV node block. It is often not possible to see the T waves which are obscured by the P waves.

The atrium contracts regularly at 200–400/min. Usually the AV node is unable to conduct all these impulses, and the ventricle receives only each second, fourth or sixth stimulus (usually an even number). There is then said to be a 2:1, 4:1 or 6:1 block.

Attacks of atrial flutter tend to start and end abruptly, and may occur with most kinds of acquired myocardial, valvular or coronary disease.

Atrioventricular nodal rhythm

When the atrioventricular node becomes the dominant pacemaker for the heart, the ventricular conduction, and therefore the QRS, is normal. However, if the impulse is conducted to the atria it will be in the reverse direction, and therefore the P waves are inverted. Depending on the relative speed of conduction through the atria and ventricles the P may occur before, after or within the SQR (Fig. 31).

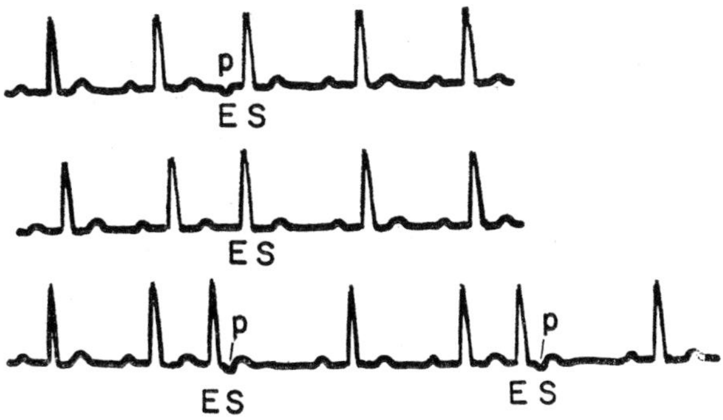

FIG **31. Nodal ectopic beats.**
Note that the R wave may precede, follow or coincide with the QRS complex.

Wandering pacemaker

The P waves may occur in varying relationship to the QRS, with a long or short P–R interval, or with the P within or after the QRS, or absent altogether, or inverted. This is due to the sinu-atrial node, the AV node or other ectopic foci in the atria becoming the dominant pacemaker intermittently.

Heart block (see Chapter IX)

Nodal rhythm or heart block may occur whenever there is interference with the normal conduction system in the region of the

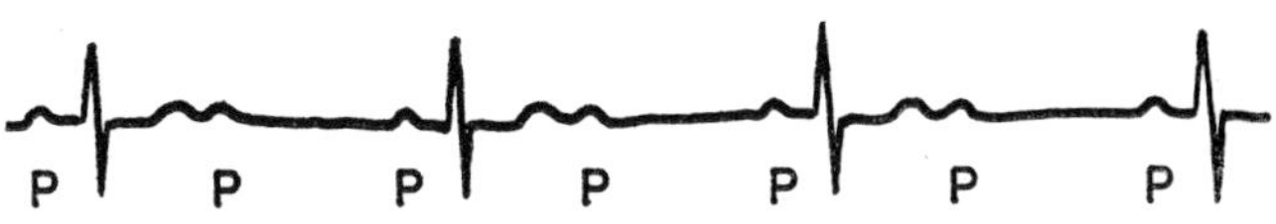

FIG **32. Second degree heart block, 2:1 block.**
Note that only every second P wave is followed by a QRS.

atrioventricular node. This may be due to ischaemia in coronary disease or surgical intervention. If it is due to swelling from local sutures the rhythm may return to normal as this subsides (Fig. 32).

Wenckebach phenomenon

The P–R interval lengthens with each beat until a beat is

dropped, i.e. the P is not followed by a QRS (Fig. 33). This is due to increasing difficulty in conduction through the AV node, which recovers during the prolonged pause when a beat is dropped.

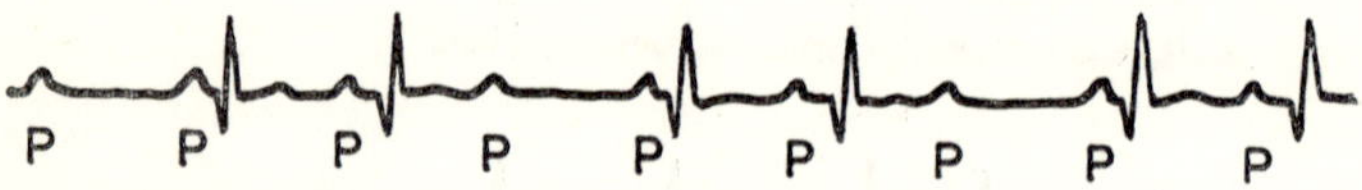

FIG 33. Partial heart block of the Wenckebach type.
Note that the PR interval is prolonged from beat to beat until a beat is dropped, after which the cycle restarts.

Ventricular extrasystole

A premature ventricular contraction or ventricular extrasystole (Figs 34, 35) occurs when the ventricle contracts early in reponse to

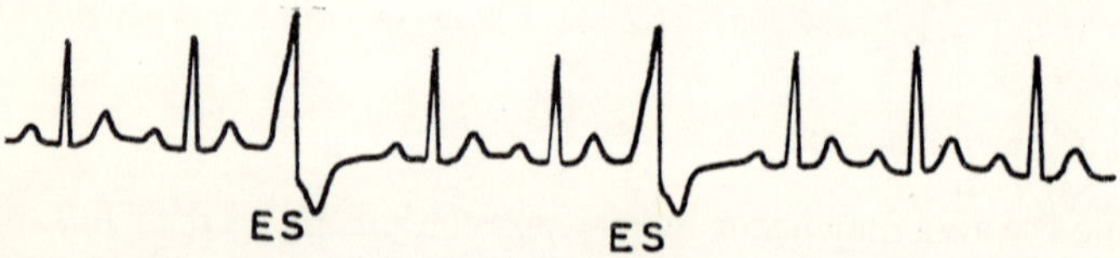

FIG 34. Ventricular ectopic beats (ES).
Note the bizarre pattern of the QRST and succeeding compensatory pause.

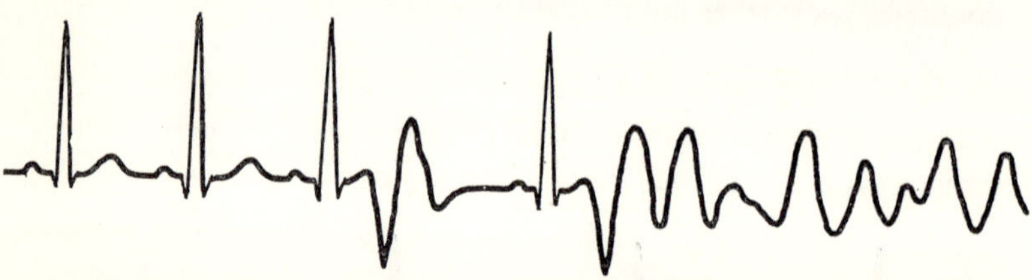

FIG 35. Ventricular ectopic beat interrupting the T wave of a preceding beat. The second beat of this type initiates ventricular fibrillation.

an impulse from an ectopic focus in the ventricle. Conduction from this focus to the ventricular muscle necessarily takes place in an abnormal direction and may occur through muscle (slow conduction) instead of through the normal conductive tissues. Consequently the QRS is abnormal in shape and widened. Each extrasystole from the same focus is the same shape and occurs at the same intervals after the previous sinus beat. After most ventricular extrasystoles there is a complete compensatory pause, i.e. the succeeding sinus beat occurs at the same time interval after the preceding one as it would have done if the beat in between had been normal. Since extrasystoles tend to occur after a long R–R interval, the combination of these two factors may result in bigeminal rhythm, i.e. each sinus beat followed by an extrasystole. This is most commonly seen with digitalis intoxication.

Occasionally single ventricular extrasystoles may be found in a normal person, but usually ventricular extrasystoles denote an irritable ventricle and should therefore be reported. If more than 5/min are seen or they occur 2 or more successively it is likely that ventricular tachycardia and possibly ventricular fibrillation may follow later.

Ventricular tachycardia

Runs of 3 or more ventricular extrasystoles are known as paroxysmal ventricular tachycardia (Fig. 36). This most commonly

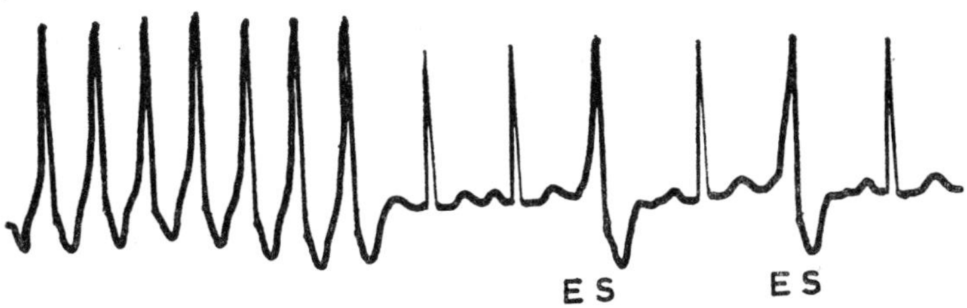

FIG **36. Ventricular tachycardia.**
Note the broad bizarre QRS complexes, resembling ventricular ectopic beats (ES) seen after termination of the ventricular tachycardia.

occurs in ischaemic myocardial disease but may occur with digitalis intoxication.

Ventricular fibrillation

This appears on the oscilloscope as an irregular wavy line with no obvious pattern (Fig. 37). Contraction and relaxation of the ventricular muscle is completely disorganized and uncoordinated. The ventricle quivers and there is no effective cardiac output. This may be a complication of myocardial disease, cardiac surgery or the administration of certain anaesthetic drugs, such as adrenaline, or intoxication with digitalis or quinidine.

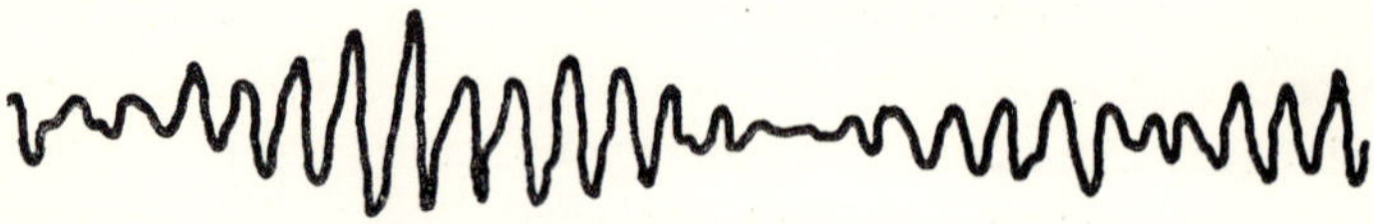

FIG **37. Ventricular fibrillation.**
Note the broad, bizarre and irregular complexes.

Asystole

A straight line appears on the oscilloscope as the heart ceases to contract.

Ventricular fibrillation or asystole indicate that there is no effective circulation. Cardiopulmonary resuscitation must be effectively instituted within 3 min if it is to be successful.

Continuous display of the cardiac rhythm can play a considerable part in reducing mortality and morbidity from dysrhythmias provided that staff are trained to observe the oscilloscope frequently and intelligently and to report abnormalities.

Treatment of dysrhythmias

Cardioversion

Two electrodes covered with electrode jelly or saline pads are placed on the chest wall and an electrical current is passed through it. The machine initiating the current incorporates an ECG oscilloscope to which the patient is attached by limb electrodes. When the operator (usually a doctor) presses the button the discharge of electricity is synchronized by the machine to occur just before the R or S wave, whichever is the larger deflection. This abolishes electrical activity in the heart for a brief period, which may allow the sinu-atrial node to resume the role of pacemaker and recommence sinus rhythm. The shock must be synchronized since a shock given in the vulnerable period, i.e. near the T wave, may provoke ventricular tachycardia or fibrillation. Although the same machine is often used for defibrillation, it must then be switched from synchronized to manual operation. In defibrillation a synchronized shock cannot be given since there are no complexes with which to synchronize it.

When cardioversion is performed on a conscious patient a light anaesthetic is usually necessary.

Drugs

Drugs such as lignocaine, procainamide, propranolol or practolol are often effective in reducing the irritability of atrial or ventricular muscle and preventing or controlling tachycardia or extrasystoles.

Atropine or isoprenaline may be used to increase the heart rate when bradycardia is causing too great a decrease in cardiac output. However, isoprenaline may sometimes cause ventricular extrasystoles.

Digitalis is used, particularly in atrial fibrillation, to decrease atrioventricular conduction and slow the ventricular rate.

Strict control of the serum potassium levels is necessary when dysrhythmias are troublesome, or likely to occur, since either hypokalaemia (too little potassium) or hyperkalaemia (too much) may affect cardiac rhythm and function. Digitalis intoxication may easily occur when the serum potassium is low. For further information see Chapters 10 and 11.

Artificial pacemaker

Artificial pacing with a transvenous pacemaker catheter electrode may be used either to remedy complete heart block or bradycardia with a low cardiac output. This is fully described in Chapter 6.

Vagal stimulation

Gentle but firm pressure over the carotid sinus or eyeball may be used by experienced people to control paroxysmal tachycardia.

Operations for myocardial ischaemia

Operations may be performed on patients with myocardial ischaemia to increase the circulation through ischaemic areas, to relieve the pain of angina pectoris, to reduce the work of the heart or to repair the damage caused by an infarct.

Early attempts to increase the myocardial blood supply consisted of stitching to the myocardium a segment of omentum (cardio-omentopexy) or a piece of lung (cardiolingulopexy). It was hoped that when the raw surface adhered blood would flow through the adhesions to the myocardium. Post mortem examinations have not shown significant vascularity in the adhesions even in patients clinically improved after operation. Another method still in use is the introduction of asbestos talc between the pericardial layers around the ventricles. This causes inflammation and results in increased anastomosis between the coronary vessels. However, results are not very good.

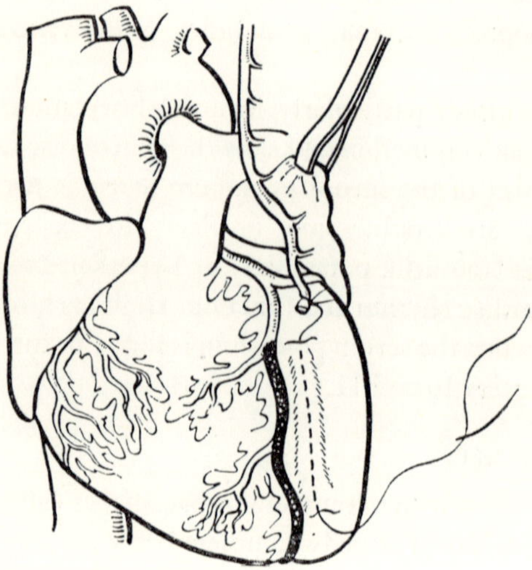

FIG 38. **Vineberg's operation.**

Vineberg's operation (Fig. 38), first performed in 1946, is a more direct attempt to combat myocardial ischaemia. A tunnel is made in the anterior wall of the left ventricle, the internal mammary artery is severed distally and its proximal end inserted into the tunnel and secured in place. Blood flows through this artery into the sinusoidal spaces in the myocardium and into the coronary system.

Coronary thrombo-endarterectomy (direct removal of the obstructing atheromatous plaque) is now sometimes performed, usually with cardiopulmonary bypass during operation. Good coronary angiograms are needed preoperatively to outline the vessels and the site of occlusion. Comparatively few patients have a single localized area of obstruction in a main vessel which would be suitable for this operation.

Dorsal sympathectomy may be performed to relieve persistent severe anginal pain. The fourth, third, second and whole or lower half of the first dorsal sympathetic ganglia are removed through a thoracotomy or collar incision at the root of the neck. Before operation the left stellate ganglion may be injected with 2% procaine through the neck and the patient exercised to see if anginal pain is less than before the injection. This is a test to see how effective the operation is likely to be. Stellate ganglion block causes a drooping upper eye lid, contracted pupil and enophthalmos (Horner's syndrome). This is temporary, but will become permanent if the upper half of the first dorsal ganglion is removed at operation. The good effects of operation are thought to be due partly to relief of pain by blocking the sensory sympathetic fibres and partly to the removal of sympathetic stimulation to the heart.

After severe myocardial infarction, some patients recover only if their circulation is assisted until the heart is able to maintain adequate circulation unaided. This has been done by fitting a pump and reservoir to a large artery. Blood is drawn into the reservoir during ventricular systole, so reducing the arterial resistance and the heart's work, and pumped back into the artery during diastole to increase circulation. A simpler method is to pass an intravenous catheter into the right atrium and through the septum into the left atrium. Oxygenated blood is withdrawn from the left atrium and pumped back into an artery, so bypassing the left ventricle. These methods are not yet in common use because of the problems of preventing clotting and haemolysis when assisted circulation is needed for days or weeks.

A ventricular aneurysm, a ventricular or atrial septal defect or a large area of fibrosis in the wall of a ventricle can result from coronary occlusion and death of ischaemic muscle. With cardiopulmonary bypass it is possible to remove an aneurysm or infarcted area of the ventricular wall or to repair a septal defect.

One of the most recent developments in this field of surgery is complete replacement of the damaged heart by another human heart from someone who has died from non-cardiac causes. The transplantation of first human heart in 1967 showed that a transplanted heart can adapt itself to maintain circulation in a different body and that many of the changes in other organs associated with cardiac failure can be reversed. However, the problem of rejection of the foreign heart by the recipient has not been completely solved. Tissue typing, similar to blood grouping, reduces the risk of rejection. Cytotoxic drugs are used to suppress immune reactions, but make the patient very susceptible to infection. There are also ethical considerations as to who should be the donors and recipients for heart transplantation. After heart transplant the patient is at first nursed in an isolated, sterile area to reduce the likelihood of infection. These patients also require all the postoperative nursing care and observation necessary after any major cardiac operation, including psychological support.

More work is now being done on vein grafts. A piece of the saphenous vein is removed, valves obliterated, and it is anastomosed to the coronary artery at two points, so that the area of coronary occlusion is bypassed. Good coronary angiograms are necessary preoperatively to define the blocked area. The technique is as for transaortic catheter angiography, but the ends of the catheters are specially shaped so that they can be manoeuvred into the right or left coronary orifices. A vein graft offers a chance of considerable improvement to a patient with severe coronary disease without many of the problems inherent in cardiac transplantation.

5
Congenital heart disease

Congenital abnormalities of the heart or great vessels occur in 5–6/1000 live births. If at all severe they may not only limit the quality and length of the patient's life, but also affect the life of the whole family. Anxiety about the child's condition, the extra care needed and possible intermittent visits to a hospital may be a strain on the parents, while other children in the family may feel deprived because they receive less attention, even though they may not be neglected.

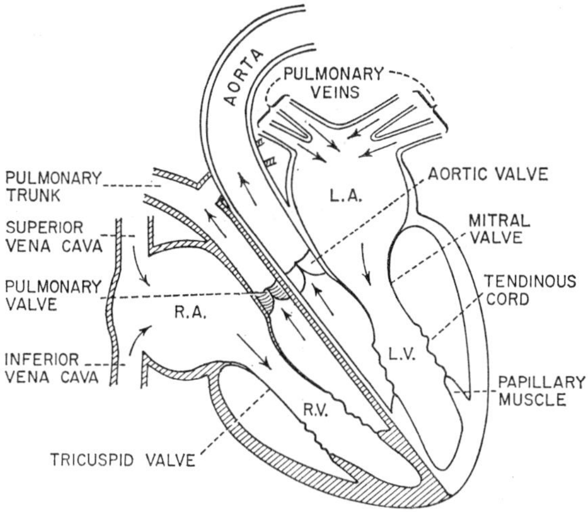

FIG **39. The normal heart.**
L.A., Left atrium. L.V., Left ventricle. R.A., Right atrium. R.V., Right ventricle.

The expression of these defects ranges from severe cyanosis, dyspnoea with consequent feeding problems and cardiac failure in infancy to minimal signs, such as abnormal cardiac sounds or murmurs on auscultation with no associated signs or symptoms.

There may be no apparent effects until adult life; indeed some mild defects are compatible with a life normal in activity and length. The public health nurse or midwife may be able to help in diagnosis by bringing to the doctor's notice any feeding difficulties, cyanotic attacks or unusual dyspnoea on exertion which she notices while in contact with the child. She will be particularly alert for these when there is any history of maternal infection, e.g. rubella early in pregnancy (before 12 weeks), or genetic factors or drug therapy predisposing to congenital abnormalities. The Local Authority 'At Risk' Register, where it exists, lists all infants known to be at risk of abnormality for any reason. Routine school examinations aid in early diagnosis.

If the defect is at all severe the child may be poorly developed physically or develop increasing dyspnoea as the pulmonary resistance rises or heart failure supervenes. The severe cyanosis resulting from some defects is associated with clubbing of fingers and toes, and a high haemoglobin and red cell count, and recurrent attacks of pulmonary infection are liable to occur where there is abnormally increased pulmonary circulation.

Many of these patients are prone to subacute bacterial endocarditis, since abnormal jets of blood caused by the abnormalities damage the endocardium or endothelium of large vessels, thus providing a suitable site for the growth of circulating bacteria. *Streptococcus viridans* may often be cultured from the blood stream after tooth extraction. It is for this reason that penicillin or other antibiotics are given to 'cover' tooth extraction or other minor procedures.

Because of the extra care they need, the limitations on their physical activity, their frequent absence from school during illness or investigations and especially the emotional impact of the diagnosis 'heart disease' on the parents, these children are in danger of being overprotected and becoming anxious and dependent. It is even more important to avoid this now that in many cases surgery offers a good chance of cure or alleviation and a normal life which may be impaired by 'cardiac neurosis'.

Nurses have an important part to play both in the hospital and in the community in cooperating with medical staff to ensure that the parents understand as much as is helpful to them about their child's defect, the investigations and treatment necessary and any necessary physical limitations. By establishing a good rapport with the parents a nurse can obtain their cooperation over dietary and other medical treatment, and at the same time provide moral support and encourage them to allow the child as normal a life as possible. This is especially important when it is desirable to postpone surgery for a few years. It is also important to establish good relationships with the child, who, being unable to compete physically with other children, may have associated much with adults and may consequently be rather precocious and need more detailed explanations than his age would normally warrant.

Causes of death

The usual causes of death from congenital heart disease are cardiac failure (right, left or both), anoxia leading to cardiac arrest or bacterial endocarditis.

Congenital heart disease may be associated with other abnormalities which make treatment more difficult and early death more likely. These include Marfan's syndrome, where the patient has arachnodactyly (thin spidery fingers and toes), is long and thin in build and may have numerous other skeletal and connective tissue abnormalities such as laxity of ligaments, scoliosis, a high arched palate and myopia and subluxation of lens, and mongolism, which is quite often associated with ventricular septal defect or Fallot's tetralogy.

Advances in treatment

Over the last twenty years or so advances in surgical and anaesthetic techniques, especially the development of cardiopulmonary bypass techniques in the 1950s, have made possible the palliation or cure of an increasing number and variety of defects. At normal temperature circulation can be stopped for 3 minutes only without risking brain damage. If the body is cooled to 31° C by iced water or a cooling blanket the circulation can be stopped for 8–10 minutes. This is long enough to repair a simple atrial septal defect, but allows little safe time to deal with any difficulties or defects found at operation.

Cardiopulmonary bypass allows the maintenance of circulation, if necessary, for several hours; while the heart is arrested or in ventricular fibrillation the operation is performed. This technique is therefore used for surgery on almost all defects except those right outside the heart (such as persistent ductus arteriosus or coarctation of the aorta) or those which can be dealt with quickly (such as isolated pulmonary stenosis).

Incidence of specific abnormalities (Campbell 1965)

Ventricular septal defect (V.S.D.)	15–20%
Atrial septal defect (A.S.D.)	10%
Persistent ductus arteriosus (P.D.A.)	10%
Coarctation of the aorta	10%
Pulmonary stenosis	10%
Fallot's tetralogy	10%
Aorticopulmonary transposition	10%
Aortic stenosis	5%
Others	15–20%

These abnormalities can be divided into the two groups of acyanotic and cyanotic conditions.

Acyanotic conditions

This group includes all those conditions where no blood reaches the systemic circulation without first passing through the lungs to be reoxygenated. There may be obstruction to flow from heart chambers, or abnormal communication between left heart chambers and systemic circulation and right heart chambers and venous or pulmonary artery circulation. The pressure in the left side of the heart and systemic circulation being greater than that in the right heart or pulmonary artery, oxygenated blood flows from the left to the right side, or from the aorta to pulmonary artery, unless there is obstruction to the normal outflow tract. These are left-to-right shunts, and the amount of shunt depends on the size of the defect and the pressures involved. Because of the extra blood supply the pulmonary circulation becomes overloaded, thickening of vessels occurs and pulmonary resistance increases. This in turn increases the strain on the right ventricle (and possibly the left) as it tries to maintain adequate circulation. Eventually this results in a right heart pressure higher than the systemic so that the shunt becomes reversed, i.e. a right-to-left shunt. This is called Eisenmenger's syndrome.

Ventricular septal defect

During fetal development the muscular septum grows upwards almost to the endocardial cushion, on either side of which are the developing mitral and tricuspid valves. The commonest ventricular septal defect (Fig. 40) is a high or membranous one (85%), but a

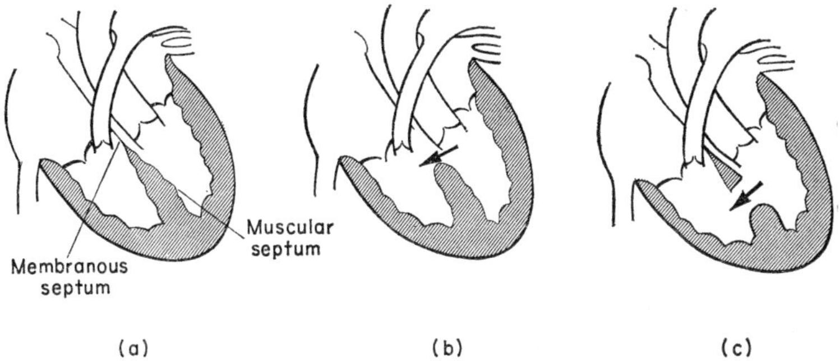

FIG **40. Ventricular septal defects.**
A, Ventricular septum. B, High or membraneous defect. C, Low or muscular defect. The septum may be almost completely absent.

low or muscular one may occur (10%). This may be very small or so large that there is almost no septum, and consequently only one ventricle. Presenting features may be palpitations, breathlessness on exertion and failure to thrive, or symptoms occurring as a result of complication, i.e. cardiac failure, pulmonary hypertension and recurrent pulmonary infections, or bacterial endocarditis.

Investigations. X-ray may show pulmonary artery dilation and increased vascularity of the lungs. Bilateral enlargement of the ventricles, especially the left, may be shown. Cardiac catheterization will usually show increased pressures and oxygen saturation in the right ventricle and the pulmonary artery, and the catheter may be seen to go through the defect. The electrocardiogram may show signs of left ventricular strain.

Prognosis. This depends on the size of the defect and shunt.

Most patients die before the age of 50 if the shunt is greater than 2:1, and some much earlier. The prognosis after surgical repair by direct suture or patch with Teflon or pericardium is good. A complete cure can result if this is done before complications supervene, ideally at the age of 3–5 years (pre-school) or certainly before 12. Heart block is a possible complication, owing to the damage to the bundle of His. If temporary this may be overcome by artificial pacing, but if heart block is permanent the outlook is much worse. Permanent pacing may be necessary.

Atrial septal defect

The atrial septum is formed in fetal development by two septa. The septum primum grows downwards to join the atrioventricular valves; the upper part perforates and forms the foramen ovale 1. The septum secundum grows down to the right of it covering the opening, but leaving another opening, foramen ovale 2. These two openings form the foramen ovale, which is necessary for fetal circulation (to bypass the lungs which are not yet functioning), but usually closes when the septa unite shortly after birth. An atrial septal defect (Fig. 41) may result from a persistent foramen ovale, early arrest in the development of the septum primum (ostium primum defect) or failure of the septum secundum to cover the foramen ovale 1 (ostium secundum defect). The latter is much more common (65% of cases) but less serious than ostium primum defect. This is because associated deformities such as split mitral or tricuspid valve cusps or communicating ventricular defects (atrioventricular canal) may occur with the latter.

Signs and symptoms. Symptoms may not occur until the age of 15 years or more with the ostium secundum defect. Increasing tiredness and dyspnoea on exertion are usually the most prominent symptoms, followed by the features of pulmonary hypertension, recurrent pulmonary infection and cardiac failure. Bacterial endocarditis is uncommon. A large secundum or ostium primum defect causes earlier and more severe difficulties.

Investigations. Chest radiograph may show right-sided enlargement of the heart and increased vascularity of the lungs. Electrocardiograms may show right ventricular strain and a right bundle-branch block pattern as the impulse takes longer to traverse

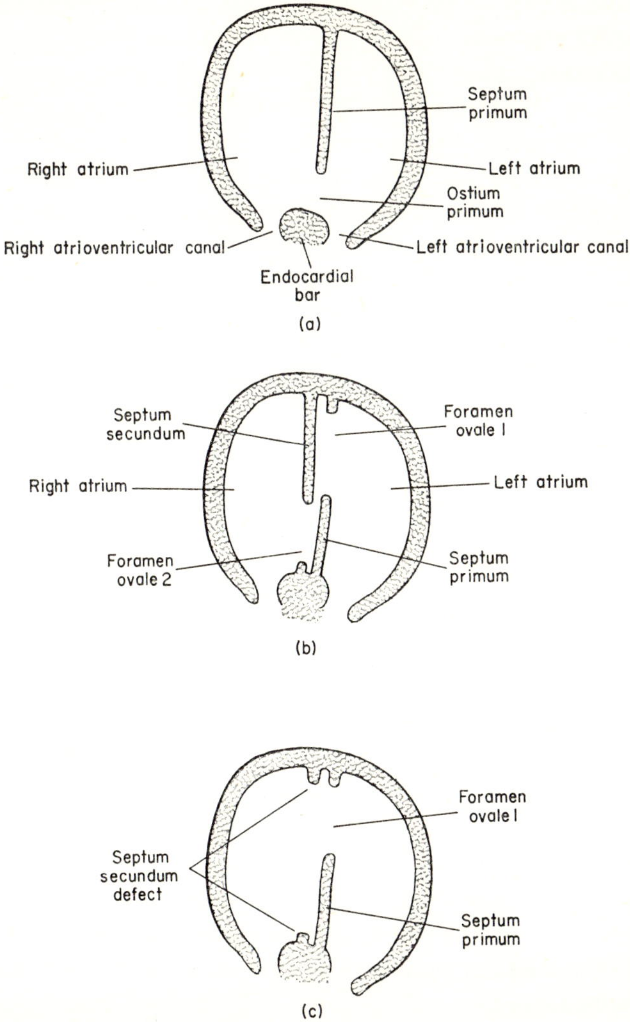

FIG **41. Atrial septal defects.**
A, Transverse section of the primitive atrium, showing its division in to right and left atria by the septum primum. B, Transverse section of the primitive atrium, showing the formation of the septum secundum and foramina ovale. C, Diagrammatic representation, showing the septum secundum type of atrial septal defect.

the enlarged right ventricle. Cardiac catheterization usually shows the catheter passing through into the left atrium, and may show increase in pressures and oxygenation in the right atrium, ventricle and pulmonary artery.

Prognosis. The patient usually dies by the age of 50, or much earlier if the defect is large or associated with other abnormalities, such as split valve cusps, a ventricular septal defect or anomalous pulmonary venous drainage into the right atrium. The results of surgical repair by direct suture or by Teflon or pericardial patch are good if the defect is of the ostium type, but repair of the ostium primum type is more difficult and results less good if there are associated defects in the valves. Damage to the atrioventricular bundle and consequent conduction defects are also more likely. The repair should be performed in childhood.

Persistent ductus arteriosus

The ductus arteriosus runs from the pulmonary artery to the aorta, usually beyond the subclavian artery. In fetal life, since oxygen is supplied through the placenta from the maternal circulation and not through the fetal lungs, most of the blood flowing through the pulmonary artery passes through the ductus to the systemic circulation. Normally the ductus ceases to function within a few hours or days of birth and is completely fibrosed after 3 months. If the ductus remains open blood from the aorta flows back into the pulmonary artery (Fig. 42), because after birth the pulmonary artery pressure is lower than that in the aorta. The condition is more common in girls.

Signs and symptoms. Signs and symptoms may occur early or late depending on the size of the ductus and the volume of the shunt. Dyspnoea and palpitations may occur with the onset of pulmonary hypertension and cardiac failure, and subacute bacterial endocarditis and pulmonary infections are likely complications. The characteristic 'machinery' or Gibson murmur increases with exercise.

Investigations. Chest X-ray may show left ventricular and pulmonary artery enlargement and increased vascularity of the lungs. In the electrocardiograms left ventricular strain may be evident.

Cardiac catheterization will show increased oxygen tension in the pulmonary artery and possibly increased pressures if the ductus is large. The catheter may be seen to pass through the ductus. Occasionally to confirm diagnosis a retrograde aortogram may be done, i.e. a catheter is passed through a peripheral artery up to the aortic

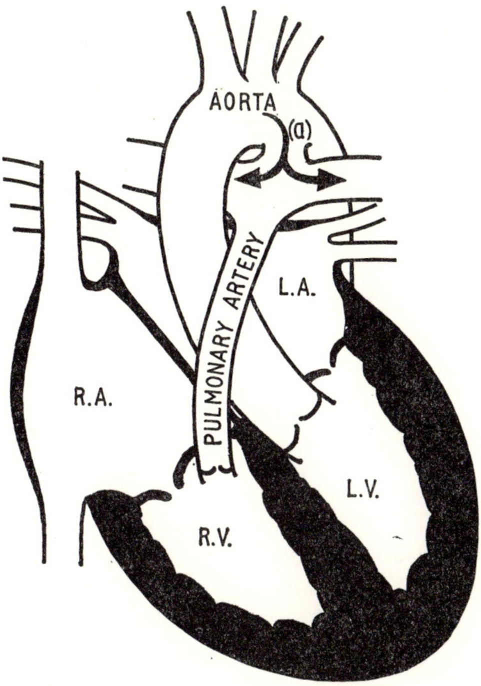

Fig **42. Persistent patent ductus arteriosus.**

arch and contrast medium injected so that it can be seen passing through the ductus into the pulmonary circulation.

Prognosis. Most patients die by the age of 50, or earlier if the ductus is large. If the ductus is ligated or, in the case of a wide ductus, divided and the ends sutured, the expectation of life is normal unless pulmonary hypertension or other complications have already developed. The operative risk is small. Bacterial endocarditis, if it occurs, is controlled by antibiotics and the ductus is then closed as soon as possible.

Pulmonary stenosis

This may be narrowing of the valve itself (80%) or infundibular stenosis, where the outflow channel from the right ventricle is narrowed just proximal to the valve (Fig. 43). The right ventricle becomes hypertrophied as it tries to maintain adequate pulmonary circulation through the stenosis.

Signs and symptoms. The principal symptom, which may not

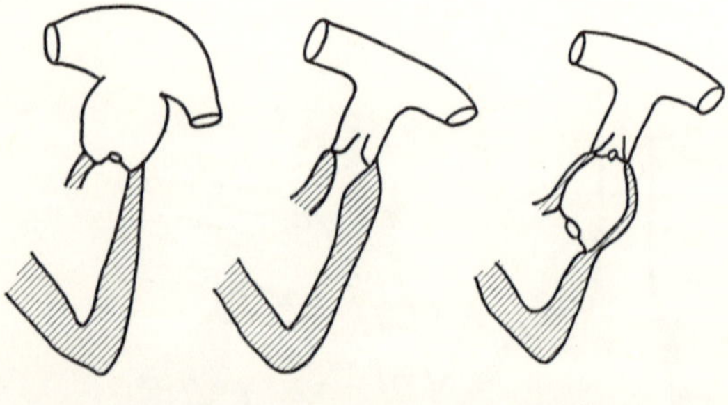

FIG **43. Congenital pulmonary stenosis.**
A, Pulmonary valvar stenosis. B, Subvalvular or infundibular stenosis. C, Infundibular diaphragm with subvalvular chamber and normal or stenotic valve.

occur until late adult life, is dyspnoea on exertion due to inadequate cardiac output. Later signs and symptoms of right heart failure may occur, depending on the severity of the stenosis.

Investigations. Chest X-ray may show diminished vascularity of the lungs and post-stenotic dilatation of the pulmonary artery, i.e. the dilatation which occurs due to the turbulence of blood beyond the narrowed valve. Cardiac catheterization will show the marked rise in pressure as the catheter is drawn from the pulmonary artery into the right ventricle. The difference between the pressures is known as the gradient, and the tighter the stenosis the higher the gradient. Electrocardiograms may show right ventricular hypertrophy and strain.

Prognosis. Prognosis depends on the degree of stenosis, as a tight stenosis will result in early onset of congestive heart failure. Once right ventricular hypertrophy and strain develop the patient is liable to die of sudden ventricular standstill during violent exertion.

Results of operation, i.e. splitting the valve or resection of part of the infundibulum, are good.

Coarctation of the aorta

Aetiology. This narrowing of the aorta develops early in fetal life in the region of the ductus arteriosus (or ligamentum arteriosum as it becomes when fibrosed after birth.) It is usually a localized constriction, though it may occasionally be elongated; since it lies below the left subclavian artery the vessels of the upper half of the body enlarge to form a collateral circulation to the lower half of the body (Fig. 44). This compensates for the diminished or even absent flow of blood down through the aorta. The condition is more common in boys.

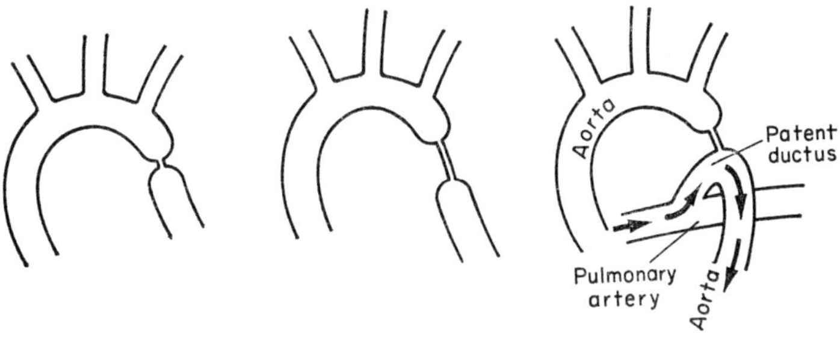

FIG **44. Types of coarctation of the aorta.**

Signs and symptoms. Sometimes the fetus or infant is able to develop sufficient collateral circulation to avoid cardiac failure and no symptoms are present in early childhood. However, the patient gradually develops hypertension in the upper limbs and head, the systolic pressure reaching 300 mm Hg or more, and left ventricular hypertrophy and failure occurs. The patient then complains of headaches, dizziness and epistaxis, and possibly palpitations and breathlessness. He may also complain of cold feet and intermittent claudication. Owing to the resistance in the smaller collateral vessels the systolic pressures are usually lower in the systemic circulation beyond the coarctation, so that the femoral pulses are absent or delayed and the blood pressure is unrecordable or lower than in the arms. Eventually cardiac failure, cerebral haemorrhage or rupture of the aorta may occur, especially during pregnancy, or the kidneys may fail. Subacute bacterial endocarditis may complicate the condition.

Investigations. Chest X-ray may show left ventricular enlargement and notching of the inferior surface of the ribs posteriorly, from pressure by the dilated intercostal arteries.

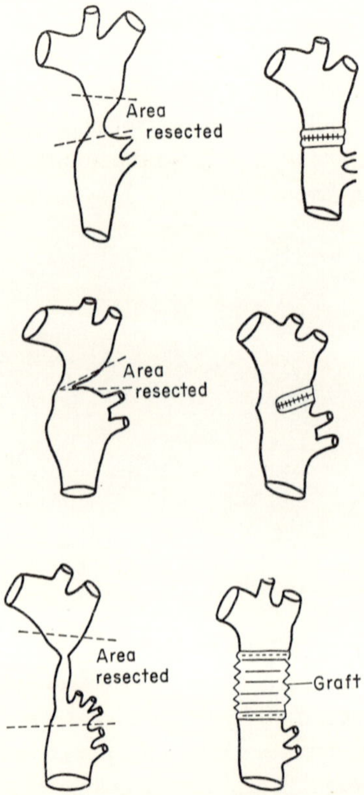

FIG **45. Operations to correct coarctation of the aorta.**

Aortography may be performed to demonstrate the coarctation.

Cardiac catheterization is performed only if there is a likelihood that persistent ductus or other lesion is also present.

Prognosis. Few patients survive beyond the age of 40 without surgical treatment (Fig. 45), which consists of excising the stricture and anastomosing the aorta or, if the stricture is long, putting in a graft (normally Terylene).

Ideally the operation is done between the ages of 8 a
before complications develop and when the aortic lu
enough to allow adequate blood flow even if the ana
not grow. The results of operation are usually good, tho
blood pressure may not fall immediately. The risks of operation
tend to increase with age after childhood.

Aortic stenosis

Aetiology. In this condition the three cusps of the aortic valve have failed to separate and may be almost completely fused along the commissures. There may be narrowing of the outflow tract of the ventricle proximal to the valve (Fig. 46).

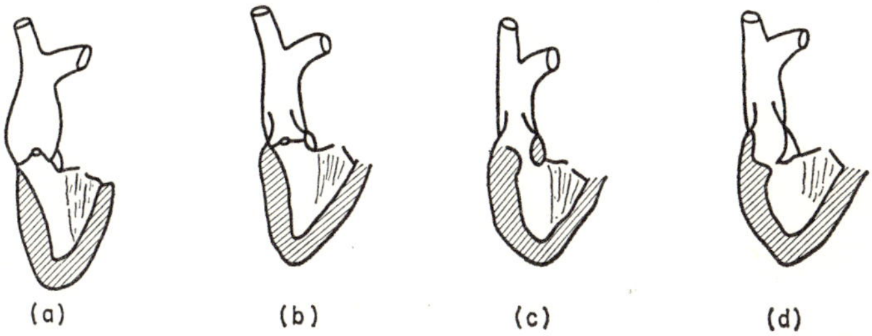

FIG **46. Congenital aortic stenosis.**
A, Valvar stenosis. B, Subvalvar diaphragm, usually a membrane with a central hole, rarely stenosis as well. C, Muscle thickening of the outflow track of the left ventricle. Note close relation to the septal cusp of the mitral valve. D, Subvalvar fibromuscular diaphragm with a chamber between it and the valve.

Signs and symptoms. Up to the age of about 15 there may be no signs and symptoms, though the patient may be rather pale and have a small pulse pressure owing to the peripheral vasoconstriction by which the body attempts to compensate for the small cardiac output. When the patient is fully grown the cardiac output becomes inadequate, and as left ventricular hypertrophy increases, increasing dyspnoea and signs of left ventricular failure occur. Calcification of the valve eventually occurs, and because of the involvement of the coronary orifices in this or because of pressure on the coronary arteries by the hypertrophied muscle anginal pain may occur.

Investigations. Chest X-ray may show left ventricular enlargement. Calcification may be demonstrated by screening. Electrocardiography may show left ventricular hypertrophy and strain.

Left ventricular puncture may be performed, i.e. a needle is passed through the chest wall into the ventricle to measure the systolic pressure and determine the gradient between that and the systemic pressure taken at the same time. Nowadays cardiac catheterization and transeptal puncture are more often performed so that a catheter can be passed through into the left atrium, down into the left ventricle and through the valve to measure pressures, but this is not without risk as serious dysrhythmias may be provoked.

Prognosis. Unfortunately, because of the gross ventricular hypertrophy, left ventricular standstill and sudden death are prone to occur, sometimes without obvious cardiac failure beforehand.

Once signs and symptoms of any severity occur the patient is likely to die within 2 years or less.

If the valve split is under direct vision with cardiopulmonary bypass technique (a 'closed split' is likely to result in regurgitation) before complications have arisen, the results are good. However, if the valve is very calcified it may be necessary to replace it by a homograft (human valve), heterograft (animal valve) or a prosthetic (artificial) valve.

Cyanotic conditions

This group includes those conditions where unoxygenated blood enters the systemic circulation (*a*) because of a right-to-left shunt, e.g. where the resistance caused by pulmonary stenosis causes blood to pass through a ventricular septal defect to the left ventricle, or (*b*) because of transposition of the great vessels leaving the heart.

Secondary effects

Polycythaemia, i.e. an increase in the number of red cells, develops to increase the oxygen carrying power of the blood. Cyanosis only appears when there is at least 5 g reduced haemoglobin/100 ml of blood in the capillaries. The haemoglobin and red cell count rise to a very high level. With any given proportion of their total haemoglobin reduced patients with polycythaemia appear more cyanosed than if their haemoglobin were normal.

Fallot's tetralogy

This consists of two basic defects (Fig. 47): ventricular septal defect and pulmonary stenosis. Overriding of the aorta and right ventricular hypertrophy result from these. Because of the narrowed pulmonary valve the pressure in the right ventricle is high. Consequently much of the unoxygenated blood passes through the septal defect into the left ventricle, or straight into the overriding aorta.

While the ductus arteriosus remains open it compensates for this by allowing some of the partially oxygenated blood to pass from the aorta to the pulmonary artery, and so through the lungs.

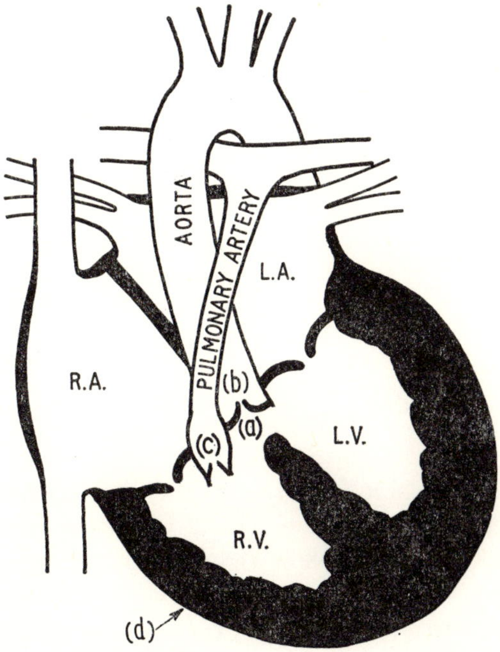

FIG **47. Fallot's tetralogy.**
a, Ventricular septal defect. *b*, Dextro position of the aorta. *c*, Pulmonary valvular stenosis. *d*, Thickened wall of right ventricle.

Signs and symptoms. The most obvious sign of this condition is cyanosis which increases with exertion. This may not be so obvious at birth, partly because of the 'safety valve' while the ductus is open and partly because of the infant's relative inactivity. Cyanotic attacks occur, the patient becoming even more cyanosed or grey and often losing consciousness. Dyspnoea, particularly on exertion, is evident, and the child adopts a characteristic squatting position to relieve this (Fig. 48). Clubbing of the fingers and toes occurs, associated with persistent cyanosis. General physical development is poor.

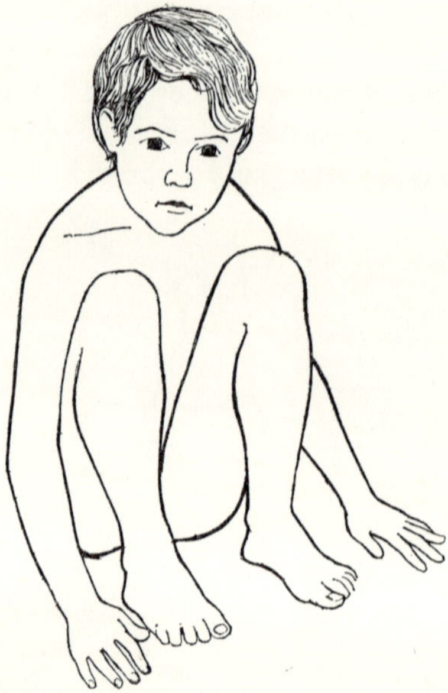

FIG 48. The squatting position adopted by a child with Fallot's tetralogy.

Investigations. Chest X-ray shows the typical 'coeur en sabot' or boot-shaped heart, and diminished vascularity of the lungs. Electrocardiograms will show right ventricular hypertrophy in most cases.

Angiocardiograms will show the radio-opaque solution entering the aorta and pulmonary artery simultaneously. This is also used to estimate the size of the pulmonary artery, which is important if a normal circulation is to be re-established surgically.

Cardiac catheterization will show raised pressure in the right ventricle. It may be difficult to pass the catheter into the pulmonary artery, but it will probably be seen to pass into the aorta, where oxygen levels will be abnormally low. Estimation of the arterial or venous blood gases will show abnormally low oxygen tensions.

Prognosis. Most patients die before the age of 20, either during a cyanotic attack, from the cerebral thromboses which are liable to occur owing to the increased viscosity of the blood (due to polycythaemia), or from right heart failure. Bacterial endocarditis may occur, patients who live more than 20 years are usually severely incapacitated.

Pott's operation (anastomosis of pulmonary artery to aorta) or the Blalock–Taussig operation (Fig. 49) (end-to-side anastomosis

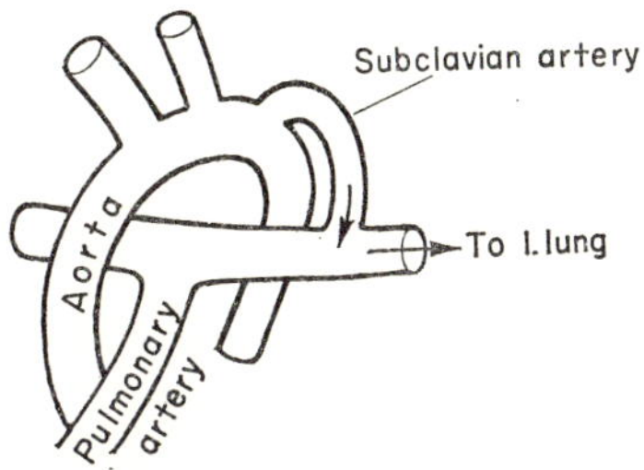

FIG **49. Blalock operation.**

of left subclavian artery to left pulmonary artery) are useful palliative procedures which relieve the cyanosis by directing more blood through the lungs. The patient's condition is often much improved for a number of years, but since one more defect has been added, strain on the heart is increased. Also as the child grows cyanosis may recur as the shunt through the anastomosis becomes too small to be adequate. Brock's operation (closed pulmonary valvotomy) may be performed as a first stage measure. The first two operations may be repeated on the other side and, since all three can be performed through an ordinary thoractomy without cardiopulmonary bypass, are a useful means of enabling the child to survive until over the age of 3 when total correction may be considered if the pulmonary artery and left ventricle are a reasonable size. Total correction consists of pulmonary valvotomy and closure of the ventricular septal defect with the aorta directed into the left ventricle. This offers the best chance of normal life, but the operative mortality in severe cases is still high. These patients tend to bleed more than average after operation because of clotting defects associated with the polycythaemia, and the increased collateral circulation which represent the body's attempt to increase blood flow through the lungs. It should be remembered that after the Blalock–Taussig operation there will be no radial pulse on the operated side since the subclavian artery has been ligated.

Aorticopulmonary transposition or complete transposition of the great vessels (Fig. 50)

Aetiology. In this condition the septum between the pulmonary artery and the aorta fails to spiral as it normally does. Consequently

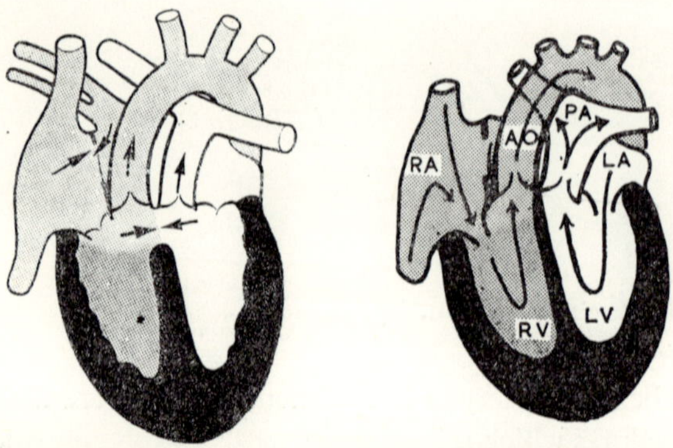

FIG **50. Aorticopulmonary transposition of the great arteries.** The aorta arises from the right ventricle and the pulmonary artery from the left. The aorta is placed anterior to the pulmonary artery, the reverse of the usual situation. Life can only be sustained if communications exist between systemic and pulmonary circulations.

the pulmonary artery leads from the left ventricle and conveys all the oxygenated blood back to the lungs, while the aorta leads from the right ventricle and conveys the unoxygenated blood back through the systemic circulation. Life can obviously only continue if there is a further defect, such as an atrial or ventricular septal defect or a persistent ductus arteriosus, which allows the blood to mix.

Signs and symptoms. Cyanosis and dyspnoea, increasing on exertion, are the most obvious signs of this condition, the smaller the additional defect allowing a shunt the bluer and more dyspnoeic the patient. The patient's general physical development is poor, and a high haemoglobin, polycythaemia and clubbing of toes and fingers are present.

Investigations. Chest X-ray will show enlargement of the heart. Cardiac catheterization will show raised pressures in the right ventricle. The catheter may be seen to pass straight through into the aorta, or if the catheter can be passed through the septum and into the pulmonary artery the oxygen tensions will be found to be higher than in samples from the aorta. Angiograms will show the aorta lying in front of the pulmonary artery.

Prognosis. Prognosis is very poor without surgery and few children reach the age of 10 years. The obvious surgical answer might appear to be the transposition of the two vessels to their correct site, but this is difficult because the coronary arteries cannot be moved and consequently the myocardium would continue to receive unoxygenated blood. There are three operations which may be performed at present.

1. *Hanlon's operation.* The heart is opened and a piece of atrial

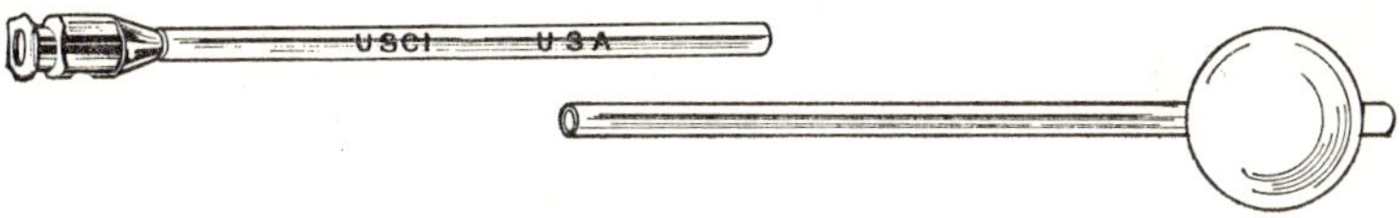

FIG **51. A Rashkind catheter.**
(By courtesy of Chas. F. Thackray Ltd)

septum resected. This is a palliative procedure, and the same result can now be achieved more simply by the use of a Rashkind catheter. Cardiac catheterization is performed transvenously. The Rashkind catheter (Fig. 51) is passed through the atrial septum by transseptal puncture, the balloon at the end inflated with a few millilitres of radio-opaque fluid, and then withdrawn through the septum. The catheter is passed through and withdrawn several times, each time with the balloon a little more inflated, until the septal defect is deemed large enough. This relatively small procedure may make possible the survival of a severely anoxic infant to an age when major surgery is possible.

2. *Baffe's operation.* In the first stage the right pulmonary veins are implanted in the right atrium and the inferior vena cava is connected by a graft to the left atrium. This often gives good results without the second stage, which consists of transferring the superior vena cava to the left atrium and the left pulmonary veins to the right atrium.

3. *Mustard's operation* (Fig. 52). The atrial septum is removed

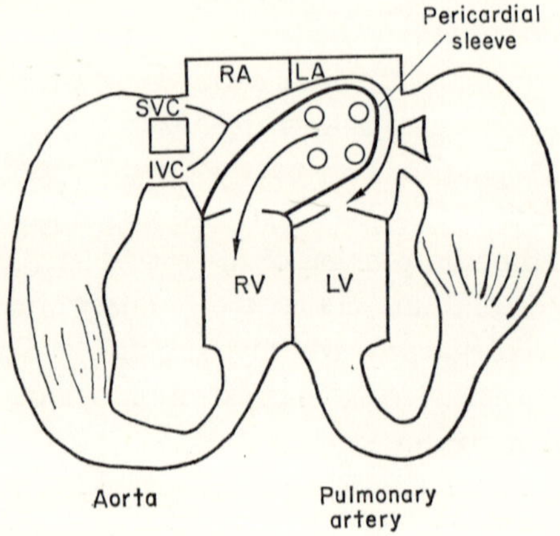

Fig 52. Mustard's operation, a corrective procedure.
The atrial septum is removed and the ostia of the pulmonary veins connected to the tricuspid valve by a pericardial tunnel.

and a pericardial tunnel inserted from the openings of the pulmonary veins across to the tricuspid valve, to redirect the flow of blood.

Other rarer abnormalities such as anomalous (abnormal) insertion of pulmonary veins or combinations of the defects described do occur, but their effects can be deduced by studying the anatomy and using the knowledge gained from a study of the commoner defects.

6

Acquired cardiac disease

Medical conditions

Early rheumatism affecting the heart

Rheumatic heart disease is one of the commonest forms of heart disease so it is important to understand something about its original cause, sometimes called rheumatic fever. Rheumatism affecting the heart is not fully understood, however; as a cause of heart disease it is now thought to be a hypersensitivity to streptococcal infection or an autoimmune reaction following such an infection.

Children between 5 and 15 years are usually affected, but sometimes adolescents and young adults may also suffer from it. The condition usually manifests itself some two or three weeks after a streptococcal infection of the throat. In acute rheumatism the symptoms are severe, but a subacute form occurs in which they are mild and may even escape detection. In each type the joints are affected. There is one type known as chorea where the nervous system is affected. The usual characteristic of this is involuntary uncoordinated jerky movements. The joints may not be affected, but it is not uncommon to find involvement of the heart.

The onset of acute rheumatism may be gradual, with increasing listlessness, loss of appetite and mild pyrexia, or it may begin suddenly, with moderate pyrexia and acute painful swellings of one or more joints. The joint symptoms may vary daily, the pain affecting one joint one day and another the next. Although red, hot and painful while affected, the joint itself appears to return to normal when the inflammation subsides. In a subacute attack the child may complain of vague joint pains often referred to as 'growing pains', and little notice may be taken of them. There may also be an erythema of the skin, and sometimes small nodules may form on the skin subcutaneously. The erythrocyte sedimentation rate is raised from the normal 10 mm to 60 or 80 mm in 1 hour.

The extent to which the heart is involved varies from patient to patient, but in all cases is of concern because of the permanent damage which may develop. The endocardium, the myocardium and the pericardium may be individually affected, but sometimes there is an association of all parts in rheumatic pan-carditis.

The danger of endocarditis is that the inflammatory process may affect the valves of the heart. After the inflammation scar tissue may cause them to become distorted and, in addition, lesions, often called vegetations, may form along them. In later life, the distortion of the valves and the presence of the vegetations may give rise to chronic valvular heart disease and to bacterial endocarditis.

Myocarditis, inflammation of the heart muscle, may produce no symptoms, but in severe forms may lead to heart failure, of which an unduly rapid pulse and irregular pulse may be the early signs, together with the changes in the electrocardiograph. Small lesions known as Aschoff nodes may occur in the myocardium and these may interfere with normal heart activity.

Pericarditis may occur in severe attacks. There may be no symptoms, but rubbing of the two pericardial surfaces may cause discomfort over the heart. Should pericardial effusion occur, it may interfere with the action of the heart.

Nursing a patient with acute rheumatism requires skill, an understanding of the patient, and a knowledge of the underlying condition. Rest plays a very important part during the active phase of the disease and to this end the patient is kept in bed until all symptoms and signs have subsided. Some doctors require the patient to lie recumbent with one pillow, but others allow him to assume a position of maximum comfort so long as his activity is restricted.

Due to a rise in temperature there may be considerable sweating, so the patient will need washing at regular intervals, and the personal clothing should be changed. Painful joints should be handled gently; they may be wrapped in gamgee and placed on a soft pillow in a comfortable position. A bed-cradle will keep the top bedclothes from pressing on the joints. The patient must be kept warm and not allowed to feel chilled; a flannelette sheet next to him provides this measure of comfort.

The diet should be light and nutritious. The patient is encouraged to drink plenty of fluid, especially as he will be losing a considerable amount due to sweating while pyrexial. If he lies in the recumbent position there may be some difficulty in drinking; to overcome this a feeding cup, straw or angulated polythene tube may be used.

The temperature, pulse and respiration should be taken and recorded four-hourly, special note being taken of any alteration in the rate and regularity of the pulse as these may indicate involvement of the heart.

The patient may find lying in bed somewhat boring and the restriction in moving about somewhat frustrating, so the nurse must use her imagination to find means of relieving him of these feelings. The provision of radio, television and books is helpful. A view of the street or road from a window relieves monotony. Visits by relatives and friends are of immense value. The nurse should be willing to sit down and talk for a while whenever her other duties permit. Young children tend to be quiet when they feel ill, but are apt to move about much more once they begin to feel better. Whereas a simple explanation may be sufficient to obtain the cooperation of older children and young adults, with a young child the nurse must be ingenious in the measures she takes to encourage him to rest. He may be able to read, but for short periods only, and indeed may sustain interest much longer and lie much more restfully if the nurse reads to him. The solving of a jigsaw puzzle could keep him occupied, with help and encouragement from the nurse whenever he becomes restless. Drawing and painting may absorb his attention, and also making paper models, dressing a doll or building with bricks and other constructional toys. Sometimes the nurse can just sit with the child near the window and talk about what can be seen outside; at other times she can draw his attention to something in the room, such as a picture, the movement of a fish in a tank or a mobile toy suspended from above. When the child is being nursed at home the parents may be able to play in similar ways, as may older members of the family, providing there is no tendency to get the child excited or physically active.

When the child is in hospital, the parents should be encouraged to visit frequently and to play quietly with the child, thus helping him to rest. Indeed, the parents will probably know the type of quiet games which the child likes to play or the quiet activities which absorb his attention.

The doctor may order a course of penicillin, especially if there is or has been evidence of streptococcal infection of the throat. Anti-inflammatory drugs may be ordered, usually salicylates and corticosteroids. Soluble aspirin is a form of salicylate frequently given, the amount prescribed by the doctor. A young adult may be given 1 g every 3 or 4 hours. It will probably lower the temperature and relieve the joint pains, but does not appear to have any significant effect on the carditis. The possibility of intolerance to aspirin or signs of overdose (salicylism) should be remembered, and any nausea, vomiting, tinnitus or deafness reported.

Corticosteroids, such as cortisone, prednisone and prednisolone, are sometimes more beneficial in suppressing the joint pains and lowering the temperature; it is sometimes felt that they control the acute inflammation of myocarditis. When corticosteroids are being administered, any signs of oedema, glycosuria and moon face should be noted and the doctor informed. Phenylbutazone may be prescribed for older patients to suppress the painful joints.

Heart failure may occur in the more severe attacks of acute rheumatism, especially among adolescents. Should it occur, the treatment adopted is that used for heart failure in other conditions and age groups, and includes rest in bed, adopting the sitting position to relieve dyspnoea, the administration of digitalis and diuretics and probably the restriction of sodium in the diet.

As the condition improves the patient feels better, the joint pains disappear and the temperature returns to normal. When the pulse rate and the E.S.R. are returning to normal, the patient may be allowed to increase his activities. The need to rest and take things easy may last for several weeks.

It is natural for the child to wish to play with older children. Within the family the parents should be advised to encourage the playing of quiet games only, and they may need to guide the play and even to curtail excitement and overactivity. In some communities the child may be able to attend a play group, in which case the play-leader should be informed of his condition and the possible need to restrict activities. Parents are advised that there may be recurrence of the condition, and should inform the doctor if there is any return of symptoms.

When the child resumes attendance at school, or when a child needing to restrict physical activities commences school, the teacher and the school medical service personnel should be informed of his condition. His welfare and progress at school should be regularly discussed by the teacher, parents, school medical officer or school nurse and the child's own doctor. Some adolescents and young adults may eagerly wish to return to school or to work with all the associated activities. They should be advised to accept the doctor's guidance on the extent to which they must limit their activities. On the other hand, any tendency to regard the patient as a permanent invalid should be avoided, and he should be encouraged to return to a normal life as soon as possible.

Bacterial endocarditis

Should there be any unevenness of the endocardium, bacteria may lodge there and cause endocarditis. This can occur in those with congenital heart abnormality, after cardiac surgery, and especially after rheumatic endocarditis where small vegetations form on the valves of the heart. The causal organism may be a *Staphylococcus* or *Streptococcus faecalis*, but more often is *Streptococcus viridans*.

The organism may enter the blood stream after upper respiratory tract infection or after minor trauma, such as tooth extraction, tonsillectomy, cystoscopy and childbirth. Under normal circumstances the bacteria which enter the blood stream are destroyed by the phagocytic action of the leucocytes. However, when the endocardium is uneven, the blood flow is slowed down in that particular area, the bacteria lodge near the uneven part and multiply. Fibrin is laid down, forming larger vegetations and also protecting the bacteria from the leucocytes. Thus the condition of bacterial endocarditis can be considered from three aspects. First, the presence and multiplication of the bacteria which set up septicaemia. Second the presence of the vegetations, some of which may break off, be carried round the blood stream and form emboli. Third, the fibrous formations on the edges of the valves may prevent their closing properly and thus interfere with the normal functioning of the heart.

Bacterial endocarditis is rare in childhood and not common in young adults. It becomes more common over the age of 30 years and recently has been very common in those between 50 and 70.

The onset of the condition may be sudden or it may be gradual and more insidious. The early symptoms and signs are those of infection with weakness and malaise, and an intermittent pyrexia of up to 40° C (104° F), alternating with rigors and sweating. The pulse rate is increased. There is anorexia and loss of weight. As the condition progresses the patient becomes anaemic and his skin takes on a brownish *cafe-au-lait* colouring. As the vegetations are broken off and circulate, signs of emboli may appear. On the skin they may cause petechiae or purpuric spots. Small painful swellings known as 'Osler's nodes' may appear on the fingertips, and splinter-like haemorrhages in the fingernails. Emboli lodging in the brain may lead to symptoms of cerebral embolism, hemiplegia or coma, and in the kidney to haematuria and pain in the loins. Other arteries may also be occluded. Clubbing of the fingers and toes may appear later in the disease.

Changes in the heart valves may interfere with the flow of blood through them and this may be heard as murmurs if a stethoscope is used. The erythrocyte sedimentation rate will be raised. Blood culture will be performed to aid diagnosis and to identify the organism causing the disease and its sensitivity to antibiotics.

The patient is nursed in bed at first and is encouraged to rest as much as possible. While in bed he should be made as comfortable as possible. If he feels chilled extra blankets should be given; similarly if he has a rigor extra warmth should be provided, but these blankets should be removed when he feels warmer or begins to sweat. If pyrexia is high, tepid sponging may be required to lower the temperature. Damp personal cothing and bedclothes should be changed and the patient's skin washed and dried. Owing to the sweating it is important that the patient drinks plenty of fluid, and he should be encouraged to eat light and nutritious food. The nurse's manner should be one of sympathy and understanding, and she should be kind and pleasant, especially when the patient does not feel well.

Temperature, pulse and respiration should be taken and recorded four-hourly, and any fluctuations noted. The skin should be observed for any presence of petechiae, the urine for any haematuria. Any complaints of loin pains, severe headache or loss of feeling or movement should be reported to the doctor, together with any other signs or symptoms suggesting embolism.

Antibiotic therapy will be ordered by the doctor to eradicate the infection. The usual treatment is large doses of penicillin, as much as 4 or 5 million units being given daily, but other antibiotics may be used if the organism is found to be sensitive to them. The treatment is prolonged and may last up to 6 weeks. The penicillin is usually given intramuscularly as this is considered to be the most reliable way of ensuring absorption and maintaining the high level of it in the blood. The amount is ordered in divided doses to be given 6-hourly. When so many injections are to be given it is important to have a good technique for giving an intramuscular injection so as to cause a minimum of discomfort. Each injection causes some local inflammation; in order to allow this to subside before another is given, it is important to rotate the sites at which the injections are given. If the upper outer quadrant of each set of gluteal muscles and each outer aspect of the thigh is used, this gives 4 sites, each of which can be used once daily. Although the patient may remember where the next injection is to be given the nurse should also have some method of recording this, remembering that in addition to a good injection technique, strict rotation of the site of injection will greatly diminish the discomfort of the patient.

As the symptoms subside and as the condition of the patient improves, he will be allowed to increase his activities, and eventually to get out of bed. He should be encouraged not to overdo things, and should not be allowed to continue any activity up to the point of exhaustion. When antibiotic treatment has been discontinued, observations should be maintained in case there is any relapse of the infection or any further embolism. Before discharge the doctor will assess the extent of damage to the heart, and afterwards will keep the patient under surveillance.

Thyrotoxic heart disease

The hormones produced by the thyroid gland, L-thyroxine and triiodothyronine, regulate the rate of tissue metabolism, that is the speed of the chemical reaction, the amount of oxygen used and the amount of heat given off. The more hormone produced, the greater the metabolic rate.

Hyperthyroidism is the term used to indicate overactivity of the thyroid gland, the increased output of hormones increasing the metabolism. The increased heat production warms the blood, and this in turn increases the heart rate. The person becomes excitable and 'nervous', which also stimulates the heart to beat more quickly. The hormones also have a direct effect upon the heart muscle by increasing its excitability.

In thyrotoxicosis, when the hyperthyroidism is causing the patient to be clinically ill, tachycardia and atrial fibrillation may occur. The fibrillating atria cause the ventricles to contract irregularly and at a high rate (120/min). If the condition is not treated, permament damage may be done to the heart, resulting in congestive heart failure. The patient may complain of palpitations.

Treatment is aimed at controlling the thyrotoxicosis by the use of anti-thyroid drugs such as carbimazole, the use of radio-active iodine, or by removal of part of the thyroid gland itself, after which the heart condition usually improves.

Propranolol may be given to control the atrial fibrillation. Digitalis helps the ventricles to beat more slowly, regularly and effectively. When congestive cardiac failure occurs it is treated along the appropriate lines.

Pericarditis

The pericardium is a fibroserous sac which envelopes the heart and the roots of the great vessel. It consists of two closely connected parts, an outer fibrous sac which is continuous with the outer covering of the great vessels, and an inner serous membrane which lines the fibrous sac (parietal layer) and covers the myocardium (visceral layer). Between the parietal and visceral layers of serous pericardium is a potential space containing a small amount of pericardial fluid which acts as a lubricant when the heart moves inside the fibrous sac.

As already mentioned, pericarditis occurs in acute rheumatism. It also occurs as a result of viral, pneumococcal and tuberculous infections, after myocardial infarction and in association with malignant conditions in the thorax.

In *dry pericarditis* there may be pain in the chest, sometimes referred to the shoulder and neck, as well as symptoms related to the condition causing the inflammation. In listening to the heart, the doctor may detect a pericardial rub. He may note changes in the electrocardiograph, and the serum transaminase may be slightly raised. The treatment is aimed at the underlying cause. The patient is encouraged to rest and he is nursed under the regimen described in the section on acute rheumatism.

In *pericardial effusion* there is an increase in the amount of pericardial fluid, and the two layers of pericardium become separated. Although the fibrous pericardium is pliable, the extent to which it can be distended is limited, so that if the amount of fluid continues to increase, it will eventually cause pressure on the heart and great vessels. This in turn interferes with the venous return to the heart, and with the distension of the ventricles as they fill during diastole. The venous pressure is raised, the cardiac output reduced and, although the pulse rate is increased, the blood pressure falls with a low pulse pressure. The heart sounds are faint and at X-ray the heart is not enlarged. The patient will probably feel weak and faint, have an anxious expression and look pallid and grey. He may express a little difficulty in breathing. This condition is referred to as *cardiac tamponade*. If the effusion continues to increase, cardiac failure will eventually occur. Cardiac tamponade may also occur when, after injury or surgery involving the pericardium, blood collects in the pericardial space.

The patient is encouraged to rest. Measures to relieve the discomfort may be instituted, but the treatment ordered by the doctor will be aimed at the underlying cause.

Aspiration of the pericardium may be performed to withdraw a little fluid for examination purposes, or, to relieve the pressure of the cardiac tamponade. The needle may be inserted to the left of the xiphisternum. Sometimes drainage of the pericardial sac may be performed, a polythene drain being inserted into the pericardial space at the side of the lower sternum to the left of the xiphisternum.

In *adhesive pericarditis*, as a result of the inflammation, the two

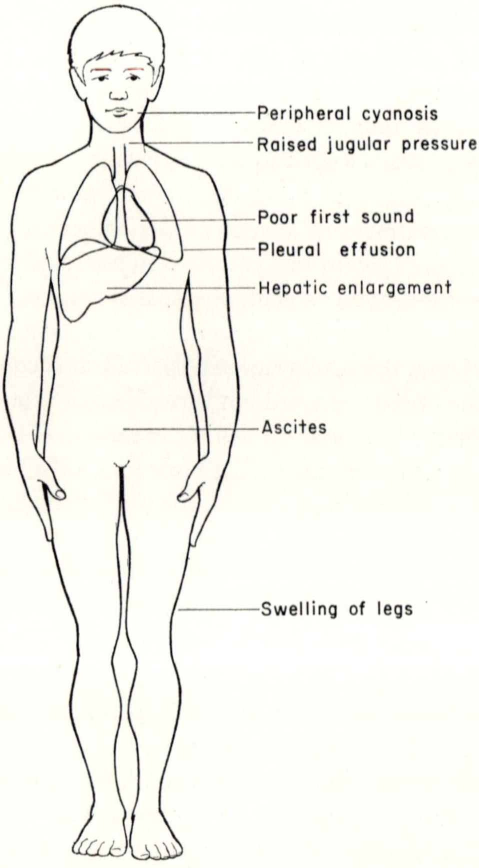

FIG 53. **Physical signs in constrictive pericarditis.**

layers of serous pericardium become adherent. The condition causes a little or no embarrassment to the heart's function. Also as a result of the inflammation, the pericardium may become adherent to nearby structures.

In *constrictive pericarditis* (Fig. 53), after inflammation, especially if due to tuberculosis, the pericardium becomes insidiously thickened and densely fibrosed. The fibrous tissue tends to contract and 'strangle' the heart. There may be desposition of calcium salts, especially near the atrioventricular groove. Due to the concentration and the rigidity, there is a restriction on the extent to which the heart is able to distend as it fills during systole. Usually filling of the right side is impaired, resulting in the venous pressure being raised to as much as 30 cm H_2O. The veins of the neck are usually noticeably distended. The collecting of blood in the inferior vena cava causes engorgement and enlargement of the liver, and ascites follows. The patient may feel and look ill. Although he may have a little dyspnoea on exertion, it is not usually present at rest. The cardiac output is reduced, the heart rate may be increased, but the arterial pressure may be reduced with a small pulse pressure. The time for the blood to circulate round the body may be increased, resulting in peripheral cyanosis, especially noticeable round the lips. Sometimes atrial fibrillation may be present. There may be some atrophy of the myocardium. Ultimately the heart fails. Treatment consists of surgical removal of the pericardium (pericardiectomy) in which the dense pericardium is removed.

Conditions amenable to surgery

Many of the adults admitted for cardiac operation have damaged heart valves as a result of acute or subacute rheumatic disease. In some patients with acute rheumatism the valves become inflamed and thickened, though there is no definite relationship between the severity of joint symptoms and the degree of cardiac involvement. As the inflammation subsides, the cusps may fuse so that the valve is narrowed (stenosis) or become thickened and irregular so that it cannot close properly (incompetence) and allows blood to flow back through it (regurgitation). Fibrosis and shortening of the chordae tendinae may cause both incompetence and stenosis by pulling down the cusps so that the valve can neither open nor close efficiently. It is the mitral valve which most commonly suffers damage, but the aortic and less often the tricuspid valves may be damaged also.

Distortion of the valves by fibrosis and subsequent calcification tends to be a progressive process, so that the full effects of damage may not be seen until years later.

Bacterial endocarditis is another important cause of valve disease, and again it is most commonly the mitral or aortic valve which is damaged. Acute bacterial endocarditis may attack normal valves, but more often the disease occurs in subacute forms and attacks valves which are already abnormal. The valve cusps may be distorted or perforated, or a chorda tendina may also be so damaged that it ruptures, perhaps during exertion, and as a result mitral regurgitation occurs. These patients may deteriorate rapidly over a few months unless the damage can be repaired.

Mitral valve disease

Signs and symptoms. Since mitral stenosis is commoner in females the typical patient with this condition is a rather thin

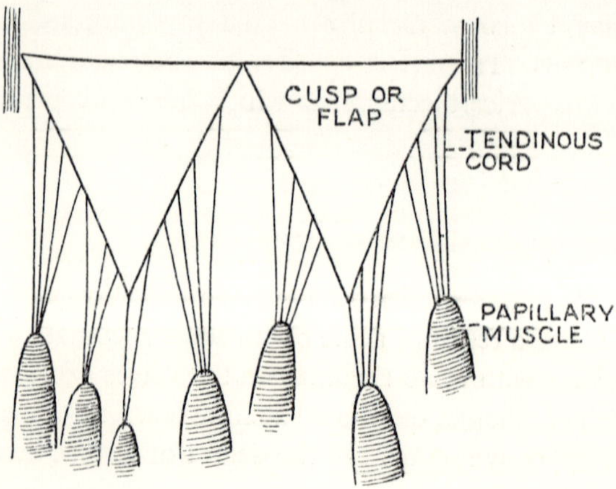

FIG **54. The mitral valve laid open.**

young woman with flushed cheeks, possibly cyanosed lips and a small pulse pressure, complaining of increasing dyspnoea on exertion and recurrent chest infection. She may also complain of attacks of breathlessness with profuse frothy and sometimes blood-stained sputum (pulmonary oedema), orthopnoea and, if the condition has persisted long, generalized oedema. When the mitral valve is obstructed the left atrium cannot empty easily but blood is

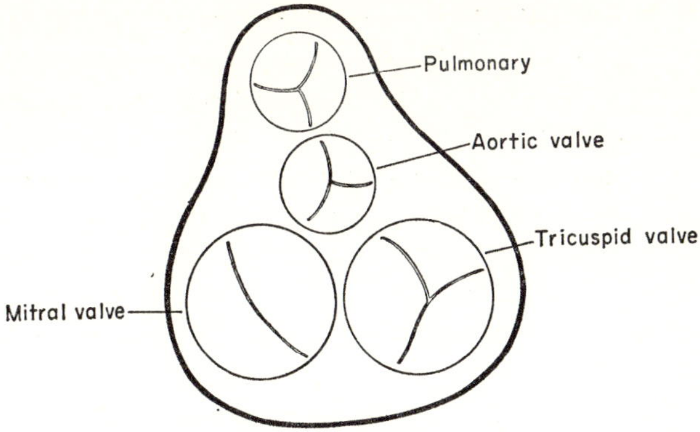

FIG 55. **Relationship of the cardiac valves, as seen from above.**

still being pumped into the pulmonary circulation by the right ventricle. Consequently the pressure in the left atrium and pulmonary vessels rises, especially during exercise which increases venous return to the right atrium. Eventually the pressure in the right atrium and systemic venous system rises. It is this sequence of events which causes the signs and symptoms mentioned so far. Clotting may occur in the enlarged left atrium, especially if atrial fibrillation (which commonly occurs) has replaced the normal atrial contractions, or round the irregular valve surfaces. If clots become detached (emboli) and pass into the systemic circulation they may reach the brain and cause hemiplegia, unconsciousness or even death, or may block a large peripheral artery, causing gangrene of the tissue supplied. Infarction or death of tissue distal to a blocked artery may occur in the kidney, giving rise to renal symptoms or even failure, or in the gut, causing abdominal signs and symptoms.

Mitral regurgitation (Fig. 56) causes similar signs and symptoms apart from the sounds heard on auscultation, since the reflux of blood through the mitral valve causes a rise in pressure in the left atrium and pulmonary circulation, but the patient's main complaint is often of tiredness.

Investigations. Oblique chest X-rays with barium swallow may demonstrate the selective enlargement of the left atrium in stenosis, while a straight chest X-ray may show general enlargement of the heart.

Cardiac catheterization may be performed to estimate the severity of valve damage either by measuring the wedge pressure in the pulmonary arterioles or by transeptal puncture to obtain left atrial pressure. Cine-angiograms may be used to provide a permanent moving film record of the radio-opaque substance being injected via the catheter into the left ventricle passing back through the valve and demonstrating reflux.

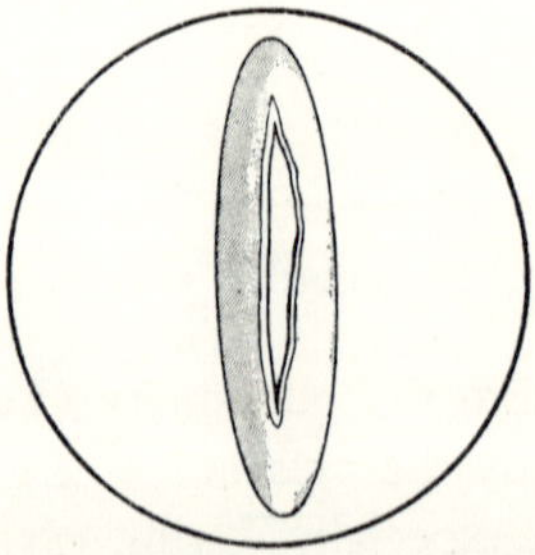

FIG 56. **Stenosed and regurgitant mitral valve. The valve cannot open normally or close competently because of rigidity and distortion.**

Cardiac disease in pregnancy. Since mitral valve disease occurs most often in young women it is relevant to consider the effects of pregnancy. The increased weight carried and the increased circulation needed to supply the fetal requirements via the placenta both put extra strain on the heart, while the pressure of increased abdominal contents below the diaphragm may impede its action. The maternal blood volume increases 30% by about the twenty-eighth week and cardiac output by 35%. These effects are likely to be most troublesome about weeks 32–36 of pregnancy, since placental function is then at its maximum and the fetus tends to be high under the diaphragm, the head having not yet become engaged in the pelvis. Such patients need extra rest during pregnancy and possibly admission to hospital at 28–36 weeks if the heart condition cannot be relieved before then. Extra care must also be taken to prevent the iron deficiency anaemia which may occur because of the demands of the fetus. If the patient is anaemic the oxygen-carrying capacity of the blood is diminished and the heart will have to work harder to supply the oxygen requirements of mother and fetus.

Treatment. The treatment for mitral stenosis which is causing signs and symptoms of a raised left atrial pressure is valvotomy or splitting of the valve along the fused edges (Fig. 57). This may have to be preceded by treatment for cardiac failure to improve the patient's condition as much as possible, and if there have been

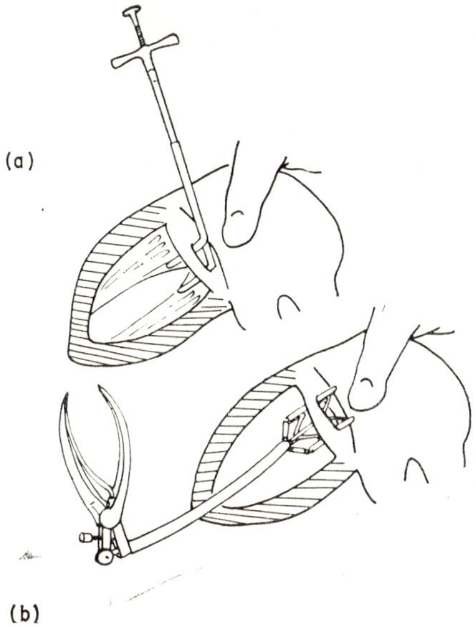

FIG **57. Opening the mitral valve with a valve splitter.**
A, Transatrial mitral valve splitter. B, Transventricular mitral valve splitter. In both cases the splitter is guided into position and the split controlled by the intra-atrial finger.

embolic episodes then anticoagulant therapy may be given. This will not dissolve the clot which has already been formed, but will prevent the formation of new loose clots which may separate and cause embolization at operation. Mitral valvotomy may be performed by splitting the valve with a finger, but more often these days a splitter is used, either a Tubbs through the ventricle or a Ronald Edwards through the atrium. This is guided by the finger and controlled so that the valve can be carefully split from 3·5 to 4 cm without any increase in regurgitation, and great care is taken to avoid the escape of the clot into the circulation. The carotid arteries are often compressed during manipulation to prevent cerebral emboli occurring. Mitral valvotomy is usually performed through an ordinary left thoracotomy and is a common and relative safe operation, overall mortality being 2–3%. It can, if necessary, be safely done during weeks 14–30 of pregnancy. If there is much clot or calcification an open operation with the aid of cardiopulmonary bypass may be preferred.

The surgical treatment of mitral regurgitation is more difficult, and usually requires operation under direct vision with cardiopulmonary bypass. It may be possible to repair the valve with a

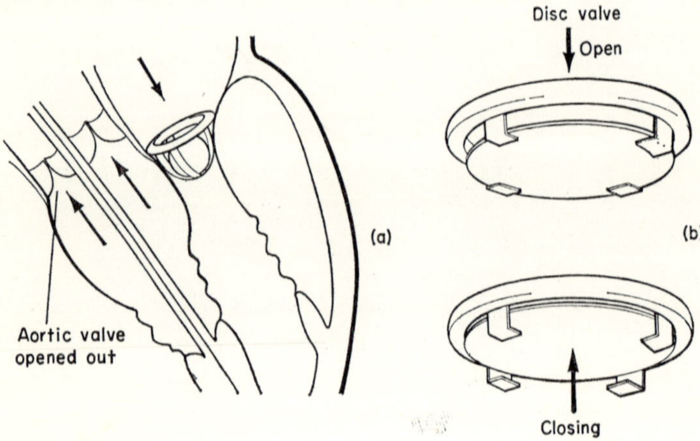

FIG 58. **Prosthetic valves.**
A, Starr-Edwards (ball and cage) mitral replacement. B, Disc type, open and closing.

Teflon or pericardial patch or by appropriately placed stitches (valvoplasty), but often the valve must be replaced by a ball valve, such as the Starr-Edwards, or a disc valve (Fig. 58). The use of homografts (human valves) or heterografts (animal valves) for mitral replacement is still in the stage of development.

Mitral valve replacement still carries a fairly high risk but without operation the expectation of life for these patients is very limited.

Prognosis. The results of surgery on the mitral valve vary considerably since they depend not only on the success of the operation, but also on the state of the heart and lungs. A young patient with mitral stenosis which has only recently caused trouble, and with no apparent impairment of myocardial efficiency, may reasonably be expected to live a normal life after mitral valvotomy and convalescence, though the valvotomy may occasionally need repeating after several years if the split was not quite adequate or acute rheumatism has recurred and caused restenosis. However, the patient who has considerable myocardial damage caused by the original disease process, or whose valve has been inefficient long enough to cause permanent damage to the heart or lungs, is unlikely to have such a happy outcome. A successful operation may nevertheless considerably improve the patient's condition and chances of a longer and more enjoyable life.

Aortic valve disease

Aortic stenosis or incompetence may result from acute rheumatism by the same process as mitral valve disease. Indeed, the mitral valve is often damaged at the same time. However, aortic valve disease alone is quite often caused by a process of fibrosis and calcification which involves the valve, the surrounding aorta and possibly extends into the left ventricle. This may be superimposed on a mild congenital aortic abnormality. Calcification is unusual below the age of 20 and may be delayed for years. Bacterial endocarditis is another cause of aortic valve disease, incompetence resulting from perforation of a cusp or from part of the valve shearing off the aortic wall so that one or more cusps prolapse through the valve.

Signs and symptoms. Usually the patient's main complaint is dyspnoea. In aortic valve disease of rheumatic origin the signs and symptoms may be overshadowed by those of associated mitral disease, apart from the characteristic heart sounds. Aortic valve disease makes it difficult for the heart to maintain adequate circulation, since stenosis obstructs the flow of blood through the valve while incompetence allows blood to flow back into the ventricle from the aorta so that less blood reaches the systemic circulation with each ventricular contraction. In order to compensate the left ventricle becomes progressively hypertrophied, and pressure of the muscle fibres on the coronary arteries combined with calcification round the coronary orifices may cause myocardial ischaemia (deficient blood supply) and anginal pain. This is a typical substernal gripping pain which occurs on exercise and may extend down the left arm.

The other compensatory mechanism to maintain circulation is peripheral vasoconstriction, the patient having cool pale extremities and a raised diastolic blood pressure and a relatively small difference between systolic and diastolic pressure, e.g. 120/90. In aortic incompetence, however, the diastolic pressure will be low since some of the blood flows back into the ventricle during diastole. This can be felt at the wrist as the characteristic 'water hammer' or Corrigan's pulse, each beat being felt as a short, rapidly decreasing pressure.

Once signs of left ventricular failure have begun to appear it is often only a matter of months before the left atrial, pulmonary circulation and then right heart pressure rise. Raised venous pressure can then be observed in the neck veins, and general oedema and enlarged tender liver occur as the right side of the heart fails.

Investigations. Chest X-ray will show enlargement of the heart, especially the left ventricle. Electrocardiography will show signs of left ventricular hypertrophy and possibly strain. Angiograms or cine-angiograms may be used to demonstrate the stenosis or degree of regurgitation. Cardiac catheterization and transatrial puncture may be performed to record the left ventricular pressure, the systemic blood pressure being recorded at the same time. The difference between the two is known as the gradient, and is a measure of the severity of the stenosis.

Prognosis. Usually symptoms do not occur until there is gross hypertrophy of the left ventricle, and in this state the enlarged ventricle is liable to cease beating suddenly. Consequently, unless abnormal heart sounds and cardiac enlargement are found during a routine examination, the patient may die suddenly without the aortic disease having been recognized. Once signs and symptoms appear deterioration is often rapid, the patient surviving 2 years or less.

Treatment. Aortic valvotomy or splitting of the valve via the ventricle as a 'closed' procedure may provide good results if the disease is of rheumatic origin. Mitral valvotomy may be done at the same time. However, if the aortic valve is calcified or incompetent, an 'open' operation with cardiopulmonary bypass is usually necessary. It may occasionally be possible to split or repair the valve (valvotomy or valvoplasty) but often the valve must be replaced by a plastic and stainless steel valve, such as the Starr-Edwards, or by a homograft (human valve.)

Tricuspid valve disease

The tricuspid valve may be damaged by rheumatic disease and become stenotic, but there is almost always associated mitral disease. The narrowed valve will prevent normal emptying of the right atrium, so that the right atrial pressure will be raised, neck veins will be engorged and there may be enlargement of the liver and oedema.

Treatment. The X-ray may show enlargement of the right atrium. The valve may be split (valvotomy) in conjunction with mitral valvotomy, but it is usually necessary to replace it or perform an annuloplasty.

Constrictive pericarditis

This condition usually follows tuberculous infection of the pericardium and has already been described earlier in the chapter. The operation of pericardectomy usually needs to be performed if the condition is to be cured.

The surgeon strips off all or most of the dense pericardium. It may be a difficult process because calcified areas may adhere firmly to the myocardium in places, and the myocardium itself may be thin and atrophic due to the constriction. Removal of the pericardium allows the heart to distend and to fill during diastole, cardiac output is increased and the circulation improves.

Before operation the patient rests and any underlying condition, e.g. tuberculosis, is treated. In order to decrease excess tissue fluid, the fluid and sodium intake may be restricted and diuretics given. Abdominal paracentesis may be performed to relieve the ascites and any pleural effusion aspirated. If atrial fibrillation is present, digoxin may be ordered.

After operation the patient is nursed along the lines of any patient who has had an intrathoracic operation. Oxygen is given if there is any cyanosis, and digoxin if atrial fibrillation persists. The restriction of fluids may be continued, intravenous fluids and blood transfusions being withheld unless there was severe loss of blood at operation.

The patient's general condition rapidly improves, but the full benefits may not be seen until several months later, when the myocardium has had time to redevelop to its normal thickness.

Myxoma

Tumours of the heart are rare but the most common is a myxoma in the left atrium attached by a pedicle to the edge of the foramen ovale. The signs and symptoms are usually those of mitral stenosis, and emboli are common. The patient may also have attacks of chest discomfort followed by unconsciousness when the tumour falls across the mitral valve and blocks the flow of blood through it. As the patient becomes unconscious and falls, the tumour falls away from the mitral orifice, circulation is restored and the patient regains consciousness.

Angiocardiograms may demonstrate the tumour but if this condition is suspected cardiac catheterization is undesirable because of the risk of embolism.

The removal of a myxoma needs open surgery with the aid of cardiopulmonary bypass and the surgeon takes great care to avoid emboli by covering the mitral valve while removing the tumour.

Neoplasms arising from surrounding structures may invade the heart, possibly giving rise to dysrhythmias such as atrial fibrillation. If the area affected is not too large, resection may be possible when the main neoplasm is resected. A piece of synthetic material may be used to reinforce the weakened area.

Heart block

To main adequate cardiac output it is necessary to have:

1. An electrical impulse.
2. An intact conduction system so that this impulse reaches the ventricular muscle.
3. Ventricular muscle which is capable of contracting.
4. An adequate circulatory volume.

Normally, the electrical impulse which stimulates cardiac contractions starts from a small mass of tissue which contains nerve cells and fibres and is situated in the right atrial wall (Fig. 59). This is known as the sinu-atrial node or pacemaker. The impulse then passes through the atrial wall to the atrio-ventricular node, the only point at which it can pass from the atria to the ventricle. From the atrioventricular node the specialized conductive tissue continues down through the interventricular septum as the bundle of His, divides into the right and left bundle-branches and reaches

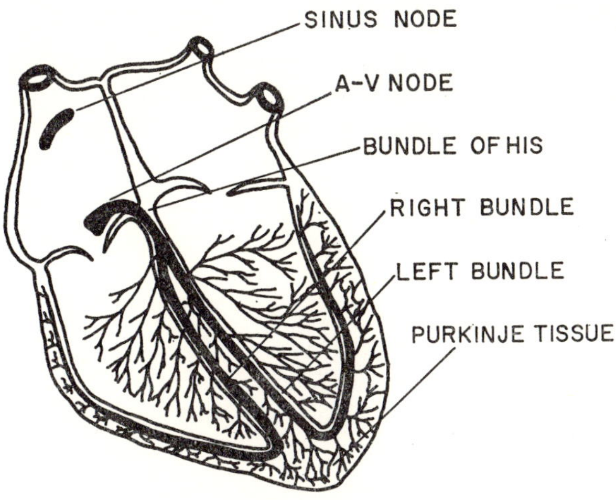

FIG **59. The pathways of conduction.**

all parts of the ventricular walls as filaments known as the fibres of Purkinje. Thus the impulse passes through the atrial wall muscle fibres, but from the atrioventricular node it normally passes through special conductive tissue which transmits it much more rapidly (5000 mm/sec) than if it passed through the ventricular muscle (500 mm/sec). This accounts for the wide QRS complex, showing slow conduction, when a ventricular extrasystole originating in the ventricle muscle is demonstrated by electrocardiogram (see Chapters 3 and 9).

Heart block is the condition in which part of the conduction system is damaged or fibrosed and fails to transmit normally some or all of the impulses. The most common cause of heart block is fibrosis of the conductive tissue which may be associated with coronary artery disease. It may also be congenital. It sometimes occurs with acute myocardial infarction, or after heart operations in close proximity to the conductive system, i.e. valve replacement or repair of a ventricular septal defect. In these cases the block may be due to local inflammatory reaction and may cease as this subsides.

In first degree heart block all impulses from the atrium are transmitted, but more slowly than usual. This shows on the electrocardiogram as a prolonged P–R interval. More severe degrees of block result in only 1 in 2 or 3 impulses being received by the ventricle, or in complete heart block (atrioventricular dissociation), when the ventricles contract 20–40 times/min unrelated to the atrial contractions. Such a slow heart rate is usually inadequate to maintain sufficient cardiac output, and heart failure may occur, or Stokes–Adams attacks. In these the heart becomes asystolic or goes into ventricular fibrillation, circulation ceases, the patient becomes unconscious and may convulse, and death will take place if circulation is not restored within 3 minutes. Recovery from a Stokes–Adams attack is often spontaneous.

Initially drugs may be tried to increase the heart rate, and avoid Stokes–Adams attacks. These include 30–60 mg ephedrine three times a day, 20 mg isoprenaline sublingually or the longer-acting drugs of a similar type, e.g. sustained action isoprenaline, given every 4–6 hours. An intravenous infusion of isoprenaline may be used to control the situation temporarily and steroid drugs may be tried. In an emergency, 0·2–0·8 ml adrenaline 1 in 1000 solution may be given intravenously.

Artificial pacemaking

In the 1950s it was found to be possible to control heart block by means of artificial electrical pacemakers, and this method has been used with increasing success (Fig. 60). It is more certain and controllable than drug therapy and often more effective.

There are 4 main methods of artificial pacemaking:

1. External electrodes are placed on the chest wall and an electrical current is passed through them at regular intervals. A considerable current is necessary and since this is painful for the patient, this method is now only used in an emergency.

2. Electrodes may be sutured to the ventricle and the connecting

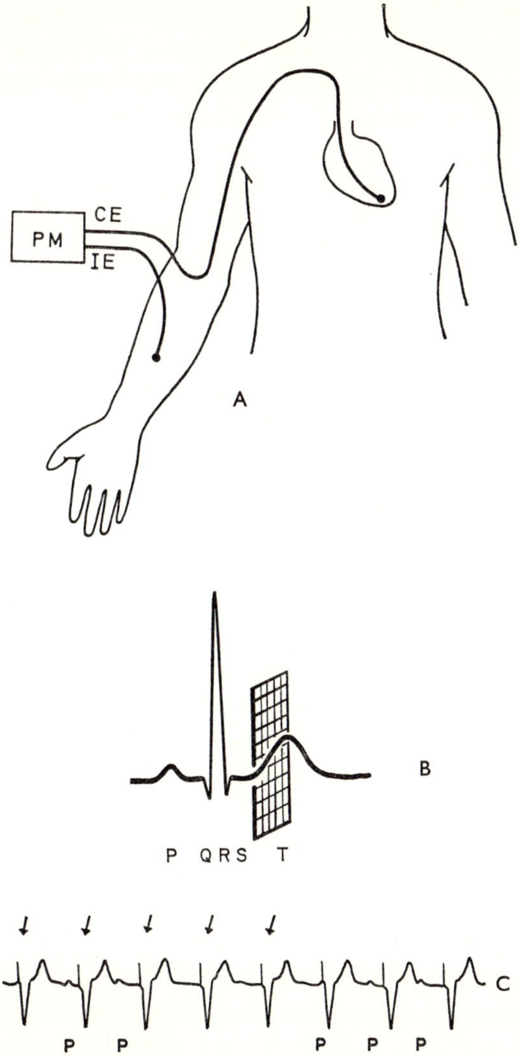

FIG 60. Cardiac pacemaking.
A, The pacemaker in position. PM, pacemaker; CE, catheter electrode; IE, indifferent electrode. B, The vulnerable period of ventricular repolarization (hatched). Electrical impulses of sufficient magnitude occurring during the upstroke of the T wave may initiate ventricular fibrillation. C, The oscilloscope trace. A thin vertical pacing impulse, indicated by the arrow, immediately precedes the broad QRS resulting from ventricular stimulation. The P wave continues independently, due to heart block.

wires passed through the skin and connected to an external pacemaker. Alternately, a pacemaker catheter may be passed via one of the jugular veins and its tip lodged in the apex of the right ventricle to transmit the impulses from an external pacemaker. Usually, X-ray screening is used during this procedure, but in an emergency the catheter may be introduced 'blind'. Since the transvenous route does not necessitate a thoracotomy, it has many advantages for patients who are in their seventh, eighth or even ninth decade as are many patients with heart block.

3. Epicardial leads or a transvenous pacemaker catheter inserted as described above may be attached to a silicone-covered pacemaker box (Fig. 61) implanted subcutaneously in the axilla or

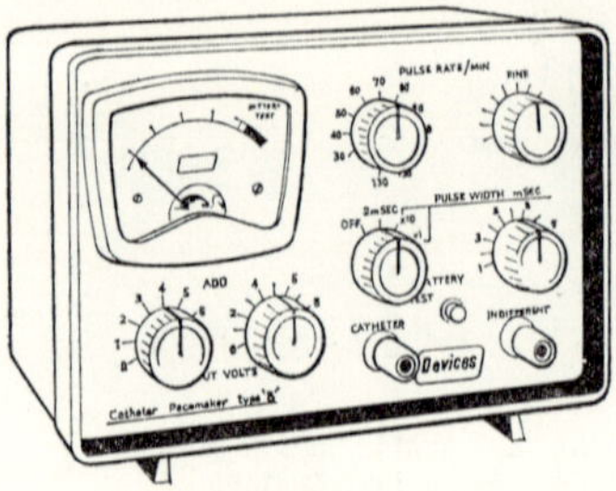

FIG **61. An external pacemaker box.**

abdomen. This leaves no part of the system outside the body, thus reducing infection risks and enabling the patients to forget about their disability more easily. The pacemaker can be implanted, batteries changed or a new box put in under local anaesthetic. At present pacemaker units are powered by 2 or 3 mercury cell batteries, and may, but not always, last up to three years. Nuclear-powered units are being tried, using plutonium 238. The patient must be well protected from radiation hazards, but the nuclear-powered unit is efficient and might be expected to last 10–20 years, well beyond the life expectancy of most patients needing it.

4. A silicone-covered induction coil consisting of 1000 turns of copper wire is implanted subcutaneously in the chest wall, and the stainless steel ends of the wire are attached to the left ventricle. The coil is ring-shaped so that tissue grows through the middle and holds it in place. Another electrode is strapped to the chest wall

over the coil, and is connected to a pacemaker unit carried in the pocket or a small bag.

It is powered by U2 batteries which are universally available and easily changed.

Each pacemaker delivers a fixed current, usually less than 1 volt, at a pre-set rate. With external units it is possible to alter the rate, and sometimes the current, to achieve the optimum cardiac output. Some pacemakers have been designed to transmit the patient's own atrial impulses to the ventricles. Others, known as demand pacemakers, will only emit pacing impulses if the ventricles fail to contract as at pre-determined rate.

For long-term pacing, a transvenous pacemaker catheter attached to a unit implanted subcutaneously is the method most often used. For the more acute situation an external pacemaker is used with a catheter or with wires sutured in an operation.

Complications

1. Failure of pacing. The heart rate will be found to be lower than the set rate of the pacemaker. If the pacemaker is an external one, it should first be ascertained that it has not been turned off, or the current reduced. Other causes of failure are disconnection of wires internally or externally, a break in the wire running through the catheter, movement of the catheter tip in the heart so that it fails to transmit impulses to the ventricle, fibrosis round epicardial electrodes, or a faulty pacemaker.

Often the pacing impulses can be seen as a vertical line on the electrocardiogram. With effective pacing each pacing beat should be followed by a QRS complex. Medical staff should be informed if this does not occur.

2. Increase in the patient's heart rate so that it surpasses the pacing rate. The heart rate will be found to be faster than the set pacing rate, and on the electrocardiogram the pacing impulse will occur in a different place in each complex. This is dangerous, because if the pacing impulse occurs during the vulnerable period, it is possible that ventricular fibrillation may be provoked.

3. Infection may occur along the track on the percutaneous wires or round an implanted pacemaker box or electrodes. All possible steps must be taken to see that this does not happen, but if it does,

the infection must be treated and the catheter, box and electrodes removed and re-sited.

After insertion of a pacemaker, the electrocardiogram is usually monitored for 24–48 hours to ascertain that pacing is effective. The patient is taught to take his pulse once or twice daily, so that after discharge he can inform his doctor if the rate rises or falls as much as 10 beats/minute. He is also required to attend a follow-up clinic every 3 months and should live within reach of medical supervision experienced in artificial pacing.

His relatives should be assured that they need not worry about the pacemaker providing he attends the clinic, and that he will be able to lead a life normal for his age and condition. They should be advised that if there is any change in the patient's condition the doctor should be informed.

Despite the fact that pacemakers are expensive and still provide technical problems, they have proved their worth in allowing a number of patients to continue to live an active and enjoyable life for a number of years. Even with a fixed rate the heart can increase its output to meet increased demand, and these patients can undertake most normal activities. A number of lives have been saved by temporary pacing in an acute situation.

7

Cardiac surgery: preparation and postoperative care

Preparation for surgery

Medical–surgical cooperation

An operation is only one incident, though a major one, in the course of treatment for heart disease. The heart has been abnormal for some time before operation and will remain so for some months afterwards, perhaps for ever. Therefore good team work between surgeons, physicians and their nursing staff is essential

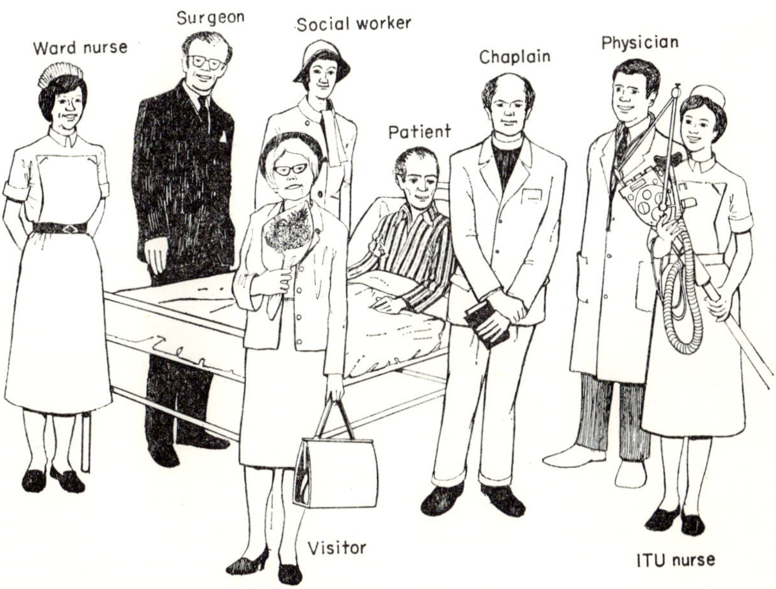

FIG 62. Interpersonal relationships.
All these people (and others) cooperate to help the patient.

all the way through (Fig. 62). Once a patient has been referred and accepted for operation all the investigations performed and the treatment given may be considered preoperative preparation, since their object is to make the patient as well equipped as possible to undergo operation.

Period in hospital before operation

Some patients may be ill enough to be kept in hospital for weeks or months having treatment and investigations concurrently and then may go straight on to operation. Others may be treated and observed for weeks, months or years as out-patients, with intermittent periods as in-patients for more intensive treatment or major investigations before being admitted for operation. A few patients may never have been in hospital before, and can be admitted, assessed and come to operation within a fairly short period. However the major of cardiac patients will probably be in hospital at least 5–7 days before operation so that certain up-to-date information can be obtained, and any necessary treatment given.

Investigations

These include:

1. Routine temperature recordings. Pyrexia may be an indication for estimation of sedimentation rate and bacteriological examination of the blood to exclude rheumatic activity or bacterial endocarditis.

2. Careful history and physical examination by medical staff. Septic spots, styes, a cold or other infection may make it necessary to postpone operation.

3. Haemoglobin estimation and white cell count to detect anaemia or infection which may need treatment.

4. Estimation of serum electrolytes, particularly if the patient has been having diuretics. Many modern diuretics cause excessive excretion of potassium or sodium and it is important to correct electrolyte imbalance before operation.

5. Chest X-ray to determine the state of the lungs, e.g. any infection or pulmonary congestion which may be improved with treatment.

6. Routine urine examination to exclude diabetes mellitus, renal failure or infection.

7. Examination of the sputum for pathological organisms and their sensitivities to antibiotics.

8. Nose and throat swabs may be taken so that any infection with organisms can be specifically treated; for example. *Staphylococcus pyogenes* may be treated with antibacterial cream to the nose, or monilial infection of the throat by lozenges.

9. Electrocardiograph.

10. Fluid intake and output record. Sometimes a daily weight record is preferred since the best kept fluid chart gives inaccurate results to some extent, because of variations such as the amount of fluid lost by sweating.

11. Respiratory function tests such as a vital capacity (VC), maximum voluntary ventilation (MVV) and forced expiratory volume (FEV) or other more detailed tests may be performed. It may be possible to improve respiratory function by the use of antispasmodic drugs and physiotherapy. Persistently poor results give warning of possible postoperative problems.

12. When cardiopulmonary bypass is contemplated, height and weight are measured if possible. This allows calculation of the surface area, upon which the rate of flow from the pump is calculated.

Special preparations

Necessary investigations such as angiocardiograms or cardiac catheterization have usually been performed previously, but occasionally they may need to be repeated.

Necessary dental treatment is also performed well before operation with appropriate prophylactic antibiotic cover.

Patients for open heart surgery may have their blood grouped and cross-matched with a number of donors, so as to ensure that an adequate amount (6–7 litres or more) of compatible fresh blood can be obtained shortly before operation. Now that the bypass machine is often primed with electrolyte solutions, only 5–6 units of stored blood may be needed. For closed heart surgery without cardiopulmonary bypass, 1–2 pints are usually sufficient, and cross-matching can be done a day or two before operation.

Drug therapy

During this time many patients continue with supportive therapy, e.g. digoxin and diuretics. However, it is considered desirable to stop diuretics if possible, as total body potassium may be depleted after prolonged administration. This is undesirable and may not be obvious, since electrolyte estimations normally show only the extracellular potassium level. If anticoagulant therapy is being given it is usually continued, according to the prothrombin index, with warfarin sodium, phenindione (Dindevan) or other long-acting drugs, until 48 hours before operation. It is then usually changed to heparin 100 mg intravenously six-hourly since this can be reversed by a calculated dose of protamine sulphate before operation.

Activity

The patient should be allowed to get up at least for toilet purposes if possible, and to be as active as is compatible with his condition. This helps to avoid deep venous thrombosis and respiratory and excretory difficulties. It also allows the patient more contact with others and less time to worry.

Physiotherapy

The physiotherapist plays an important part in preparation by teaching breathing exercises to improve respiratory function and leg exercises for the postoperative period. The patient's posture may need attention, since this tends to be poor in chronically ill people and may impede breathing. General exercises may be given to patients who are confined to bed or to those with hemiplegia.

Psychological preparation

The final period before operation is usually spent in the cardiac surgical ward, and presents an excellent opportunity for the nursing staff to get to know the patient and establish good rapport. This is vital for the best possible postoperative recovery, but it may not be easy. Previous hospital visits may have provided happy memories and fostered confidence, or unfortunate experiences and anxiety.

The young patient, particularly, may be thoroughly bored and exasperated by long periods of hospital routine when he longs for normal life. Family care or financial matters may worry the parent, while the single person wonders who will look after him until he is fit again. Added to this may be the irritability and emotional instability resulting from such physical causes as prolonged illness, lack of peaceful sleep and cerebral hypoxia. Above all there is the prospect of a heart operation, to most people an awesome prospect, especially since many may know that the operation they are to have has only become possible comparatively recently.

Anxiety may show as irritability and aggressiveness, or as withdrawal, depression and reluctance to communicate, all of which nurses find difficult to deal with unless they understand the causes. Overconfidence and flippancies may cover a cry for reassurance which may be missed unless the nurse is alert. Hypnotics at night, sedatives by day and, if necessary, oxygen may help. However, perhaps the best tranquillizer is an understanding nurse who responds to the unspoken as well as the spoken needs, who takes time to explain, to encourage and to make the patient feel part of the team for his recovery. Nowadays it is common for cardiac patients to be nursed postoperatively in an intensive care unit for the first days, which makes it essential that information about them should be passed on to provide continuity. A member of the intensive care staff should visit the patient. The patient appreciates knowing that there will be one familiar face, while the nurse is able to explain postoperative procedures, teach the use of any special apparatus such as the Bird or the Bennett respirator, and assess the patient's mental and physical condition. Contact with a patient recovering from a similar operation can be a great morale booster. It should not be forgotten that the best person to help in fear of pain or even death may be the Hospital Chaplain, priest or minister of the patient's own faith. The medical social worker, too, may be able to settle home worries.

Relatives

If the husband, wife or close relative can balance their natural anxiety with confidence that the patient's welfare is of paramount importance to the hospital staff, they will be more cooperative.

The surgeon will usually explain the operation and its risks to next-of-kin, but relatives may turn to the nurse for further explanation and she must know what she may tell them. Nursing staff must also gain their cooperation over restrictions such as diet or visiting and this is usually given willingly if the reasons are understood. People are often delighted to help in such ways as enquiring at intervals about the patient's condition and arranging for other friends and relatives to ring them rather than the hospital. It may be necessary to arrange accommodation near the hospital for relatives who live some distance away, but it is debatable whether it is a good thing for them to live in the hospital for long. This may sometimes be wearying for the relatives without being of great help to the patient.

Immediate preparations

The consent form for operation is signed by the patient or by the parent in the case of a minor.

The skin is shaved, from neck to waist, back and front, or from neck to knees if bypass technique is to be used, since the femoral vessels may be cannulated. Other skin preparation varies according to the surgeon, but may consist of a daily bath or bed-bath with hexochlorophane soap. Bowel function should be regulated as necessary several days before operation. A good night's sleep before operation is ensured by a hypnotic drug. The last meal is usually given the night before operation, but fluids may be given up to 4 hours preoperatively.

On the day of operation, the patient is bathed, dressed in clean linen and the bed made with clean linen. He or she is then persuaded to pass urine just before the premedication is given at the prescribed time. This may be 10 mg morphine only. Dentures and jewellery are removed. Calmness and a comfortable position are of great importance during preparation and transport to theatre. The anxious patient who is orthopnoeic and has been made to lie too flat on a trolley is much more likely to have pulmonary oedema and provide complications for the anaesthetist. Cardiac arrest in the anaesthetic room is an anxious but not unknown situation when dealing with severely ill cardiac patients.

Postoperative care after closed heart surgery (Fig. 63)

These operations are usually performed through a left thoracotomy, though a sternal incision may be used, particularly for pericardectomy when good access to the whole heart is needed.

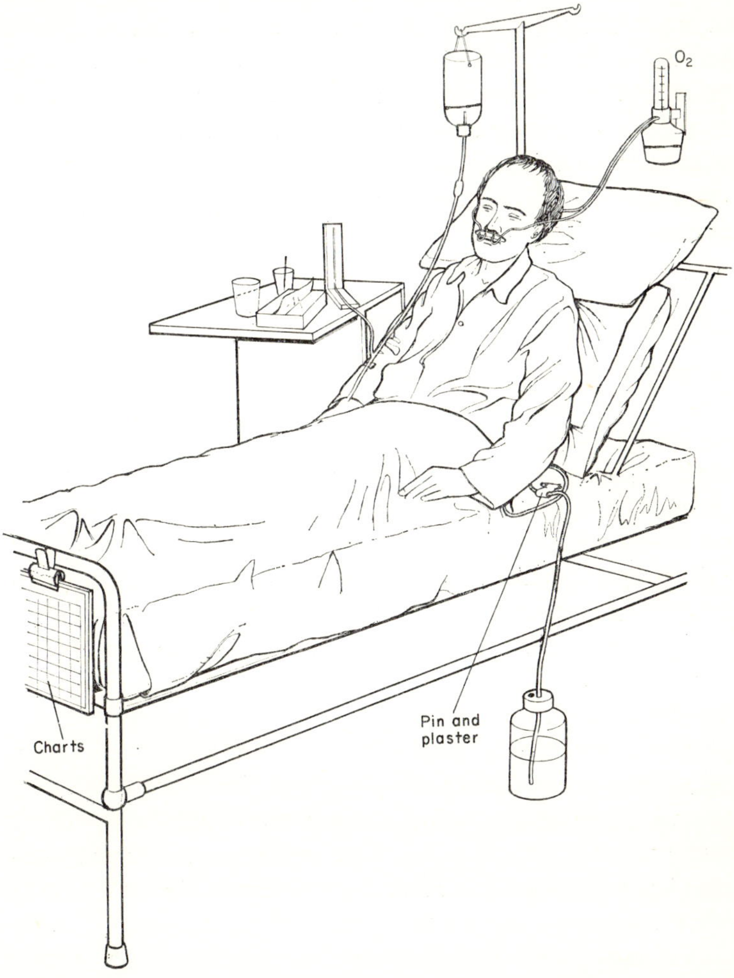

FIG **63. Postoperative care after closed cardiac surgery.**
The patient is propped up in a good position, with the tube pinned so that it drains freely into the bottle; spare tubing is coiled on the bed. Drink, sputum carton and tissues should be within easy reach of either arm.

All necessary equipment for postoperative care must be prepared while the patient is in theatre. On return from theatre, the patient is settled comfortably into bed, oxygen therapy continued, and lifting sheets or other surplus linen removed. The patient's colour, heart rate and blood pressure are checked and recorded. The rate of transfusion and the amount of drainage via the intercostal tube are checked. Usually the patient is conscious on return from theatre and will need the prescribed analgesic almost immediately. Details of blood loss in theatre and blood replacement should be recorded and pulses in all four limbs are checked and recorded as palpable or impalpable.

Routines vary a little according to the surgeon, but the following is a sample routine:

1. *Blood pressure and heart rate* are recorded half-hourly at first. If stable and satisfactory after the first 4 hours these recordings can be taken hourly and, overnight, at two-hourly intervals. The importance of recordings should be balanced against the disturbance to the patient. If it is steady and regular, the pulse may be counted and charted; the apex beat must be checked with a stethoscope and compared with the pulse from time to time, to be certain that any discrepancy between them is noticed. These records may be discontinued the day after operation or may continue, according to the patient's condition. An abnormally high or low blood pressure or heart rate should be reported at once. The expected range is known from the preoperative records and from information from the medical staff.

2. *Temperature, pulse and respiration* are recorded four-hourly and after the first week or, when persistently normal, twice daily. *The patient's colour and the rate, depth and character of respiration* are observed frequently during the immediate postoperative period. Dyspnoea, rapid respirations, moist sounds in the chest and blood-stained sputum should be reported. Peripheral coldness and cyanosis should also be reported.

3. *Oxygen therapy* is continued, 4–6 litres/min of moistened oxygen being given intranasally until the following day. It is then reduced, discontinued or continued as necessary. Nasal cannulae are usually well tolerated by the patient, but must be passed into the nasopharynx (about 5–6 cm) to be efficient. Oxygen must be

moistened to avoid drying of the mucosa. A mask or tent may be used, but may be less well tolerated. For infants or young children a tent is necessary.

4. *Position* is usually flat at first, the patient being propped up gradually after an hour or two. If orthopnoea is evident the patient is propped up immediately. The 'jack-knife' position with both feet and head raised is useful. It allows good drainage, helps respiration and also increases venous return, so helping to maintain adequate blood pressure. By the following day the patient can usually be nursed alternately in the right lateral and upright positions, always supported in good position by pillows. After removal of the intercostal tube, the left lateral position is also used. This helps lung expansion, relieves pressure areas and helps the patient to relax. While changing the patient's position, limb pulses should be checked.

5. The *intercostal tube* is kept patent and drainage observed; the bottle is marked at the level of the fluid put in the underwater seal bottle so that the amount of drainage is obvious. Tubing should be fixed to the bed with strapping and pin so that the fluid drains down into the bottle. Excess tubing should be coiled on the bed between the pin and the patient, so that he can move without pulling on the tube. If the fluid level in the tube ceases to rise and fall with respiration (that is, to swing) the tube may be kinked or blocked. This should be remedied by unkinking or milking the tube. When the lung is fully expanded the swing may cease. Some surgeons like suction applied to the drainage bottle. The tube should never be removed from the fluid without occluding the tube or pneumothorax may result. The bottle should never be lifted above the level of the patient's chest unless the tube is clamped, or fluid may be syphoned into the chest. When drainage is minimal (usually 24–48 hours after operation) the tube is removed. The stab wound stitch inserted at operation is tied as the tube is removed. Air must not be allowed to enter. The amount of drainage is recorded, the original amount of fluid in the bottle being subtracted. If the lung surface has been torn at operation (due to pleural adhesions from a previous operation or pleurisy) air may be expelled via the tube ('blowing'). A tube will be left in the chest while this continues and

it must never be clamped for longer than a few seconds or a tension pneumothorax may occur.

6. *Fluid replacement* is continued intravenously at first. Blood loss is often not completely replaced, because of the risk of overloading the circulation. Intravenous fluids, usually 5% dextrose, are given only at the rate ordered for the same reason. Fluid is given orally starting as soon as possible and increasing as tolerated. Light diet can usually be given on the day after operation.

7. The *physiotherapist* will visit the patient intermittently to give passive and active leg movements, deep breathing exercises, and to help the patient to cough. She will also give arm exercises and correct the patient's posture. There is a tendency to hold the affected side rigid which results in backache and a stiff shoulder. Good posture and the avoidance of respiratory or venous thrombotic complications are the combined responsibility of nurse, physiotherapist and patient, and mutual cooperation and good relationships are essential.

8. Sufficient *analgesics* must be given to keep the patient comfortable enough to rest and cooperate, without depressing respiration or consciousness. Intramuscular morphine 6–10 mg every 4–6 hours may be given for 24–48 hours, then a milder analgesic such as 30–60 mg dihydrocodeine bitartrate or later 500–1000 mg paracetamol. The experienced nurse must be able to assess accurately the patient's need for and response to analgesics since comparable individuals may vary considerably. Hypotension is not necessarily a reason for withholding analgesics, since excessive pain may cause hypotension.

9. *Drugs* such as digoxin or diuretics are often continued after operation, though dosage may be adjusted. Many surgeons prefer not to give antibiotics unless there is a specific indication.

10. *Ambulation* may start about the fourth day, sometimes earlier or later, according to the surgeon's wish and the patient's condition. The important thing is that activity should increase gradually as tolerated, and that the patient does not sit immobile in a chair thus encouraging thrombosis.

11. *Sutures* are removed about the tenth day.

Investigations

These usually include a daily chest X-ray until the lung remains expanded, thereafter less frequently. Haemoglobin is estimated about the second day after operation, and at least once again before discharge. Serum electrolytes will be estimated if diuretics are given, and if anticoagulants are used the dose is controlled by estimation of the prothrombin index.

Most patients are in hospital 2–3 weeks after operation, sometimes more. An out-patient appointment is arranged and a letter to the general practitioner written by the medical staff, since follow-up care is very important.

Unless home circumstances are exceptionally good, convalescence should be arranged, particularly for women. It is almost impossible for the average housewife and mother not to do too much if she goes straight home. A supply of any necessary drugs should be given to the patient on discharge, with full instructions on when to take them.

Postoperative care after cardiopulmonary bypass

The operation

Circulation can be stopped for only 3–4 min without the risk of permanent cerebral damage. A body temperature of 31° C allows 10 min without circulation, since metabolic oxygen requirements are reduced by 50% at this temperature. Operations such as valve replacements or repair of many congenital abnormalities take longer than this, and circulation must be maintained by a cardiopulmonary bypass machine (Figs 64, 65).

A sternal split approach is employed to allow good access. The venae cavae are cannulated and blood flows to an oxygenator where it is exposed to oxygen. It is pumped by a roller pump through a filter and debubbling chamber, through a heat exchanger, which allows cooling or warming of the blood, and back into the femoral artery cannula or upper end of the aorta. The machine is filled before use with heparinized fresh blood, electrolyte solution or a mixture of both.

The haemodilution technique reduces the need for fresh

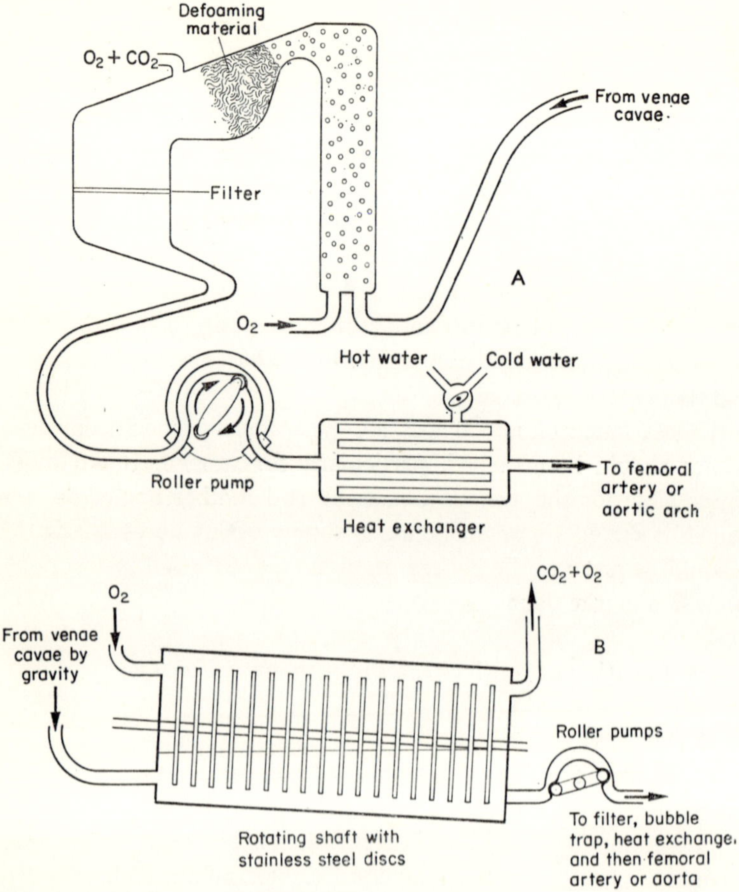

FIG **64. Cardiopulmonary bypass equipment.**
A, Bubble bag type. B, Rotating disc type.

heparinized blood which must be used within 24 hours. Special donor sessions are necessary to obtain it. The water solution also improves perfusion by reducing the tendency to sludging of blood in the tissues.

If the coronary orifices are in the region of operation, cardiac circulation may be maintained through coronary artery cannulae. However, because of the technical difficulties which sometimes occur, and the possibility of damaging the coronary vessels, some surgeons now cross-clamp the aorta and leave the heart anoxic and

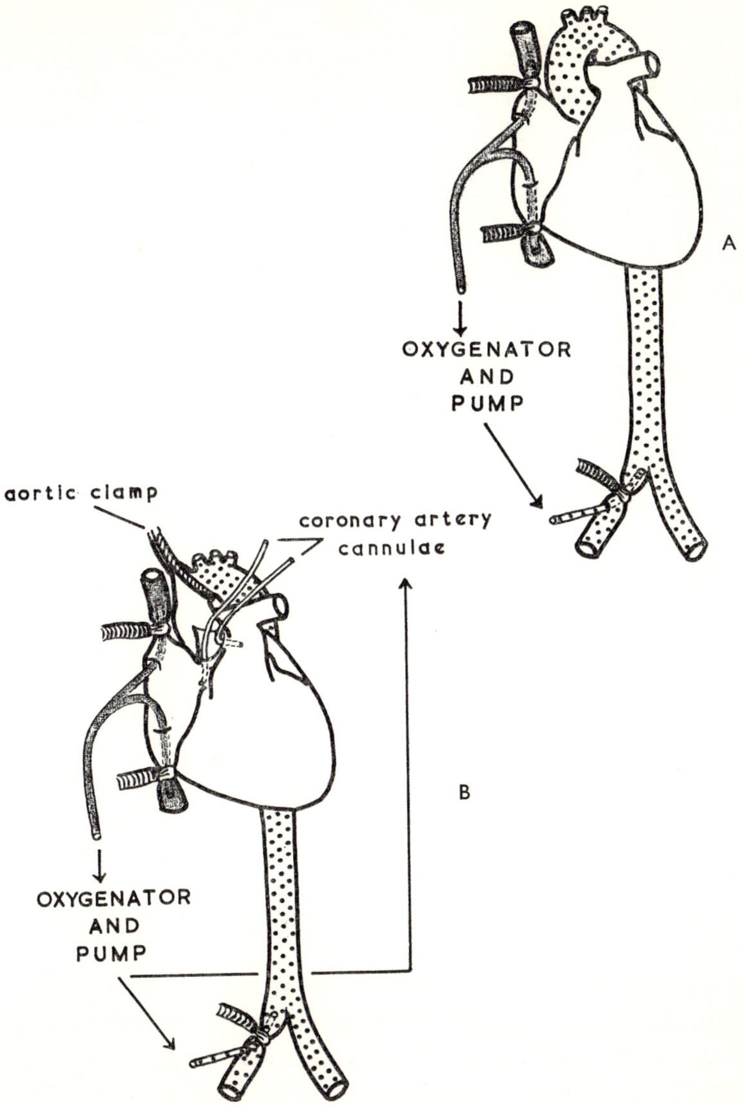

FIG 65. **Cardiopulmonary bypass.**
A, Venous blood drains from the cannulae in the venae cavae into an oxygenator, and is then returned to the aorta or femoral artery by a pump. The aortic valve prevents regurgitation of blood into the left ventricle. B, The bypass utilized for aortic valve surgery. The aorta is clamped below the innominate artery, permitting a dry operating field. The coronary arteries are perfused through special cannulae.

limp. This makes the operation easier. The oxygen and other metabolic requirements of a completely inactive heart are much less than if it is fibrillating.

Before the start of bypass circulation a calculated dose of heparin is given, and this is reversed by the appropriate dose of protamine sulphate when normal circulation is resumed. Each machine is designed to reduce haemolysis (by mechanical damage to cells) to a minimum, and frequent blood gas and acid–base balance estimations are done to make sure that circulation to the tissues (perfusion) is adequate and indicate any necessary correction. Effective heart action may be stopped during operation and at the end of bypass electrical defibrillation is usually necessary to start it. Arterial and venous cannulae and a urethral catheter are used during operation to allow observation of arterial and venous pressure and urine output, and are left in position postoperatively. Drainage tubes are left in the mediastinum and pericardium and if the pleural cavity has been opened this is drained. For convenience all chest tubes are drained into two bottles.

Return from theatre

All necessary equipment for postoperative care is prepared during the operation.

The patient is usually lifted into bed in theatre semiconscious. A clear airway and good supply of oxygen must be maintained during transport. At least two nurses are needed to receive the patient from theatre. A chest X-ray is taken. Oxygen administration is checked and continued. ECG electrodes are attached for monitoring. Venous pressure, arterial pressure and heart rate are checked. Drainage tubes are attached to measuring cylinders calibrated at 10 ml intervals, and suction of 25 mm Hg applied by a mechanical pump. Rates of drainage and transfusion are noted. The arterial line is attached to the meter and the urethral catheter to a precision volume urometer. The amount of intravenous fluid in progress is recorded. Blood and urine for electrolytes are sent to the laboratory as soon as possible. Throughout all this and for the next few hours the patient must be closely observed for any change in condition. By this time the patient is usually awake and needing reassurance and analgesia; 2·5–5 mg morphine intravenously are usually

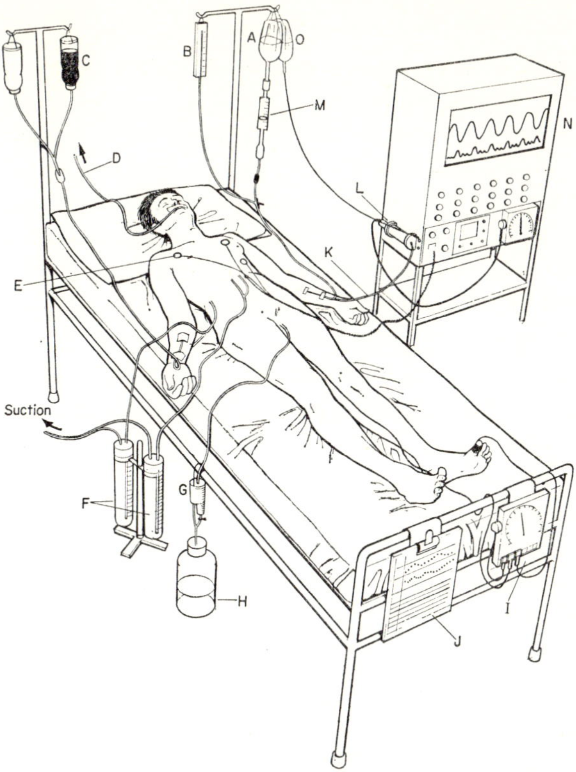

FIG **66. Postoperative care after cardiopulmonary bypass.**
A, Fluid reservoir. B, Ruler for venous pressure. C, Blood transfusion. D, Oxygen. E, ECG electrodes. F, Measuring cylinders attached to mediastinal and pericardial drains. G, Urometer attached to urethral catheter. H, Winchester bottle. I, Thermometer with leads to toe and rectum. J, Chart. K, Cannula into radial artery. L, Pressure transducer (Head) attached to taps and radial artery cannula. M, 100 ml burette in infusion line. N, Oscilloscope. O, Fluid reservoir to flush the arterial line. Bedclothes are omitted for clarity.

effective. Body temperature should be recorded as soon as possible as it may be abnormally low; if so, the patient should be kept covered with warm blankets until it is normal. An abnormally cold patient tends to bleed as cold inhibits normal coagulation. It is helpful to record the peripheral skin (toe), core (rectal) and ambient air temperatures half-hourly/hourly so that any coldness of the extremities due to poor peripheral perfusion is demonstrated. Usually as the patient's condition improves and becomes stable over the first few hours, the skin and core temperatures approach to within 1–2° C of each other. Postoperative routine varies in different cardiac units, but the basic principles are the same.

Oxygen therapy is continued with 6 litres/min moistened oxygen intranasally. This is usually continued 2–3 days or more after valve replacement, but may be reduced earlier if the patient's condition warrants it. If a greater flow than 6–8 litres is indicated a mask is necessary. Some surgeons prefer a mask or tent, or artificial ventilation via an endotracheal tube routinely for 24 hours. Blood pressure, heart rate and venous pressure (Fig. 67) are recorded every 15 min for 3–4 hours, then half-hourly if recordings and the patient's general condition are stable and satisfactory. If all is still well after another 6 hours recordings may be hourly, then two-hourly after 24 hours, and gradually reduced in frequency. This depends entirely on the patient's condition.

Blood loss from the drainage tubes is recorded each 15 min at first, added to the cumulative total and balanced with total blood replaced. Recordings are less frequent as drainage diminishes. Drainage tubes must be milked vigorously at intervals (frequent at first) to ensure adequate drainage and remove clot; they are removed after 24–48 hours when drainage is minimal.

Blood is transfused to replace loss, plus such amount as is sufficient to maintain a satisfactory blood pressure without an excessively high venous pressure. The acceptable level of venous pressure varies according to the patient's condition. After valve replacement a patient may need a venous pressure of 15–20 cm H_2O if preoperative pressure was high. After atrial septal defect repairs 2–5 cm Hg may be the aim, and it may be difficult to keep it above 0 cm initially. If haemodilution was used during the operation, urine output will usually be increased and extra blood transfusion required to prevent anaemia. Platelets may be transfused when they are available, but with improvements in bypass techniques they are not always necessary. Blood transfusion can usually be discontinued after 24–36 hours.

Fluid balance is recorded separately, the cumulative totals and balance of intake and output being recorded hourly and later 2-hourly for 24–48 hours. Ordinary intake and output records are normally adequate after this. Daily weighing may be useful but

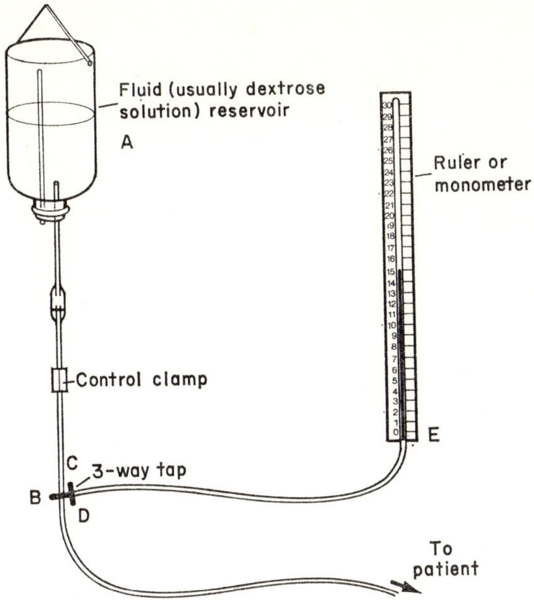

FIG 67. A method of recording the central venous pressure. With the three-way tap in the position shown fluid will flow to the patient at the rate set by the control clamp. To record the venous pressure, turn the tap so that B points to the fluid reservoir and C to the ruler. Allow fluid to flow up the tube attached to the ruler. Turn the tap so that B points to the patient's tube and D to the ruler. Raise and lower the ruler to ensure that fluid will flow to and fro freely between the patient's and ruler tubes. Rest E on the patient's sternoclavicular angle with the ruler vertical and allow the fluid to settle to an almost stationary level in the tube (there will be a slight rise and fall with respiration). Read the figure against the fluid level; this is the venous pressure, usually required in cm H_2O (though the fluid in the tube is usually Dextrose solution). The cannula in the patient must be in a large vein to obtain an accurate recording, e.g. the subclavian, femoral or venae cavae. If fluid will not flow freely to and fro as the ruler is raised and lowered the cannula may be kinked, e.g. at elbow, axilla or groin, or the filter at the top of the ruler tube may be wet. After recording the venous pressure the nurse must ensure that the tap is turned as shown to allow fluid to flow only to the patient and that the flow is controlled at the correct rate. Some units measure venous pressure from the mid-axilla rather than the sternoclavicular angle, but the patient would have to be lying on his back for this to be done. Venous pressure may be measured by a pressure lead and displayed on an oscilloscope.

involves disturbing the patient unless bed-weighing apparatus is available. Fluid replacement is calculated according to the size of the patient and any other factors affecting his needs, e.g. excessive sweating. For an average adult it is usually about 1500 ml of 5% dextrose from the time of operation to the next morning. Potassium is added as necessary to maintain the electrolyte balance. The fluid must be given evenly during the period ordered (*a*) because of the danger of overloading the circulation and (*b*) because rapid infusion of fluid with a high potassium content (which may be used) can provoke cardiac dysrhythmias. Small amounts of fluid may be given orally, increasing gradually if well tolerated and if the abdomen is not unduly distended. Some patients can take a light diet the day after operation; most can take fluids. Fresh fruit juice is a pleasant and safe way of giving some extra potassium. Urine output is measured hourly, specific gravity checked 4-hourly and the 24-hour urine output is collected. It may be necessary to test for blood, glucose or other abnormal constituents intermittently.

Position. After the first hour or two the patient can usually be propped up a little, and later raised further, always well supported in a good position, to an angle of 30–45°. The ill cardiac patient should not be sat up suddenly, since this may disturb the circulatory equilibrium. If the blood pressure is low the 'jack-knife' position may improve drainage and the patient's comfort and respiratory function while maintaining blood pressure (Fig. 68). Pressure areas are treated as usual, the patient being moved gently without pulling on any tubes. By the day after operation, or sometimes before this, the patient can usually be turned to a recumbent or semirecumbent lateral position intermittently, to relieve pressure areas and encourage expansion of each lung in turn. Movement of feet and legs is encouraged, passively if necessary. During change of position and at intervals in between peripheral circulation in the limbs and all possible sites of bleeding, e.g. the femoral area, should be observed.

Respiratory function must be observed carefully and increase in cyanosis, dyspnoea or moist sounds in the chest noted and reported. Deep breathing and expectoration should be encouraged. A 'triggered' respirator with mouthpiece, such as the Bird or Bennett (Fig. 69), is useful to assist deep breathing with little

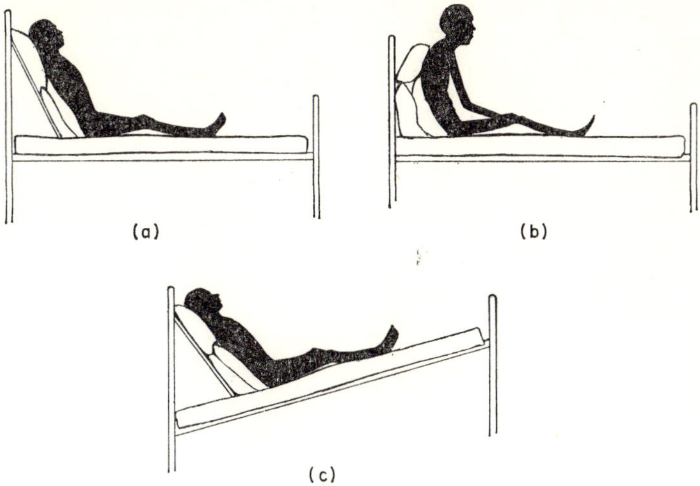

Fig 68. **Various positions.**
A, Good position, back straight. B, Bad position, patient slumped. Back-ache and poor lung expansion result. C, 'Jack-knife' position.

effort by the patient and to loosen viscid secretions by good humidification. This may be used for 5–10 min/hour, starting soon after return from theatre, and then more or less frequently as the patient's condition and need for rest demands. The patient must be taught the purpose and use of the machine *before* operation. The rise and fall of the chest and air entry heard by stethoscope indicate the efficient use of the machine. The Bennett respirator, with mouth mask and nose-clip if necessary, is useful for the patient who is unable to cooperate by closing his lips on the mouthpiece; and the terminal flow control is useful to compensate for slight leaks. Controls must be adjusted to air dilution. 100% oxygen is a totally absorbable gas and to use it may encourage alveolar collapse.

Drugs are often given intravenously at first to ensure their effect when peripheral circulation is poor and to reduce disturbance of the patient. Routine drugs include:

1. Morphine 5 mg intravenously as often as necessary for relief of pain.

2. Although it is not always considered necessary, intravenous calcium gluconate 10% in 10 ml may be ordered to be given slowly

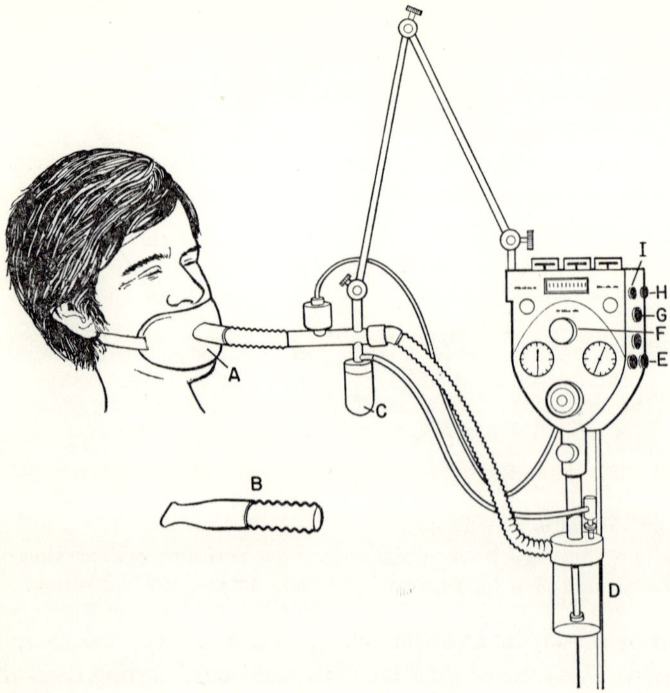

FIG 69. **A patient using a Bennett respirator for assisted deep breathing.**
A, Mouth mask. B, Mouthpiece. C, Nebulizer. D, Puritan nebulizer. E, Nebulization controls. F, Pressure control. G, Oxygen dilution control. H, Sensitivity control. I, Terminal flow control.

for every bottle of blood transfused. Sodium citrate in stored blood given in large amounts reduces the amount of circulating ionized calcium.

3. Antibiotics are always ordered, but the routine varies according to the unit policy or the patient's specific needs or allergies.

4. Digoxin is usually given intramuscularly or later by mouth because of the danger of provoking dysrhythmias by giving it intravenously. It is ordered only when the serum potassium level is known. A hypolakaemic patient is liable to digitalis intoxication.

5. Anticoagulant therapy is started within 24 hours after removal of drainage tubes, if a prosthetic valve has been inserted, because of the risk of clot forming on the valve. Warfarin sodium is given and dosage controlled to maintain a prothrombin level of 30–40%.

Phenindione is less often used because of the possibility of renal failure with long-term use; patients with mitral prosthetic valves usually have anticoagulant therapy for life, and those with aortic prostheses for at least 3–6 months.

6. Diuretics such as frusemide, 40–80 mg daily or more, may be ordered if there is evidence of fluid retention. Intravenous doses may be necessary in acute situations.

7. Soluble aspirin 600 mg orally or as aspirin suppositories may be ordered to be given four-hourly if the temperature rises above 38·5° C (101° F) because pyrexia increases the cardiac work. Giving aspirin to a patient having anticoagulants increases the risk of bleeding, and the anticoagulant dosage may need altering.

8. After the day of operation, as the intravenous fluids and their potassium content are reduced, potassium supplements are usually given by mouth.

9. Chlorpromazine 10 mg intravenously may be ordered after certain operations to control excessive hypertension. A hypertrophied left ventricle which has been used to an incompetent valve not infrequently maintains a blood pressure of 180/100 mm Hg, or more, until it adjusts to the competent valve again. Such hypertension may be dangerous.

Electrocardiographic monitoring is continued for as long as necessary—usually 2–5 days. Electrodes stuck to the chest wall minimize interference by muscle movement and may give a more reliable oscilloscope recording. Limb electrodes, if used, should be removed and replaced on a different area four-hourly to prevent soreness from prolonged pressure. The electrode jelly used for the routine ECG, while efficient for short recordings, may cause soreness if left on too long. Teepol 1–10 or a non-irritant jelly or cream are more suitable. The nurse cannot be expected to be a diagnostic expert on electrocardiograms, but she should be able to note and report significant changes in pattern, rate and rhythm. She should learn to note premature ventricular contractions, since an increasing number of these may be an early warning of trouble ahead. She should also recognize ventricular fibrillation. The experienced nurse will also learn to recognize such conditions as heart block. A rhythm strip is recorded daily for the first few days.

Investigations at first include:

1. Daily haemoglobin and packed cell volume, white cell count and platelet count. Serum electrolytes and urea are estimated daily or more frequently; the prothrombin index daily if anticoagulants are to be given.

2. Urine electrolytes and urea are estimated from a specimen of the 24-hour collection, or may be estimated more frequently.

3. Routine urine examination is also performed. Daily (portable) chest X-ray to assess lung expansion and detect signs of pulmonary oedema.

4. If there is any sputum, a specimen should be sent for bacteriological examination.

5. Blood gas and acid–base balance state daily or more often is indicated to assess respiratory and circulatory efficiency.

The arterial line may be used to obtain blood but the specimen must be *undiluted* blood. For blood gas estimation, 5–10 ml of blood in a heparinized syringe are needed. All air must be expelled and the syringe capped immediately, labelled with ward and patient's name, put in a beaker of ice and sent to the laboratory. Heparinized dextrose is injected to clear the line after drawing specimens or when blood leaks back into it. The solution, heparin 50 mg in 1 litre of 5% dextrose, is kept attached by infusion set to a tap on the line so that there is less risk of infection entering. *No air bubbles* must pass through the line—they would become air emboli in the arterial circulation.

Basic nursing care to keep the patient clean and comfortable, technical care and treatment, plus medical staff visits, occupy a considerable amount of time. Care must be planned to allow the ill patient as much rest as is compatible with good treatment.

By the end of 48 hours the drainage tubes, transfusion and possibly infusion equipment and catheter have been removed. The arterial line is removed if arterial specimens are no longer required. Digital pressure must be maintained for 5 min by the clock when this is done to stop haemorrhage. At this stage the patient can be left in peace more, and will often sleep for long periods.

Visiting on the day of operation is not often helpful either to the patient or to his relatives, and is therefore discouraged unless individual circumstances warrant it. The surgeon will usually speak with the next-of-kin after the operation, either by telephone or in person, and they are encouraged to keep in contact with the ward by telephone. (Note that the telephone bell in the intensive care unit must be muted.) After this, short visits by someone close to the patient are enjoyed and help to keep the patient in touch with the outside world.

It is not very unusual for patients to have *bad dreams* or to become confused within a few days after operation due to the physical and psychological stress sustained. This usually passes with reassurance and conversation to orient them to time and place.

After 2–5 days, or sometimes more, the patient returns from intensive care to the cardiac ward. This is progress, but the patient is still ill and must increase activity only as his condition allows.

Ambulation may begin on the fourth day after septal defect repairs, or the seventh day after valve replacement or operations of similar severity, but this depends on physical progress. Gradual increase of activity is important, avoiding long periods sitting in a chair without leg movements. The patient begins to enjoy listening to the radio, reading, chatting with other patients and other quiet occupations, but overtiredness must be avoided. Those who felt well before operation may need reassurance that it is natural to tire easily at first.

Nurses must always be alert for the onset of complications such as cardiac dysrhythmias, which may occasionally occur even at this stage. These may be fatal if not promptly and efficiently treated. Dyspnoea or sacral or ankle oedema may indicate the need for a temporary increase in diuretics and possibly increased digitalis therapy.

Sutures are removed on the tenth day, but wounds may be left uncovered earlier when dry.

Diet may or may not be restricted as regards salt (sodium) content, but should be temptingly served. Good nutrition is an important factor in tissue repair and resistance to infection.

Adequate convalescence at home or elsewhere, careful out-patient follow-up and good liaison with the general practitioner are important, especially for those patients needing permanent anticoagulant therapy. An adequate supply of drugs and clear instructions on dosage and side-effects to be observed should be given on discharge.

After operations such as valve replacement patients should be warned that although the damaged valve has been replaced, the overworked heart needs time to recover. Full benefits of the operation may not be felt for a year or more. The nurse may understand this better by looking at serial X-rays showing gradual decrease in heart size towards normal over 12 months or more.

Care of children after cardiac surgery

Children should normally be nursed in children's units where staff are experienced in their care, surroundings are suitably designed and they are in the company of other children. However, this is not invariably best, especially when they need specialized care, for example after cardiac surgery.

If a child must be nursed in a ward with adults then the influence of other patients is worthy of attention. Many children with heart conditions have spent much time in the company of adults because of their physical limitations, and appreciate their company. It is unwise, however, to allow a young child to become too attached to a patient who will shortly undergo surgery and be unable to cope with his attentions. Adults may help to provide amusements, but too many sweets and too much sentimentality must be avoided, a certain amount of discipline being necessary for the child's well-being. In this respect, men, though fond of children, often cause less problems than women. Physically the child may be classified as a neonate or as a child. Intravenous fluids may be calculated in the same way as for an adult, but the amount given will be very much smaller, which means care in spreading it evenly over the 24 hours. Blood transfusion particularly must be very carefully controlled as even 50 ml extra blood given quickly may overload a young child's circulation. Special giving sets with a 30 ml chamber are used so that administration can be accurately controlled (Figs 70, 71). Drug doses also will be much smaller. $\frac{\text{Age}}{\text{Age} + 12}$ gives the fraction of the adult dose needed as a rough guide, but children's toleration of some drugs differs from adults' which may alter the proportionate dosage.

Because of the small tracheobronchial tree, which easily becomes blocked with secretions, more children than adults may need

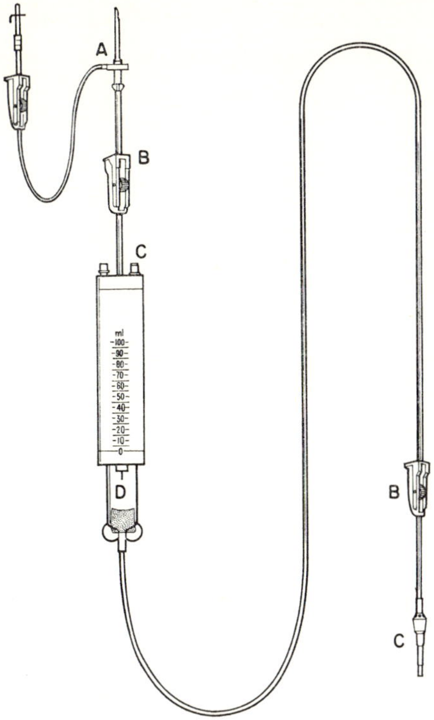

FIG 70. **Paediatric infusion set with minidrip.**
A, Connector with integral airway. B, Control clamp. C, Additional drugs may be inserted here. D, Minidrip tube meters 60 drips/ml.

tracheal aspiration and possible artificial ventilation after open heart surgery. A tracheostomy may be difficult to manage or undesirable, and can often be avoided by use of a Jackson-Rees nasotracheal tube. With or without a tracheal tube loosening of secretions by humidification is important.

In other respects a child cannot be considered as a small adult, partly because of his limited experience of life and different concept of time. The younger the child the shorter his view of the past and future; 24 hours without mother may make a young child feel quite forsaken. For this reason frequent visits by immediate relatives are usually allowed and in some hospitals the mother may be able to share a room with her child except during the immediate period of operation.

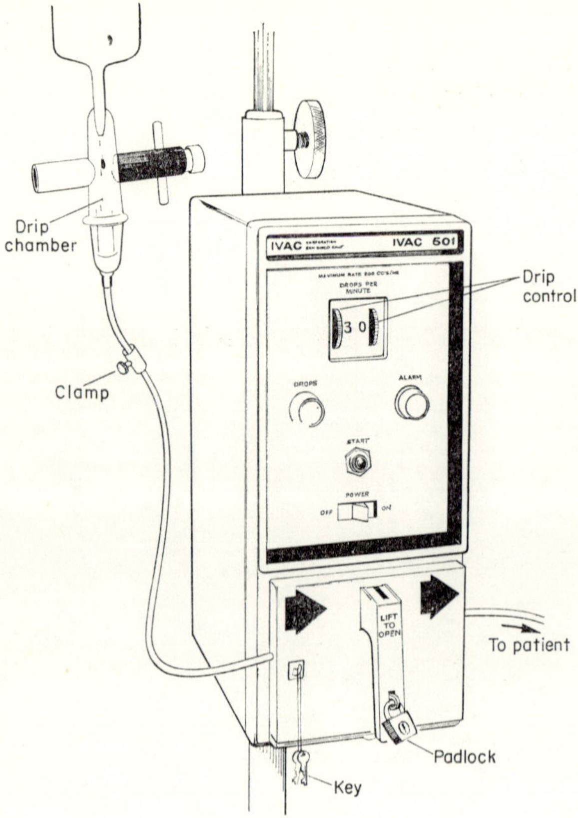

FIG **71. A controlled infusion pump.**
The drip chamber must be vertical to allow the drops to be detected by the 'electronic eye'. Opening the machine without first closing the clamp allows free fluid flow. The padlock prevents pointless opening.

The child's expectation of the nurse

As few nurses as possible should be concerned in a child's care so that nurse and child get to know each other. The nurse must be someone to love, trust and obey so that she can provide security during the potentially traumatic hospital experience even when parents are absent. This means that she must always mean what she says and not promise that 'it won't hurt' unless this is true.

Explanations of treatments, investigations and operations should be as explicit or simple as the child's understanding demands. They may be given by a nurse, parent or both, but there must be no

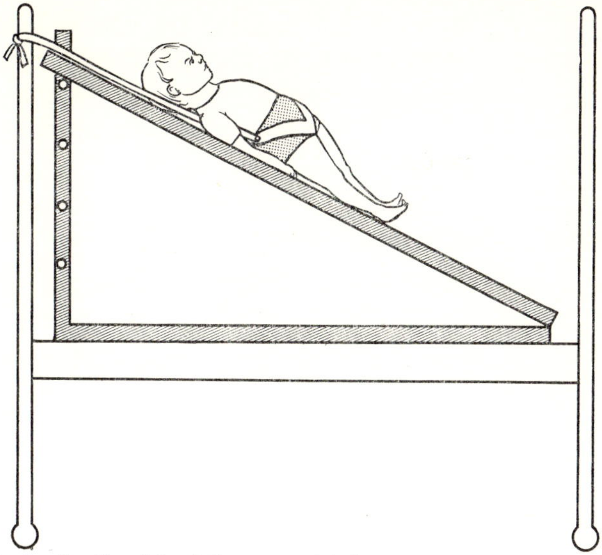

FIG 72. **An inclined bed for use with infants in cardiac failure.**

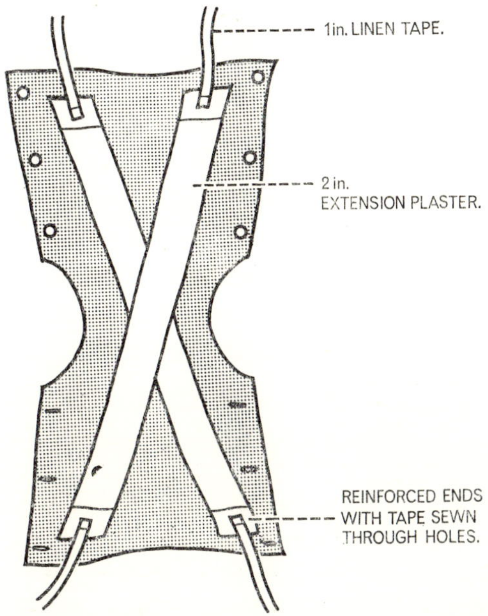

FIG 73. **A good and simple method for supporting babies in an upright position.**
This design, making use of ordinary plastic pants, was made by a staff nurse in her first post-registration year.

apparent contradictions. New experiences can often be introduced preoperatively by play, for example, the 'space flight' with oxygen and ECG monitor for older children or the 'little house' oxygen tent for younger ones. Children often accept strange things remarkably well from those they trust.

The parent's expectations of the nurse

Parents must always be made to feel part of the team contributing to their child's recovery. They rely on the nurse as a friend for explanation or simplification of information about treatments, investigations and operations, for guidance on how to help the child and for reassurance and support especially in trouble. Visits by a confident and well informed parent play a large part in keeping the child happy and contented. Friendly nurse–parent relationships seen by the child increase his confidence too.

Doctors' expectation of the nurse

Medical staff will initiate or order treatment such as intravenous therapy, bed rest or restricted activity, but rely on the nurse to maintain it.

Sedation may help at times, but most important is distraction of the child's attention by talking to him or some quiet activity. Listening to stories is a favourite pastime, whether read by the nurse, parent, teacher or recorded. Some children will be amused for long periods by fish in a tank or pictures on the wall. The convalescent but restricted child may enjoy drawing, jigsaws, simple handicrafts or even writing letters, but often needs frequent change of occupation to keep him amused.

Oral drugs and medicines are preferable to injections from the child's point of view, but must reach the stomach to be effective, which means they must be pleasantly flavoured or camouflaged, or easily swallowed pills so that the child will take them .

Nurses will also be expected to cooperate in helping the parents to an accurate understanding of the child's present and future physical capabilities. This will avoid overambitious activity too early or unnecessary restrictions on a normal life.

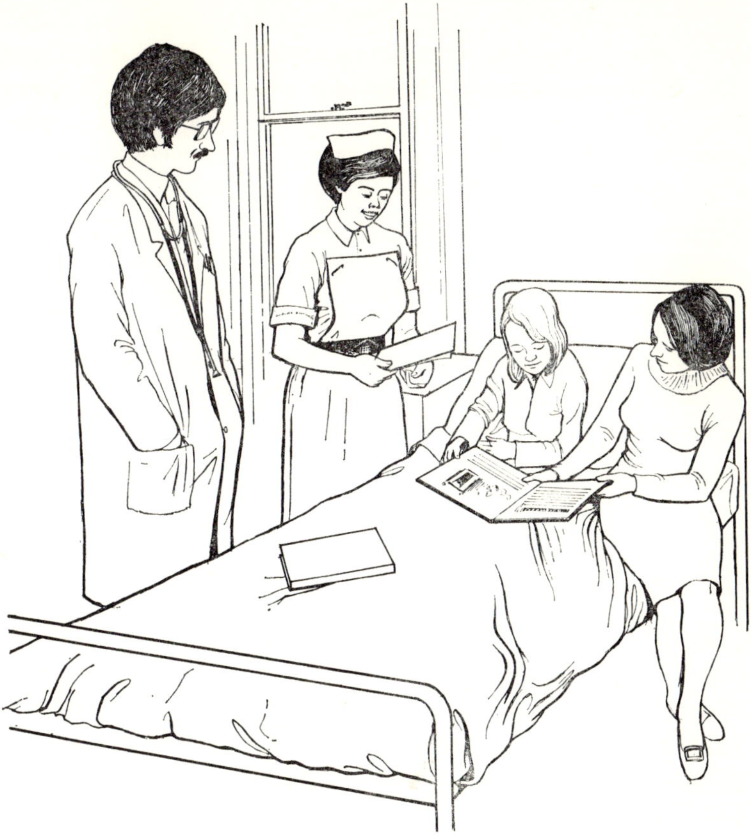

FIG **74. The parents should help to keep the child occupied.**

Postoperative complications

There are few fields of surgery where the patient's survival and good recovery depend so vitally on early diagnosis and prompt treatment of complications as they do in cardiac surgery. The cardiac nurse must be observant, alert for possible complications and knowledgeable about their treatment. She will then know when to send for medical aid, how to deal with emergencies and what to prepare for treatment by medical staff. She will also be sufficiently self-confident to sustain the patient and provide reassurance throughout difficult situations.

Bleeding

After closed heart surgery (without cardiopulmonary bypass) this is not usually a problem, only adequate blood replacement being needed. After open heart operations blood loss may be considerable, particularly after operations to correct cyanotic conditions.

Treatment. Adequate arterial and venous pressures are maintained by blood transfusion. The tubes are milked frequently to remove clot and avoid cardiac tamponade. The body temperature is not allowed to become subnormal; if it is then warm blankets are applied.

Drugs ordered may include intravenous administration of:

1. Calcium gluconate 10%.
2. Protamine sulphate 25 mg.
3. Hydrocortisone 100 mg.
4. Vitamin K 10 mg.
5. Σ-aminocaproic acid (Epsikapron) 6%, 100 ml over half an hour.

The latter is an antifibrinolytic drug, and any clot formed after its administration is very tough and may need surgical removal. An extra dose of protamine sulphate may be ordered if it is thought that the heparin given during operation has not been completely counteracted. Transfusion of fresh blood may be ordered, or extra platelets if the platelet count is low, or intravenous fibrinogen.

If excessive bleeding persists after a few hours, is uncontrollable or tamponade is developing, the chest may be reopened in theatre and clot evacuated. Often there is no obvious bleeding point.

Cardiac tamponade (Fig. 75)

This is not usually a problem after closed heart surgery through a left thoracotomy since drainage is allowed into the pleural space. After open heart surgery it may occur. If drainage is inadequate, i.e. the tubes are blocked by clot, blood collects in the pericardial or mediastinal space and compresses the heart. This leads to less blood entering the heart (and consequently a high venous pressure) and so less blood being pumped out by the heart, with consequently

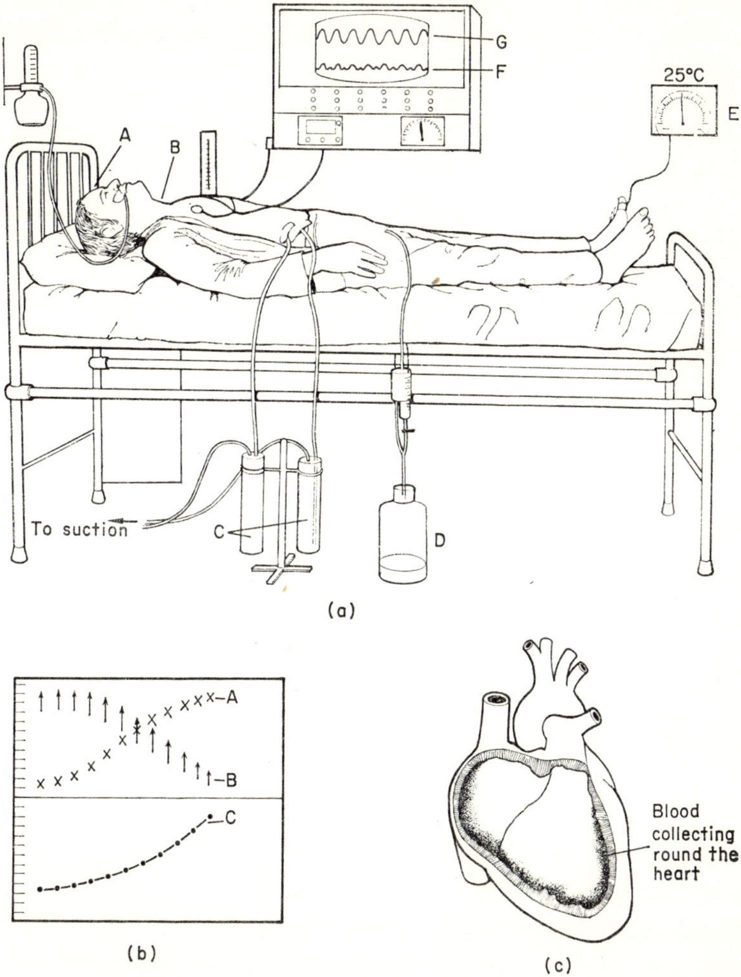

FIG **75. Cardiac tamponade.**
a, The patient's condition. A, Pale, sweating, anxious appearance. B, Neck veins distended, high venous pressure. C, Drainage diminished, profuse or clotting. D, Low urine output. E, Low peripheral temperature and peripheral cyanosis. F, Tachycardia. G, Low blood pressure and pulse pressure (arterial). *b*, The appearance of the chart. A, Venous pressure rising. B, Arterial pressure falling. C, Heart rate rising. *c*, The cause of the condition is blood collecting round the heart.

low blood arterial pressure. Rising heart rate and central venous pressure with falling blood pressure should always lead to suspicion of cardiac tamponade. The development of this condition and deterioration in the patient's general condition may take place rapidly, e.g. in half an hour, or slowly, e.g. over many hours.

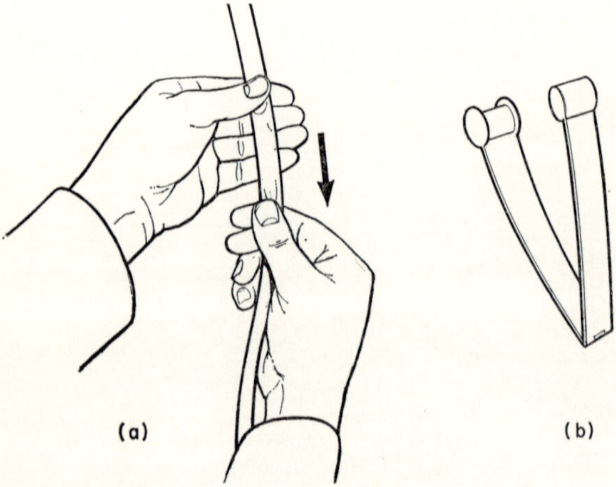

FIG **76. Milking the tube in cardiac tamponade.**
This can be done with the fingers and thumb (A) or with rollers (B). The tube is compressed as the hand is drawn down it, thus squeezing down any fluid or clot in the tube. The upper hand prevents pull on the tube where it enters the patient.

Treatment. The tubes are milked vigorously to remove all possible clots (Fig. 76). If this does not result in increased drainage, a rise in blood pressure and fall in venous pressure, then medical staff should be informed. They may wash through the tubes with warm sterile saline or evacuate the mediastinal clot surgically.

Retention of secretions and respiratory failure

Many cardiac patients have pulmonary hypertension and recurrent bronchitis before operation. Many have cardiomegaly (enlarged heart), which reduces the space available for the lungs. These patients are particularly liable to respiratory problems after operation when pain, comparative immobility and postoperative weakness tend to reduce respiratory excursions. Dehydration increases the viscosity of secretions and makes expectoration more difficult.

Tachypnoea (rapid respirations), pyrexia, cyanosis, dyspnoea or diminished chest movements may all be indications of this complication. Loose secretions may be heard as the patient breathes, or felt if a hand is placed on the chest wall, e.g. when moving the patient.

Treatment. Analgesics given should be sufficient to control the pain without depressing respiration or reducing the patient's ability to cooperate. Deep breathing as taught by the physiotherapist should be encouraged for 5 min every hour when the patient is awake.

Change of position on to alternate sides or sitting up increase respiration during movement and encourages expansion of each area of lung in turn. It is difficult to make a patient comfortable lying on an intercostal tube, and this is avoided unless there is a collapsed area in the opposite lung. Orthopnoeic patients must be supported in a good position, i.e. with the back straight to allow maximum expansion of the lungs. Inhalation of moisture-laden air or oxygen from a humidifer or ultrasonic nebulizer will loosen secretions and facilitate expectoration. Increased oral intake, if permitted, will assist this process. Manual support over the wound helps the patient to cough effectively. Increased use of a 'triggered' respirator may be necessary to assist deep breathing and provide good humidification.

Further treatment may include:

1. *Bronchoscopy* to remove plugs of mucus and secretions from a collapsed lobe and to allow re-expansion.

2. *Tracheostomy* to reduce dead space (the area through which air passes without benefit to respiratory function) and to facilitate removal of secretions. The aims of aspiration via tracheostomy are to remove secretions efficiently without introducing infection, damaging the mucous membrane unnecessarily or making the patient hypoxic. Intermittent manual inflations of the lungs with a Waters' bag may improve lung expansion.

3. *Artificial ventilation* to reduce respiratory acidosis and to improve oxygenation. Indications for this are shallow or laboured respirations, cyanosis (hypoxia), sweating, restlessness and possibly

coma (carbon dioxide retention) and abnormal blood gas estimation results, such as falling oxygen tensions and rising carbon dioxide tension.

Heart failure or low cardiac output syndrome

This may be of acute onset or develop more slowly. The venous pressure will be raised, the blood pressure low, peripheral circulation and urine output poor, the patient dyspnoeic, pale or cyanosed. Generalized oedema may appear. Pulmonary oedema may occur if the left side of the heart fails. In the immediate postoperative period it may be difficult to differentiate between tamponade and cardiac failure. Medical staff may order rapid transfusion of 100 ml blood. In tamponade the venous pressure will rise rapidly and the blood pressure fall. In heart failure the venous pressure will rise more slowly and the blood pressure will not fall unless the condition is critical.

Treatment. The patient's activities should be restricted; in acute failure he should rest as much as is compatible with necessary care. Oxygen, diuretics and digoxin may be ordered, or if they are already being administered, the dosage may be increased. Isoprenaline 2 mg in 500 ml dextrose administered intravenously at a prescribed number of drops/min may produce a marked improvement. If it is desired to reduce the amount of fluid given, then the strength of isoprenaline may be increased.

Acute cardiac failure may necessitate artificial ventilation:

1. To reduce metabolic acidosis when cardiac output is low, by removing the effort of respiration (effort requires extra oxygen consumption) and by providing a high oxygen tension.
2. To combat pulmonary oedema by constant positive pressure in the alveoli, thus counteracting the raised pressure in the pulmonary circulation which causes exudation of fluid into the alveoli.

Cardiac dysrhythmias

The onset of or increase in rate of atrial fibrillation is common after cardiac surgery. After open heart surgery ventricular extrasystoles, tachycardia or even ventricular fibrillation may occur during the first few weeks, owing to the effects of operation on an abnormal myocardium. Hypoxia or hypokalaemia increase the risk of dysrhythmias. Recurrent dysrhythmias after long-term diuretics are sometimes thought to be due to decreased intracellular potassium. In this situation extra potassium may be given immediately or as an infusion, possibly with dextrose and insulin to cause it to enter the cells, e.g. potassium chloride 4–6 g in 1 litre dextrose plus 20 units soluble insulin given each 12 hours, or an immediate dose of potassium chloride 0·5–1g may be given intravenously by one of the medical staff. This may be followed by an injection of 20 units of insulin and 25–50 g of dextrose.

Treatment. This is the same as for dysrhythmias unconnected with surgery (see Chapters 4 and 6). If isoprenaline is used intravenously in the treatment of heart block or hypotension it is essential that it is given at the rate ordered, e.g. 9 drops/min of a solution of isoprenaline 1 mg in 1 litre dextrose 5%, and a careful watch is kept for developing dysrhythmias. It is wise to use a special administration set, giving for example 50 drops/ml so that the dose can be more accurately controlled. Better still a controlled infusion pump, which can be pre-set to a specified number of drops/min should be used (see Fig. 71).

Arterial embolus

Cerebral embolus. This is caused by air entering at operation, or by clot, and may cause unequal pupils, hemiplegia, semiconsciousness and restlessness or coma. The patient may be aphasic, incontinent, and respiration may become inadequate.

Stellate ganglion block (i.e. injection of 2% novocaine into the stellate ganglion through the neck) may be tried, to dilate cerebral vessels and allow the clot to pass into a smaller vessel where less damage will result. Intravenous mannitol 12·5% 100–200 ml or urea 40–80 g may be given to produce diuresis and prevent cerebral oedema.

The temperature should be kept near normal; cooling may be necessary if the patient becomes pyrexial. Artificial ventilation may be needed. Tracheostomy may be necessary for aspiration of secretions.

Good nursing and physiotherapy are vital. This comprises maintenance of airway, prevention of pressure sores or atelectasis by frequent change of position, prevention of deformities by passive exercises (Fig. 77) and good positioning of paralysed limbs, maintenance of adequate nutrition (usually intragastric tube) and care of excretory functions. If the patient is conscious but aphasic the nurse must seek to reduce her (the patient's) anxiety and frustration by reassurance and by patience and ingenuity in communication. Often patients can answer simple questions by a nod or other movement, or use a set of word indicators.

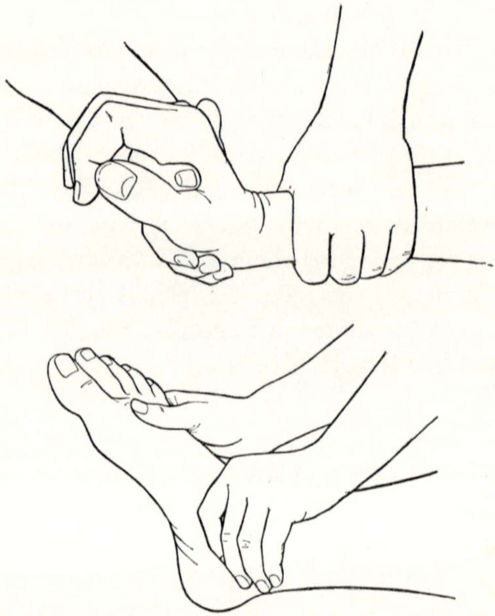

FIG **77. Passive exercises to prevent stiffness and deformity.** A, The lower extremity. B, The upper extremity.

Embolus to a limb. This will cause coldness, pallor, absence of pulses, pain or tingling distal to the embolus and possible loss of function. A saddle embolus lying over the bifurcation of the aorta will cause these signs in both legs.

Mesenteric embolus. This will give rise to acute abdominal symptoms, pain and distension. Surgical removal of limb or mesenteric embolus should be carried out as soon as possible, unless the area deficient in circulation is small and collateral circulation develops.

Renal failure

This may occasionally occur after open heart surgery, particularly if there has been a prolonged period of hypotension.

Urine output of less than 30 ml/hour in an adult leads to consideration of renal failure. Urine from a 24-hour collection is sent to the laboratory for microscopic examination, protein and sugar content, and electrolyte and urea. Urinary urea is normally more than 1100 mg/100 ml, though it is often less than this in the first 24 hours after cardiopulmonary bypass. If renal failure has occurred urinary urea concentration will be low and the blood urea and potassium increasingly raised.

Treatment. First it is necessary to make sure that the catheter is not kinked, blocked or displaced.

Treatment to correct obvious causes of oliguria, e.g. haemorrhage, hypotension, dehydration or hypoxia, will be ordered by the medical staff. 100 ml of 12·5% mannitol may be given intravenously. This will usually produce a diuresis of 40–60 ml within an hour even if the patient is dehydrated, unless there is renal failure. If renal failure is confirmed the fluid intake will be restricted, e.g. to 800 ml plus the output equivalent for the previous 24 hours, and calorie and electrolyte requirements carefully controlled. Peritoneal dialysis or haemodialysis may be required, though the latter holds considerable risks after cardiac surgery, because of the danger of haemorrhage.

Psychological disturbance

Any cardiac operation may precipitate this, but it is more common after the more serious heart operations. This kind of operation involves considerable psychological stress for the patient. Often months or years of illness and anxiety precede the operation, which may be viewed by the patient with fear as well as hope.

Postoperative care may necessitate strange surroundings and frequent disturbance for observations or treatment. Stress can be lessened by orientation to time and place by conversation, a view of the outside world in daylight or darkness, a clock and as much sleep as possible. Lights at night should be dimmed when possible and activities performed quietly. Good preoperative teaching, nurse–

patient rapport and short visits by husband, wife or immediate family help. However, nightmares, strange dreams or a feeling of unreality are not uncommon a few days after operation, and the patient can be reassured that these will pass. Occasionally severe psychological disturbance may occur. Warning signs are excessive anxiety which cannot be allayed by reassurance, confusion, inability to sleep and increasing restlessness. The patient may occasionally become violent.

Treatment. Prompt treatment with adequate sedation, e.g. promethazine (Sparine) 25 mg three times a day may prevent development of the condition beyond the early stages. The nurse must be alert for hypotension resulting from sedatives, hypoxia which will increase restlessness and cardiac dysrhythmias provoked by the patient's excessive activity.

Many patients recover quite quickly, but a few may take weeks or months.

Abdominal distension, gastric dilatation, paralytic ileus

Abdominal distension or persistent vomiting may occasionally occur and should be reported. Abdominal distension impedes cardiac and respiratory function.

Treatment. Gastric aspiration, restriction of oral fluids, administration of intravenous fluids and use of a flatus tube may be indicated. Careful electrolyte control is necessary. Cardiac surgical patients are liable to develop any of the common postoperative complications such as urinary retention, constipation, deep vein thrombosis or wound infection. Care is necessary to avoid these, and to observe and treat them should they occur.

Late complications

Three later complications may occur.

Post-valvotomy syndrome

This consists of pyrexia, visible neck pulsation, and a pericardial rub 2–6 weeks after operation. It is thought to be due to the resolution of the residual haemopericardium.

Soluble aspirin, 0·6 g given three times daily is usually effective, and steroids even more so, though these should be reserved for those patients not responding to aspirin.

Valve incompetence

The cardiac tissue to which a new valve is sewn is often poor and occasionally sutures may cut through so that blood leaks back round it. The signs and symptoms are those of incompetence and heart failure, sometimes severe.

Infection of a replaced valve

This is a rare but serious complication which often does not become evident until some months after the operation. The patient becomes very ill, showing all the signs of bacterial endocarditis and heart failure.

Treatment consists of controlling the cardiac failure as far as possible, eliminating the infection using appropriate drugs and replacing the valve with another one. Broad-spectrum antibiotics may be effective unless the infection is monilial, in which case amphotericin 0·25–1 mg/kg body weight may be ordered to be given intravenously over 6 hours daily. Amphotericin may cause renal failure.

The hazards of the condition, of repeat valve replacement and of possible toxic drugs are considerable.

Most postoperative open heart patients have numerous possible routes of entry for bacteria, e.g. arterial and venous lines, wounds, drainage tubes, urethral catheter and possibly endotracheal tube. All staff concerned in their care should be aware of the gravity of infection of these patients, and the importance of preventing it.

8 Vascular conditions

The arteries

The arterial walls consist of an outer layer of fibrous tissue known as the tunica adventita, an inner lining of endothelial tissue known as the tunica intima and, between these, the tunica media, containing elastic and muscle fibres (Fig. 78). The tunica media of the large arteries contains a higher proportion of elastic than of muscular tissue, enabling them to recoil when distended by the

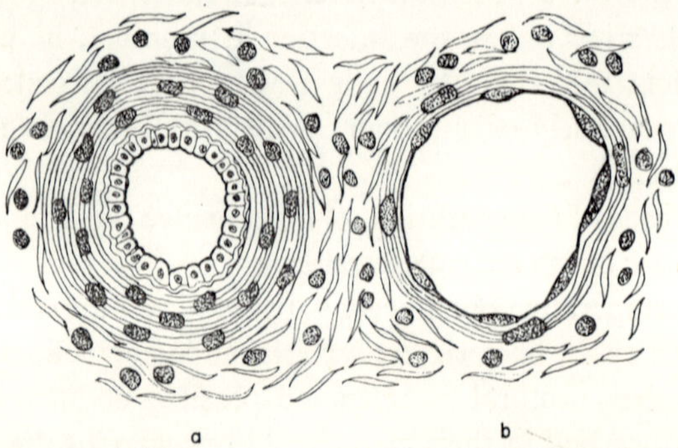

FIG 78. The structure of the artery and its companion vein.

blood ejected from the heart at systole. That of the arterioles is composed mainly of plain muscle fibres arranged in ring (circular) formation. The arrangement of the muscle fibres in rings means that when they contract the vessel narrows (vasoconstriction) and when they relax the vessel widens (vasodilatation).

Vasoconstriction in a localized area reduces the flow of blood to the part and may lead to ischaemia. Generalized vasoconstriction results in a raised peripheral resistance and a rise in blood pressure. Conversely, vasodilatation to a local area results in a better blood supply to that area, and generalized vasodilatation in a fall in blood pressure. Vasoconstriction is brought about by the sympathetic nerves, the terminal neurone of which releases noradrenaline and adrenaline, the chemicals actually stimulating the muscle fibres. Adrenaline and noradrenaline from the adrenal glands and angiotensin (formed when renin from the kidney acts upon plasma proteins) also bring about vasoconstriction.

The nerves

The vasomotor centre in the medulla oblongata controls the state of constriction of the arterioles. The centre itself is influenced by the higher centres of the brain as well as by impulses from the baroreceptors of the carotid sinus and aortic arch. Between the vasomotor centre and the muscle of the arterioles are three neurones. The uppermost originates in the centre, and passes down the spinal cord. It forms a synapse with a nerve emerging from the spinal cord alongside a spinal nerve in the thoracic lumbar regions. This nerve, called a preganglionic fibre, enters the sympathetic chain of ganglia lying alongside the vertebral column. It forms a synapse with a postganglionic fibre which passes to the muscle supplied.

Parasympathetic nerves also emerge from the spinal cord, passing out to ganglia which commonly lie in or on the organ supplied, where they also form a postganglionic fibre before actually reaching that organ.

Impulses of both sympathetic and parasympathetic nerves pass down fibres in the spinal cord, through a synapse, and along the preganglionic fibre to the appropriate ganglion (Fig. 79). Transmission of the impulse from the pre- to the postganglionic fibre across the synapse in the ganglion is achieved by the release of the chemical acetylcholine, which crosses the ganglion and stimulates the postganglionic fibre.

The impulse passes along the postganglionic fibre to the organ or muscle stimulated. At this point there is a difference, in that the parasympathetic fibre releases acetylcholine which stimulates the organ into activity, whereas the sympathetic fibre releases noradrenaline (Fig. 80) and some adrenaline. Nerves releasing

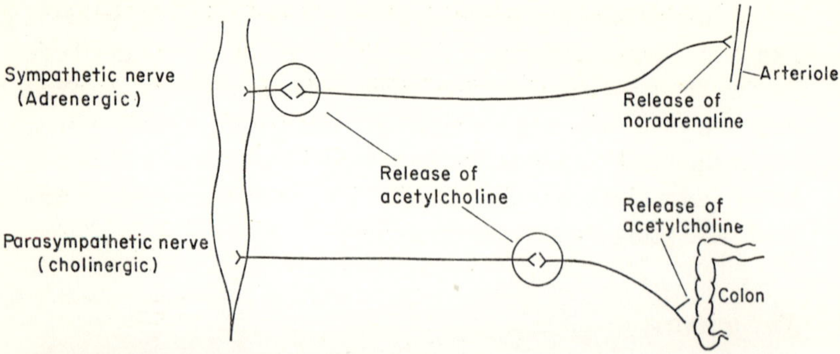

FIG 79. The site of the ganglion in relation to the organ supplied by sympathetic and parasympathetic nerve fibres, and the chemical transmitters released at the site of the ganglion and at the organ stimulated.

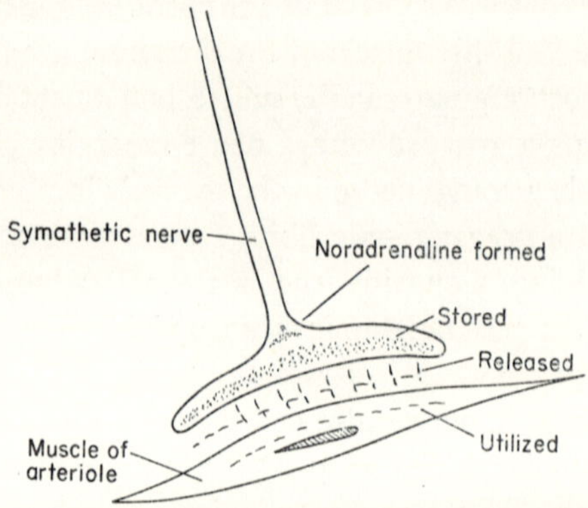

FIG 80. Formation, storage, release and utilization of noradrenaline at the junction of the sympathetic nerve and the muscle of the arteriole.

acetylcholine are called cholinergic, while those releasing noradrenaline and adrenaline are called adrenergic.

The formation of noradrenaline in the sympathetic and postganglionic nerve fibre is a complex process involving enzymes; the immediate precursor of noradrenaline is dopamine. Noradrenaline is stored in the nerve until required, some of it being converted into adrenaline. On stimulation of the nerve both substances are released, the amount of noradrenaline being greater than that of adrenaline. Together they are sometimes referred to as adrenaline-like compounds.

The response of plain muscle fibres to stimulation by noradrenaline or adrenaline may result in contraction, or it may result in relaxation of the muscle, depending upon the type of receptor found in the muscle cell. These are of two main types, the alpha-(α-)receptors which cause contraction, and the beta-(β-)receptors which cause relaxation of plain muscle. The plain muscle of the arterioles supplying the skin and intestines contains α-receptors, that of the arterioles supplying skeletal muscle contains both α- and β-receptors, while that of the bronchioles contains β-receptors only. Noradrenaline tends to affect mainly α-receptors and will cause constriction of all arterioles with an immediate rise in blood pressure. Adrenaline affects both α- and β-receptors, so that its release will cause constriction of most arterioles (α-receptors), but also relaxation and dilatation of those supplying skeletal muscles (β-receptors); the subsequent rise in blood pressure is less marked and less rapid in onset than that following noradrenaline release. Adrenaline causes relaxation and dilatation of the bronchioles (β-receptors), whereas noradrenaline does not.

The adrenaline-like compounds released are slowly destroyed by monoamine oxidase, so that supplies at the synapse must be replenished by further release. Ephedrine, by inhibiting the action of monoamine oxidase, potentiates the action of adrenaline and noradrenaline.

Although the majority of noradrenaline released is destroyed, some appears to be stored in the tissues affected, this store being depleted by reserpine.

Unlike the plain muscle of the arterioles, the muscle of the myocardium is a special form of striated involuntary muscle. It contains β-receptors which, when stimulated, result in increased rate and force of heart contraction. These receptors can be stimulated by adrenaline, and to a lesser extent by noradrenaline. However, the coronary arteries and arterioles contain β-receptors which, when stimulated, result in relaxation and consequent vasodilatation.

Arteriosclerosis and atherosclerosis

Almost from birth the arteries (and arterioles) begin to deteriorate or degenerate, at a rate which is imperceptible at first, but obviously increases rapidly after middle age. Occasionally it does happen that some elderly people have good arteries, while early degeneration takes place in some young people.

There are two main degenerative conditions of the arteries (and arterioles) themselves, arteriosclerosis and atherosclerosis.

In *arteriosclerosis* calcification of the tunica media takes place, making the arteries hard and less elastic. Usually the radial artery

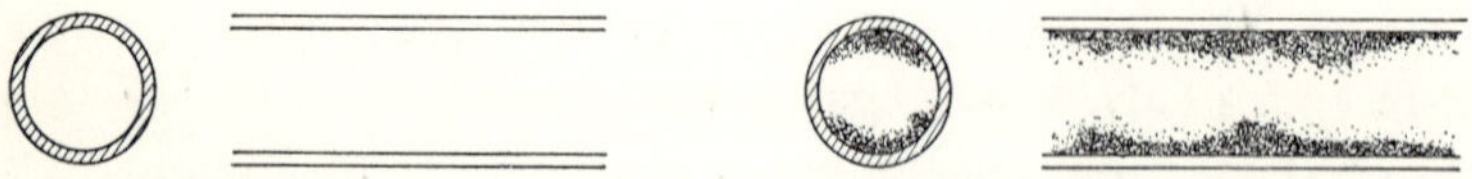

FIG 81. Narrowing of the lumen and roughening of the tunica intima of an artery by the formation of atheroma in its walls.

at the wrist feels elastic and compressible, but in arteriosclerosis it feels more like a hard tube. The vessel tends to get smaller and it cannot dilate when the need arises, thus the amount of blood to the part is diminished and ischaemia occurs.

In *atherosclerosis* the endothelial lining of the artery is replaced by patches of fatty material known as atheroma, which gradually invade the tunica media and replace the elastic muscle tissue. In addition lime salts tend to be deposited in the fatty patches. Thus as the patch increases in size the lumen of the arteries is narrowed, diminishing the amount of blood which can flow along them. Moreover, the atheroma is rough and there is a tendency for blood to clot and further obstruct the blood flow (Fig. 81).

The exact cause of these conditions is not fully known. There is a tendency for them to occur in members of the same family, and also in people with diabetes mellitus. They also seem to be associated with smoking, with overeating and obesity and with lack of exercise. It is sometimes thought that a prolonged diet containing large amounts of animal fat and cholesterol (eggs, liver, cream, butter) may contribute to its onset. The usual amount of cholesterol in the blood is 100–300 mg/100 ml of blood. People who have an abnormally high cholesterol content are prone to atherosclerosis.

As the lumen of the arteries affected by arteriosclerosis and atherosclerosis is narrowed, the parts supplied by those arteries receive a diminished blood supply, and as the ability to dilate and constrict is lost, the extra blood required in exercise cannot be supplied. Ischaemia of the heart results in angina pectoris and of the legs in intermittent claudication. The rigidity and narrowing of the arteries increases the peripheral resistance and the blood pressure is raised. The arteries become brittle and are likely to rupture if the blood pressure becomes excessively high.

There is no cure for these conditions. Patients suffering from them should take care of their skin and avoid injury. They are advised to avoid anything which may tend to vasconstriction, such as exposure to cold and smoking cigarettes. Moderate exercise is recommended. Diabetes mellitus should be treated. If overweight, the patient is advised to reduce weight. A diet low in animal fat and cholesterol may be ordered, and attempts to lower any high cholesterol content of the blood include foods containing corn oil, and the administration of a drug known as clofibrate. The doctor may order vasodilator drugs such as tolazoline in doses of 25 mg three times daily. Alcohol in small amounts might also be of value.

Thrombo-angiitis obliterans, sometimes known as Buerger's disease, is a recurring inflammation of the arteries. Those of the lower limb are usually affected, but the condition does occur in the upper limb and other parts. The walls of the artery are inflamed and become thickened, gradually occluding the lumen so that less blood flows through. Clots may form and even further obstruct the flow of blood. Often there is involvement of the nearby veins and nerves, so that in addition to signs and symptoms of ischaemia such as intermittent claudication, there may also be a severe burning pain in the affected limb. The condition progresses slowly, although there may be a remission from symptoms. Coronary and cerebral thromboses are likely to occur, as is ulceration and gangrene of the toes. The cause of this condition is not definitely known, but it is sometimes attributed to tobacco smoking. Usually men between the ages of 25 and 45 years are affected.

There is no specific treatment; the patient must stop smoking. The doctor may order vasodilator drugs, and sympathectomy is performed on some patients. Care of the skin is important; tight clothes, garters and suspenders are avoided as these tend to obstruct the easy flow of blood. Injury of the area must be avoided; special attention must be paid when cutting the nails and, indeed, the services of a chiropodist are advisable. Amputation is necessary when gangrene occurs. As much exercise as possible should be taken. Sometimes special Buerger–Allen exercises may be prescribed, which are intended to ensure flushing of all blood vessels and improvement of the collateral circulation. Basically, they are performed with the patient lying flat, the leg raised in the air until the foot becomes pale. It is then lowered below the level of the bed until the foot appears red. Both these actions take about 2 min each. The patient then rests with the legs and feet in a horizontal position.

Raynaud's phenomenon usually occurs in young women. There is abnormal stimulation of the vasoconstrictor nerves brought on by exposure to cold and by emotional upset. There is spasm of the digital arteries so that the circulation may become sluggish, when the hands become cyanosed, and the arteries may become empty of blood, in which case the fingers and even the hands too become white and look 'dead'. There is numbness and tingling rather than actual pain. As the spasm passes off and the blood flow returns to normal, there may be a reactive vasodilatation causing the skin to become red. Attacks may be slight, but in some patients ischaemia causes changes in the skin resulting in ulceration and gangrene of the fingertips or tips of the toes. These are most likely to occur in winter.

The patient is encouraged to keep warm and avoid the cold. She should wear adequate clothing over the whole body, but especially gloves and socks for the hands and feet. She should avoid standing about in cold weather; moderate exercise such as walking is helpful. She should give up smoking, and avoid situations which may precipitate emotional upset. Vasodilator drugs may be ordered in an attempt to prevent attacks, and in severe cases sympathectomy may be performed.

Hypertension

A common cause of disability and death among adults is hypertension (high blood pressure) producing, as it does, uncomfortable symptoms and often resulting in congestive cardiac failure and cardiovascular accidents.

The blood pressure

Fluid exerts pressure against the walls of the container in which it is standing, as can be seen when a hole is made in a tin containing water—the water passes out in a steady stream.

Blood pressure can be defined as the pressure exerted by the blood against the walls of the vessels (arteries, capillaries, veins) containing it. Blood is moving along the vessels, being pushed from behind by the heart's pumping action, so that the pressure is higher than if it were merely standing. Variations occur in the blood pressure, but under normal circumstances it is kept within fairly steady limits. The pressure of the blood in the capillaries and veins is fairly constant, but in the arteries there is momentary fluctuation when the heart contracts (systole) giving the blood a push and thus raising the pressure. When the heart relaxes (diastole), the pressure of the blood returns to its previous level. An adequate blood pressure is essential to make sure that the supply of blood reaches all parts of the body, uphill against gravity to the brain, for the formation of the tissue fluid and for the glomerular filtration upon which kidney function depends.

The blood pressure is maintained by the interaction of three sets of factors, the blood itself, the heart and the blood vessels. There is a considerable degree of compensation, so that a diminution in the part played by one brings about an increase in that of the other two.

Control of the blood pressure seems to originate in the baroreceptors situated in the carotid sinus, the walls of the arch of the aorta and the subclavian artery. These are sensitive to the blood pressure and send information to the cardiac and vasomotor centres of the medulla oblongata, which in turn send impulses to the heart and the muscles in the walls of the blood vessels.

The amount of blood in the circulation is one factor determining the blood pressure, sudden loss of a large quantity of blood resulting in a fall in blood pressure. In an attempt to compensate for this, the heart beats more quickly and the arterioles constrict. The viscosity of the blood caused by the cells and the plasma proteins entails a high pressure to push the blood along. It will be realized that a dilution with saline will allow the blood to flow more easily, resulting in a lowering of the pressure which would be needed to push on normal blood.

The heart is the prime mover behind the blood. It affects the blood pressure in two ways, first by the amount put out by the ventricles when they contract (stroke volume), and secondly by the frequency with which they contract (rate). When resting, the average young adult's heart puts out some 70 ml of blood each time it contracts. If the heart contracts 70 times in a minute, it will be seen that the volume of blood put out by the heart in that minute will be nearly 5 litres (4900 ml). This is referred to as the cardiac output. When necessary, the heart may beat more frequently and the ventricles may contract more firmly putting out more blood with each contraction. The ability of the heart to do this is of importance in exercise and exertion.

The blood vessels commence as one large artery leaving the heart, but soon branch into smaller arteries, then into arterioles and finally into the minute capillaries. Each division presents a junction which tends to form an obstacle in the path of the blood flow. In addition, the vessels are smaller, so that pressure is required to propel the blood by the obstacle and down the narrower tubes. This is referred to as the peripheral resistance, and the blood must be under sufficient pressure to overcome this. Another factor is that the walls of the vessels themselves are pressing on the blood—the walls of the large arteries being mainly elastic, so that after distension by the sudden input of blood following systole, they recoil and press on the blood. The walls of the arterioles contain mainly muscle fibres influenced by nerves from the vasomotor centre, and may relax, causing vasodilatation and lowering of the pressure on the blood, or contract, causing vasoconstriction which will press on the blood as well as narrow the arteriole and raise the peripheral resistance.

Measurement of the blood pressure is usually that of the larger arteries, although pressure in the veins (venous pressure) can be estimated. The arterial blood pressure is usually measured in the brachial artery using a sphygmomanometer, and the figure given indicates the number of millimetres of a column of mercury which are required to press on that artery from the outside and stop the blood flowing along it. Both systolic and diastolic pressure are measured; a typical blood pressure recording might be 120/80 mm Hg.

During childhood the systolic pressure gradually increases, ranging from 75–90 mm Hg in infancy to 90–100 mm Hg in childhood and 100–120 mm Hg during puberty. The systolic pressure remains around 120 mm Hg for several years, tending to rise gradually from the age of 25 years onwards by about 0·5 mm Hg each year, so that by the age of 50–60 the normal systolic pressure might be in the region of 135–140 mm Hg.

Women usually have slightly lower blood pressure than men.

As already indicated, the pressure remains fairly constant, but is subject to minor variation, a rise being noticeable on exercise and on changing from a lying position to a standing position. There is also a rise as a result of emotions such as fear, excitement and worry and also a small rise after meals. During rest, and especially during peaceful sleep, the systolic pressure falls to its lowest level.

The diastolic pressure is a measure of the peripheral resistance, and in particular shows the extent to which the arterioles are in a state of vasoconstriction.

The difference in the reading of the systolic and diastolic pressure is referred to as the pulse pressure.

Authorities differ as to when the blood pressure is to be regarded as unusually high. Some believe that a reading of 150/90 mm Hg should be the point at which the condition should be suspected, but others regard a diastolic pressure of 100 mm Hg or even 110 mm Hg as the figure to consider.

Causes of high blood pressure

In the majority of patients with a high blood pressure the cause of it is not really known, but in others it can be traced to some other primary condition. Secondary hypertension occurs when there are tumours of the adrenal gland, such as phaeochromocytoma, in which there is a sustained release of too much adrenaline or noradrenaline resulting in a continued rise in blood pressure. A high blood pressure is also found in Cushing's syndrome, in coarctation of the aorta and in toxaemia of pregnancy. A reduction in the supply of blood or damage to the kidney causes the release of a chemical called renin which combines with the plasma proteins to produce angiotensin, which in turn stimulates constriction of the arterioles with subsequent rise in blood pressure.

Essential hypertension is the term used when the direct cause cannot be identified. Usually, in maintaining the blood pressure within normal limits, the body's controlling mechanism brings about constriction (or dilatation) of the arterioles. In hypertension it has been suggested that the limits are set at too high a level, with the resultant increase in vasoconstriction. For some time the blood vessels and the heart can accommodate the extra pressure, but eventually are affected adversely by it. There may be a tendency for arteriospasm, arteriosclerosis or rupture on the part of the blood vessels, and of eventual failure on the part of the heart.

Apart from the ageing process, there seems to be a hereditary tendency to develop hypertension. Obesity and emotional tension are also factors which contribute to its occurrence.

Symptoms

Of itself a high blood pressure produces few symptoms, the condition usually being discovered at medical examination. However, as other structures are affected by the continued high pressure, symptoms of interference with the function of that structure begin to appear. Headache, dizziness and tinnitus, especially after bending, together with nose bleeding, are some of the early discomforts about which the patient may complain. He may also complain of palpitations as the heart becomes more affected. Arteriosclerosis of the coronary arteries may give rise to angina and even thrombosis, while the onset of left ventricular failure may produce breathlessness and oedema. The kidney itself may be affected, leading to kidney failure; this becomes a vicious circle because the ischaemic kidney itself brings about a rise of blood pressure. The eyes may be affected, spots before the eyes being one symptom, while the use of the ophthalmoscope will reveal retinal oedema and haemorrhages. As the brain is affected there may be more severe headaches, with emotional irritability and perhaps mental changes. Strokes may occur as a result of cerebral haemorrhage or thrombosis. In severe attacks hypertensive encephalopathy may occur, with vomiting, convulsions, paralysis and even coma.

The cause of this condition is variable. In benign essential hypertension it may go on for 20 years. However, there is a form known as malignant essential hypertension, usually seen in younger men, which may prove fatal in 2 or 3 years or even less.

Treatment

In mild hypertension, little treatment may be required. The patient is encouraged to adjust his life according to his condition, in view of the possible end results if it progresses or is aggravated. He is advised to avoid anything which may cause even a temporary rise in blood pressure. He is advised to take things easy and not to rush about. He should avoid anything which will cause anxiety or overexcitement. While he may take exercise with moderation, he should have plenty of rest, relaxation and sleep. To assist in this the doctor may order tranquillizing drugs or sedatives to assist in learning to manage a 'quiet life'. If there is any tendency to overweight, he will be advised to correct this with the appropriate diet. Some patients may be advised to avoid large amounts of salt (sodium chloride) with food.

Later, the doctor will order hypotensive drugs to control the hypertension and prevent any harm it may cause. He will assess the patient's condition before prescribing, and then keep him under surveillance to note the effects of the drugs. This stabilizing process may be carried out at home, but sometimes the patient may be admitted to hospital.

The drugs in common use at present include guanethidine, and its derivatives bethanidine, methlydopa and propranolol, which are described in Chapter 11. These drugs are given with the intention of lowering the blood pressure, so one effect may be to produce a hypotension (blood pressure lower than normal) which may be particularly noticeable when the patient rises from a lying to a standing position; he may feel dizzy or actually faint. Side-effects include dry mouth, constipation or diarrhoea, abdominal distension and fluid retention. Some actually cause depression. The nurse should know the possible effects and side-effects of any hypotensive drug she is giving, and should note the patient's reaction toward it, reporting any untoward signs or symptoms to the doctor.

Venous thrombosis

Venous thrombosis or clotting of the blood in a vein may occur:

1. When there is injury or inflammation of the wall of the vein.
2. When there is increased coagulability of the blood as in dehydration and in an increased number of platelets after operation.
3. When there is slowing or obstruction of the blood flow through the vein.

Thrombophlebitis means inflammation of the vein accompanied by formation of a clot. *Phlebothrombosis* means the formation of a clot in a vein in which there is little or no inflammation.

Thrombophlebitis is more commonly found in superficial veins, for example, in varicose veins of the legs or after intravenous infusion in the arm. There is local pain and tenderness. The vein looks a mottled colour; it feels swollen and often hard. Malaise and a slight rise in temperature may also be present. The clot is usually attached to the wall, so there is little risk of embolism occurring.

When this condition occurs in varicose veins of the leg, a pad of felt or sorbo rubber is placed over the affected vein. This is covered and supported by a crêpe bandage or elastic strapping extending from the toes to beyond the level of the thrombosed vein. Should pain be present, analgesics may be ordered; for this phenylbutazone is sometimes prescribed as it not only relieves the pain but also has an anti-inflammatory action. Anticoagulants are not usually ordered. Resolution of the thrombus may take up to three weeks.

Phlebothrombosis, sometimes referred to as deep vein thrombosis, usually occurs in the deep veins of the legs. Blood flowing freely through smooth-walled veins does not clot so long as the balance between clotting factors and fibrinolytic (clot dissolving) factor is normal. Three main factors contribute to deep vein thrombosis:

1. *Venous stasis*, such as occurs in the calf and thigh veins when the muscles are inactive or when there is pressure on the calf or behind the knee which slows circulation. This stasis is increased if the veins are varicose and the valves ineffective.

2. *Damage to the vein walls* may also result from prolonged pressure, or prolonged acute flexion at a joint, e.g. behind the knee.

3. Increased *coagulability* of the blood. It is known, for example, that after an operation or accident, the platelet count, plasma fibrinogen and stickiness all increase, and reach their maximum on the seventh to tenth day. Other patients at risk include the elderly, the obese, pregnant or post-partum women, the diabetic and those with myocardial infarction or cardiac failure.

Pelvic operations may result in local clotting in the pelvic veins. Preventive measures, such as leg exercises and early ambulation, prevention of pressure on veins and raising the foot of the bed to increase venous return, may be of value. One measure which is thought to be valuable in preventing the occurrence of deep vein thrombosis is the administration of 500 ml of low molecular weight dextran intravenously over 8 hours in each 24. This is used for patients particularly at risk, e.g. for 3 days after operation. It makes the red blood cells less likely to stick together and form rouleaux, which may be the base for further clot formation.

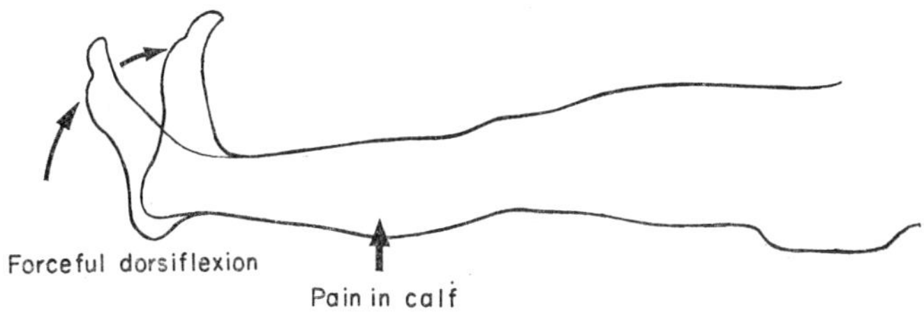

FIG 82. **Homans' sign may indicate deep thrombosis in the calf of the leg.**

Despite all these preventive measures, venous thrombosis may occur. There may be no apparent signs or symptoms. Indications may be swelling and oedema of the affected limb, and pain in the calf muscles, especially when the foot is forcibly dorsiflexed (Homans' sign; Fig. 82). There may be mild pyrexia and tenderness when the calves are gently pressed. The presence of thrombosis can be confirmed by venograms, i.e. X-rays taken after the injection of a radio-opaque fluid into the veins of the leg. Filling defects in the demonstrated venous system may indicate the site of thrombosis.

The clot is not attached to the wall of the vein; part of it may be detached and, passing through the right side of the heart to the lungs, cause pulmonary embolism.

The patient with deep venous thrombosis is required to rest in bed. The foot of the bed is elevated. Firm elastic stockings or bandages may be applied to the legs, ensuring that there are no twists, turns or creases which may result in uneven support.

Some doctors feel it advisable to discourage any activity on the part of the patient, but instruct the nurse or physiotherapist to carry out passive movements for him. Others, however, advise active exercises after application of the support, feeling that with the circulation of the blood promoted there is less likelihood of the thrombosis extending. The patient is allowed up when the pain and swelling have subsided and the temperature returned to normal, usually after a week to 10 days.

Anticoagulant therapy may be started with heparin intravenously followed by phenindione or warfarin orally. This does not dissolve the clot but prevents the formation of fresh clot which is more likely to break off and embolize.

If a small embolus has occurred, or there is a danger of major pulmonary embolism because of the extent of thrombosis, attempts are sometimes made to prevent this by surgical intervention. The inferior vena cava may be tied off, or sutures strung across it to form a network and catch any large emboli. However this may result in oedema of the leg and embolization via collateral vessels. A more satisfactory operation is embolectomy, i.e. direct removal of clot from the femoral or other veins as described for arterial embolectomy. Pulmonary embolectomy may be performed to remove a large embolus, but since the patient is very ill the mortality rate is high (though rather better results are obtained if cardiopulmonary bypass technique is used).

The advent of streptokinase, a clot-dissolving enzyme, offers new possibilities in treatment. Many doctors now prefer to use this type of drug as an intravenous infusion or, for greater effect, directly into the affected vessels. To reach the pulmonary artery it is necessary to use cardiac catheterization techniques. Although not without risk even in skilled hands, this is a much less drastic procedure for an ill patient than embolectomy.

The responsibilities of the nurse with regard to venous thrombosis are:

1. To try to prevent it.
2. To report any sign that it has occurred.
3. To report immediately any signs of pulmonary embolism, to give emotional support to the patient and to give oxygen and take emergency measures to deal with acute circulatory failure as necessary.
4. To give accurately and to time any drugs ordered.
5. To watch for, report, and if necessary, control any adverse effects of treatment, e.g. bleeding. This may appear as external bleeding from wounds, haematuria or melaena, concealed internal bleeding, or even cardiac tamponade if the chest has been opened. The antidotes to drugs in use must always be readily available.

Pulmonary embolism

This can be a serious and possibly fatal complication of any serious illness, accident or operation which causes a patient to be confined to bed. More rarely it may occur in people who have remained ambulant.

Pulmonary embolism probably occurs more often than is realized, because if the embolus is small it may cause no symptoms.

The typical picture of a major pulmonary embolism is that the patient becomes restless and anxious and may ask for a bedpan. He rapidly develops dyspnoea, pain in the chest, tachycardia, pallor or cyanosis and possibly circulatory collapse and cardiac arrest. It most commonly occurs about 10 days after operation, just as the patient is performing some activity such as getting out of bed or physiotherapy. If the patient survives then infarction of a portion of lung will cause changes in chest X-ray appearances, and possibly cough and haemoptysis. Signs of the strain on the right ventricle caused by the pulmonary artery obstruction can sometimes be seen on the electrocardiogram. The site of the embolus may be demonstrated by pulmonary arteriograms. Xenon scans may be performed but are less reliable. A radio-active fluid containing xenon is injected intravenously, and the chest area scanned by a machine which can detect the presence of xenon. The scan or picture produced shows blank areas to which the blood stream failed to carry the xenon.

Major pulmonary embolism is a terrifying event for the patient. By keeping him as calm, confident and comfortable as possible, as well as being efficient in treatment, the nurse can not only reduce his distress, but also reduce his oxygen requirements. In view of the limited supply of oxygen available to the tissues (because the blood flow through the lungs is limited) this may improve the chance of survival. Treatment by anticoagulant and fibrinolytic means has already been described.

Arterial surgery

In many countries an increasing number of people can expect to live to old age. In the older age groups arterial disease is common, and atherosclerosis is becoming commoner in the 35–50 age group. With improved operative, anaesthetic, and resuscitative techniques now available a number of these people can be saved from premature death or disablement.

The commonest acquired arterial conditions suitable for operation are:

1. *Arterial obstruction* (Fig. 83). This may occur suddenly by an embolus from the left atrium or heart valves or walls. It may develop gradually with narrowing of the arterial lumen, e.g. arteriosclerosis and atheromatous plaques. Clotting takes place on the roughened surfaces and completes the obstruction.

2. *Aneurysm* formation due to weakening of the elastic layer of the artery walls by atherosclerosis, infection such as syphilis, or occasionally trauma. An aneurysm is a dilated area of artery. It may be saccular or fusiform in shape.

3. *Trauma*. This may be an opened wound caused by a penetrating injury, or an artery may be ruptured by a crush injury or fracture of a long bone.

Arterial obstruction

Signs and symptoms depend on the site of the occlusion and whether it takes place suddenly or progressively. Sudden occlusion of an artery will cause coldness, pallor, pain, paraesthesia and loss of pulses distal to the occlusion. Gangrene will result unless the embolus is removed. Nerve damage may result from prolonged ischaemia even if circulation is restored in time to prevent the death

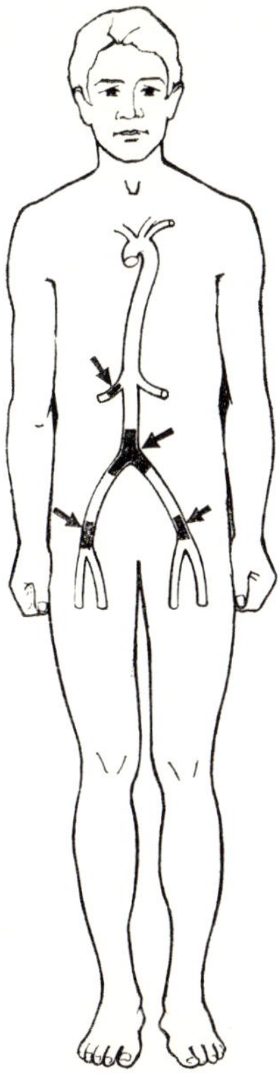

FIG **83. Common sites of aneurysm or obstruction.**
Obstruction tends to occur at or near an arterial bifurication or branching.

of other tissues. For example, a temporary or permanent paraplegia may be caused by a saddle embolus (across the bifurcation of the aorta into the iliac arteries) in situ for more than 12 hours, even though the legs are saved by embolectomy.

Progressive arterial obstruction is commonest in the lower limbs. It causes coolness and discoloration below the obstruction, diminution or lessening of pulses and pain which may at first occur only during exercise when tissue demands for blood are increased. This pain is called intermittent claudication. As circulatory obstruction increases pain will occur even at rest, and the extremity will become gangrenous unless an adequate collateral circulation develops (through other vessels).

Blocked lower femoral or popliteal vessels cause pain in the calf muscles. With obstruction of circulation at the aortic bifurcation and in the femoral arteries, pain will be felt in the buttocks and femoral pulses will be absent (Leriche syndrome).

There are other less common sites of arterial occlusion. Hypertension and renal failure may result from blocked or narrowed

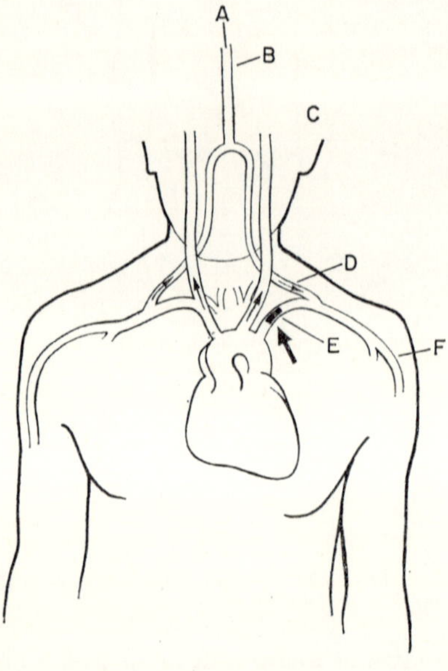

FIG **84. The 'subclavian steal' syndrome.**
A, Circle of Willis. B, Basilar artery. C, Internal carotid artery. D, Vertebral artery. E, Block in subclavian artery. F, Subclavian artery.

artery. If mesenteric or carotid arteries are affected, abdominal pain or cerebral symptoms respectively may be caused. A block in the subclavian artery between its junction with the aortic and vertebral artery causes the 'subclavian steal' syndrome (Fig. 84). When exercises of the arm increase demands on the circulation, extra blood cannot be drawn from the aorta. Blood is therefore 'stolen' from the cerebral circulation via the cerebral artery and the patient becomes dizzy or unconscious.

Aneurysm

This may be felt as a pulsatile swelling in the abdomen or leg, or seen on X-ray as a pulsating shadow in the region of the aorta. Cerebral aneurysms do occur, but these will not be discussed here as they are neurological. Dyspnoea or a hoarse voice may be due to compression of the trachea or recurrent laryngeal nerve, or of a bronchus by a thoracic aortic aneurysm. Pain may be a prominent symptom of a thoracic or abdominal aneurysm and it becomes more severe if the aneurysm leaks or erodes bone.

The dangers of an aneurysm are progressive enlargement and rupture, or thrombosis and embolism.

A dissecting aneurysm occurs when blood penetrates behind an atheromatous plaque, so that an increasing area of intima is dissected off the arterial wall. This forms a sac which blocks the arterial lumen causing pain, often severe, and inadequate circulation below the dissection. A thoracic dissecting aneurysm shows on X-ray as an increasingly wide mediastinal shadow and if branch vessels are involved other signs appear. For example, involvement of the left subclavian artery will cause a diminished or absent left radial pulse, and a difference in blood pressure.

Trauma

Arterial bleeding from an open wound will be obvious and will need immediate control by local pressure and elevation of the part if possible, followed by surgical repair.

A concealed arterial rupture will cause pain and swelling due to haematoma, and loss of circulation and pulses distal to the injury. For example, with a ruptured popliteal artery posterior tibial and dorsalis pedis pulses will be absent and there will be a tense, painful swelling behind the knee.

Preoperative assessment

Where there is injury, a leaking or dissecting aneurysm or a large embolus, the need for operation may be obvious and urgent, with a minimum of preoperative investigation. Other patients are mostly middle-aged or elderly, with generalized arteriosclerosis apart from the local lesion. Many are heavy smokers with chronic bronchitis. Careful investigation is necessary to assess the patient and reduce the risks at operation. The following investigations should be made:

1. The *medical history* taken will include the present condition and any other renal or cardiovascular disorders. The degree of pain must be assessed carefully in relation to the patient's work and social conditions. Incipient gangrene or pain at rest makes operation imperative, but otherwise it may be justifiable only if claudication occurs during normal daily activities and is not improved by taking vasodilator drugs and ceasing to smoke cigarettes (nicotine is a powerful vasoconstrictor). Frequency or difficulty in micturition should be noted since this may indicate prostatic enlargement. This may have caused inefficient excretion of urine and kidney damage, and may cause postoperative problems.

2. *Physical examination* includes general physical condition, cardiac abnormalities, respiratory state, presence or absence of pulses (radial, femoral, popliteal, posterior tibial and dorsalis pedis) and blood pressure. An electronic blood flow detector such as the Doptone may be used to detect the site of occlusion. The probe or microphone is smeared with a water-soluble jelly to ensure good contact and applied firmly along the course of the artery where it is sufficiently near the surface. The sound of blood flow is amplified, so that its absence can be detected. Since this can be done without disturbing the patient much, it can be a useful investigation where, for example, a femoral embolus is suspected postoperatively.

3. *Urine and sputum specimens* are sent to the laboratory for examination so that abnormalities can be detected and infection and antibiotic sensitivities of any organisms determined.

4. *Haemoglobin*, white cell count and blood group are ascertained.

5. *Serum electrolytes and urea* are estimated (operation risks are increased if the blood urea is raised).

6. An *electrocardiogram* is necessary to exclude recent coronary occlusion, ischaemia or cardiac dysrhythmias.

7. An *aortogram* to define the lesion, its extent and the state of the arteries distal and proximal to it is desirable.

8. A *chest X-ray* is performed.

9. An *intravenous pyelogram* is sometimes performed to estimate kidney function.

Preoperative care

Patients for elective operations will usually be in hospital for at least 48 hours preoperatively for investigations and preparation. Older patients who have been independent all their lives may find it difficult to adjust to hospital life. The nurse may need to be very patient in helping them to adapt to the strange surroundings, people and the physical indignities such as use of a bedpan or shaving of the pubic area.

Breathing exercises are taught by the physiotherapist, and the patient MUST be persuaded to STOP SMOKING.

Moderate activity is desirable to prevent venous thrombosis. Diet should be varied and nutritious and should include plenty of fluids, but fluid may have to be limited if there is any question of a cardiac failure.

Drugs ordered may include vasodilators such as tolazoline (Priscol) 25 mg three times daily or cyclandelate (Cyclopasmol) 25–50 mg four times a day. Digoxin may be ordered to improve cardiac function. Appropriate drugs will be ordered to combat any urinary or chest infection, and in any case a broad-spectrum antibiotic is usually given from 48 hours before operation. Avoidance of infection is vital to the success of arterial surgery.

Local preparation includes shaving a wide area of skin over and around the site of operation. The patient is bathed twice daily with antibacterial soap, e.g. chlorhexidine soap, paying special attention to the skin folds.

The operation consent form is signed by the patient. Blood is cross-matched 24–48 hours before operation. Ten units of blood should be available for aortic operations, less for others. If transfer to the intensive care ward is likely, this must be explained to the patient and relatives.

A good night's sleep must be ensured, if necessary, by sedation. On the day of operation the patient is given no food or fluid for at least 4 hours before the operation. He is bathed and dressed in clean linen; all removable prostheses and jewellery are removed.

The patient should pass urine just before the premedication is given.

Common arterial operations

1. *Simple suture* of a ruptured artery.

2. *Embolectomy*. This consists of incising the artery at the site of obstruction and removing the embolus. A Fogarty catheter (Fig. 85) may be passed into the artery, inflated and withdrawn to

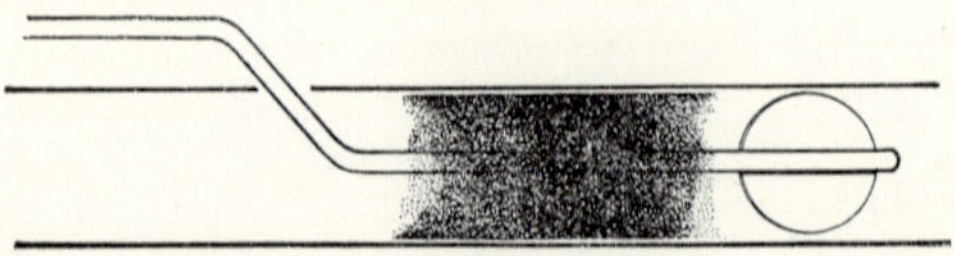

FIG 85. **The use of a Fogarty catheter to remove clot.**

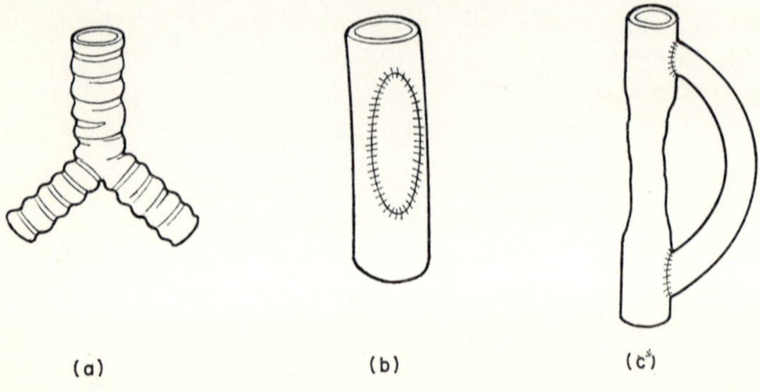

FIG 86. **Bypass or replacement graft.**
A, Dacron Y graft. B, Vein patch. C, Vein bypass graft.

remove remaining pieces of clot. A solution of heparin may be used to flush through the artery from one incision to another and so remove small pieces of clot.

3. *Endarterectomy or disobliteration.* The artery is incised, the plane of cleavage found and the atherosclerotic core removed, so that the arterial lumen is restored.

4. *Bypass or replacement graft* (Fig. 86). This is performed when the vessel is too narrow, fibrotic or calcified for endarterectomy, or in the thoracic aorta. Three kinds of graft may be done. (*a*) Crimped grafts of Dacron, a synthetic material, are usually con-

sidered most satisfactory for the aorta. Y-shaped grafts are used in the aortic bifurcation, and grafts with suitable side arms are fashioned when essential branches of the aorta are involved. The grafts are usually pre-clotted, i.e. a small amount of blood is allowed to soak the graft and clot, thus preventing leakage when full blood flow passes through it. (*b*) Vein grafts may be used below the inguinal ligament or in other peripheral arteries, where a reduced blood flow increases the risk of clot formation in a synthetic graft. The saphenous vein, for instance, may be removed, all branches tied off and the vein used to replace or bypass a length of femoral artery. It must be reversed so that the blood flows through the valves in the correct direction. A vein patch may be used to increase the lumen of an artery. (*c*) Homografts (human artery from a cadaver) are not often used now, partly because of the difficulty of obtaining and preparing them, but chiefly because aneurysms or calcified deposits tend to form in them after a few years.

5. *Operations on aneurysms* (Fig. 87) include the following. (*a*) A saccular aneurysm can sometimes be removed and the side

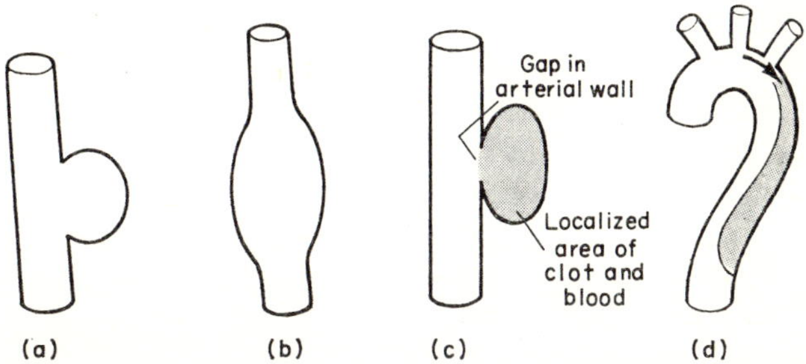

FIG **87. Types of aneurysm.**
A, Saccular aneurysm. B, Fusiform aneurysm. C, False aneurysm. D, Dissecting aneurysm.

hole in the artery repaired by suture. (*b*) A fusiform aneurysm is usually removed or obliterated and a replacement or bypass graft inserted. Occasionally, if removal of the aneurysm would be too hazardous or complicated the area may be bound round with synthetic material to reinforce it, or the aneurysm may be packed with wire. (*c*) A dissecting aneurysm is drained back into the lumen of the artery by incising the intima at the distal end of the sac. All free edges of intima are then firmly sutured to arterial wall. Cardiopulmonary bypass may be necessary during some operations on the thoracic aorta. A modified perfusion technique may be used to maintain kidney and spinal cord circulation during operations involving the lower thoracic aorta.

Postoperative care

All operations on the thoracic and abdominal aorta are major procedures with risk of considerable blood loss. Often the general condition of the patient is poor. This is even truer when the reason for operation is a leaking aneurysm. In addition to the prepared postoperative nursing equipment, the requirements for cardiopulmonary resuscitation should be readily available when the patient returns from the operating room.

Thoracic operations. Postoperative care is as described after cardiac surgery, including the special care needed after cardiopulmonary bypass if this has been used.

The patient must be observed carefully for signs of haemorrhage. Hypertension may need control by antihypertensive drugs.

Abdominal operations. After operation the patient is lifted carefully back into bed, the bed-clothes arranged over a cradle. The patient must be adequately covered, but the feet and legs easily uncovered for observation. Electrocardiogram electrodes are attached so that the cardiac rhythm can be observed. Adherent electrodes on the chest are preferable. If limb electrodes are used, the retaining straps must not be tight enough to impede circulation.

Initially the patient may need artificial ventilation for 12–24 hours. Otherwise, 5–6 litres/min of humidified oxygen are given intranasally for 2–3 days or as the patient's condition indicates.

Heart rate and blood pressure are recorded half-hourly for 12 hours, hourly for 12 hours, then less frequently unless there are indications for more frequent recordings. Pulses in the affected limbs are checked at the same time, as are the colour and surface temperature of the extremities. It is essential to report any deterioration in circulation or pulse absent for the first time. Either may indicate recurrence of arterial obstruction. Blood transfusion is

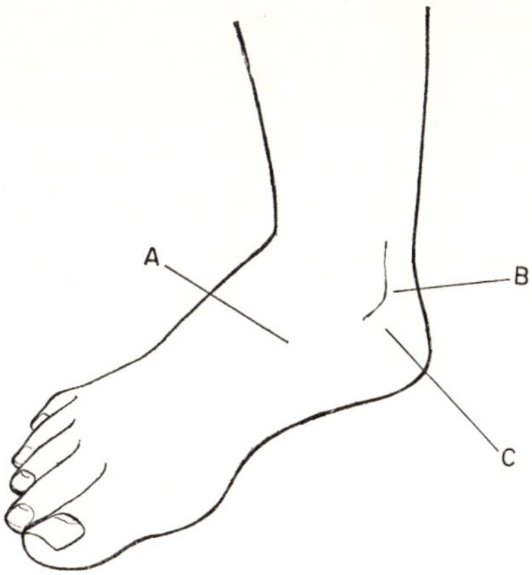

FIG 88. **Foot pulses.**
A, Dorsalis pedis. B, Internal malleolus. C, Posterior tibial.

continued as necessary. In view of the patient's condition and the difficulty of measuring blood loss accurately, the venous pressure is often used as a guide to the amount of blood needed. If the blood pressure is adequate compared with the preoperative recording, the patient pink and warm, the peripheral circulation good and the venous pressure 5–8 cm of water, then blood is not needed. A good blood pressure must be maintained to avoid clotting in the graft, but the bed foot should not be raised as this will diminish circulation to the legs. Excessive transfusion may cause pulmonary oedema.

The intravenous infusion fluids ordered may include low molecular weight dextran, a plasma expander, in the first 24 hours. This helps to maintain good peripheral flow. The infusion is then continued with $2\frac{1}{2}$–3 litres (more if the patient is dehydrated) of dextrose and electrolyte solutions each 24 hours. The regimen is adjusted according to the serum electrolytes, the amount of gastric aspirate and the patient's state of hydration. An intragastric tube is left in situ and aspirated hourly at first, less often as the aspirate decreases.

Little or no fluid is allowed orally at first, as paralytic ileus is a common complication. Mouth care is therefore particularly important.

A flatus tube must be passed when necessary to prevent abdominal distension causing tension on the long abdominal suture line. When peristalsis returns, the patient passes flatus and gastric aspirate decreases, fluids by mouth are increased and intravenous fluids decreased. Finally the gastric tube and infusion cannula are removed and the patient is allowed a light then normal diet. Calorie, protein and vitamin intake should be increased as soon as possible. A well nourished patient recovers more quickly.

Rectal suppositories or an aperient may be necessary before normal bowel habits are resumed, though diarrhoea may be troublesome after paralytic ileus. Urine output should be measured hourly or two-hourly immediately after operation and any haematuria reported. Renal failure may occur if there has been any ischaemic period for the kidneys because of the operative procedures or hypotension.

Analgesics are given as necessary to allow the patient to rest and cooperate in treatment. Morphine 5–10 mg intramuscularly, repeated every 4–6 hours, is usually sufficient, or intravenous administration may be ordered to ensure that it is effective. Milder analgesics may be used after the first 48–72 hours.

The patient is nursed flat after operation, but may be turned towards alternate sides. He may sit up when the surgeon allows it, but this may not be until after 24–48 hours. If the graft lies across the hip-joint, flexion at the hip may kink the graft and reduce circulation through it. This will encourage clotting in the graft and impair leg circulation.

Careful attention to pressure areas is necessary, especially the heels. They may be protected by foam pads and can usually be massaged every 1–2 hours without disturbing the patient much. An alternating pressure point or 'ripple' mattress may be used.

Breathing exercises and leg movement are important and should be practised for 5 minutes in each hour during waking hours. The patient should be taught to support the wound with his hand to make coughing less painful and more effective. Humidified air or oxygen inhalations may be given to loosen tracheobronchial secretions, and use of a triggered intermittent positive pressure respirator, such as the Bennett physiotherapy model, for 10 minutes at intervals of 1–2 hours, helps to keep the lung well aerated while the patient is relatively immobile.

Drains may be left in the operation area draining into either dressings or a vacuum bottle. Dressings should be changed when wet, and the negative pressure renewed in the vacuum bottle at intervals to maintain mild suction. Drains are usually shortened after 24–48 hours and removed when drainage is minimal.

Sutures are removed after 10 days or when the wound is healed. The patient may be allowed to get out of bed after 7 days, but should be discouraged from sitting immobile in a chair for long periods since this increases the risk of deep vein thrombosis. Activity is gradually increased.

Some surgeons order anticoagulants over the immediate postoperative period to reduce clotting at the suture line. With small vessel surgery, anticoagulants permanently may be desirable.

Postoperative controls include:

1. Chest X-ray to exclude postoperative retention of secretions, pneumonitis, atelectasis or pulmonary embolus.

2. Daily serum electrolyte estimations until the results remain stable.

3. Haemoglobin and packed cell volume estimation daily for the first few days to detect anaemia and to determine the state of hydration. The haemoglobin is estimated again before discharge so that the treatment for anaemia can be given if necessary.

4. Blood gases and acid-base balance estimation if acidosis or hypoxia is thought likely.

5. Urine electrolytes and urea estimation for the first few days so that any renal failure is detected early.

The patient is usually discharged after 3–4 weeks and is given an appointment to the outpatients department.

Arterial operations in the limbs. After these operations there is usually little disturbance of the patient's general condition. The main points in postoperative nursing care:

1. A careful watch for haemorrhage and prompt action to control it by pressure and elevation of the part, and to obtain help.

2. Careful observation of circulation through the affected limb by checking the pulses and observing the colour of the extremity at frequent intervals.

Varicose veins

A varicose vein is one which is dilated. The wall of a vein has a thin tunica media containing a small amount of plain muscle which, under the influence of the sympathetic nerves, is usually in a state of slight contraction or tone. The state of contraction enables the vein to maintain its shape and, by exerting a little pressure, takes part in the venous return of blood to the heart. Interference with the flow out of the vein causes the blood inside to increase in amount, and eventually the pressure will overcome that exerted by the vein wall, causing dilatation. Such varicosities occur at the lower end of the oesophagus as a result of obstruction to the portal vein and at the lower end of the anal canal (haemorrhoids).

The commonest site of varicose veins is in the leg, where the long and short saphenous veins are affected. The veins of the legs contain valves which ensure the onward flow of blood towards the heart (Fig. 89). Should these valves become incompetent, the blood pools in the veins and dilatation (varicosity) occurs (Fig. 90).

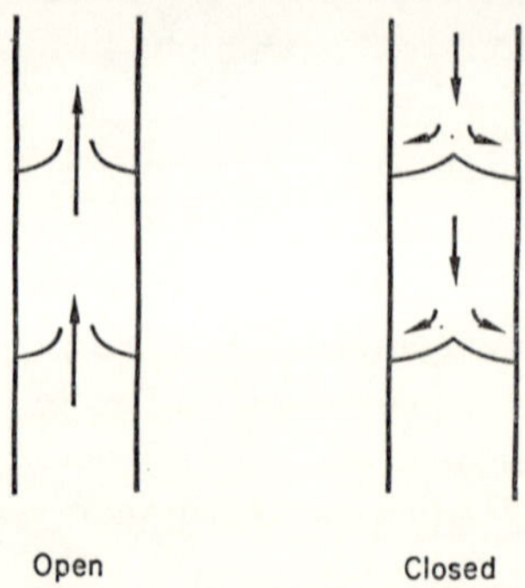

FIG 89. The action of the valves in the veins in ensuring that the flow of blood is towards the heart only. In the closed position the wall of the vein is strong enough to withstand the lateral pressure of the blood.

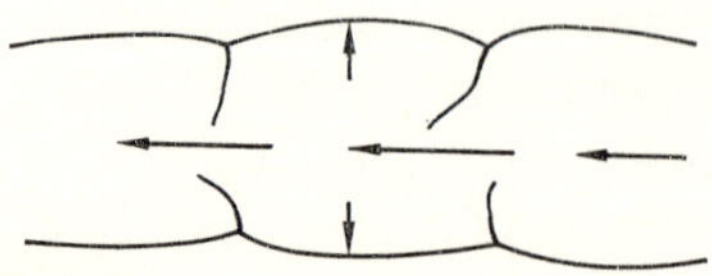

FIG 90. A varicose vein.
The valves are unable to close and the weak walls cannot withstand the lateral pressure of the blood.

The vein becomes swollen and unsightly. The legs may become oedematous due to venous congestion, and the legs feel heavy and even painful. The congestion diminishes the supply of fresh blood to the tissues so that injuries do not heal quickly and ulceration may occur. When cut, varicose veins bleed profusely.

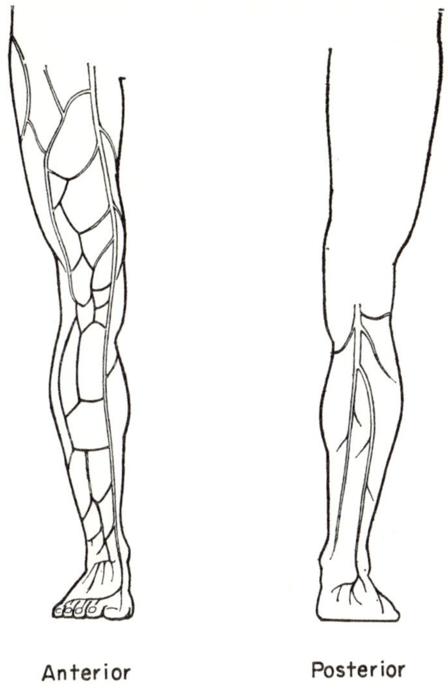

FIG **91. The long and short saphenous veins of the right leg.**

When the patient lies down and raises the leg, the blood drains out of the veins and the leg returns to its normal size, but when he stands up they fill and it dilates again. Even if a finger is placed on the distal end of the vein or a tourniquet is tied round the leg whilst the patient is lying and kept there on standing, the defective valves allow the blood to flow down the vein and dilate it once again. The blood tends to be static and thrombosis may occur.

The patient suffering from varicose veins is advised not to stand still but to move about, as contraction of the muscles of the legs squeezes the veins and plays a considerable part in the venous return. Walking is an exercise to be recommended, but should it be necessary to stand still the patient should transfer his weight from one leg to the other and flex the knees, stand on his toes and even move his toes inside his shoes.

The wearing of an elastic stocking or elastic bandage applied evenly from the toes up to the top of the leg prevents dilatation of the vein and relieves discomfort to some extent. It should be removed at night and applied in the morning before getting out of bed.

Sclerosis of the tunica intima of the vein is achieved by the injection of irritant chemicals such as 1–1·5 ml mono-ethanolamine (Ethamolin) 5% or 0·5–1 ml sodium tetradecyl. After injection a sorbo pad is sometimes placed over the vein and kept in position for about 10 days with an elastic or crêpe bandage firmly and evenly applied. The patient should walk about as usual. Repetition of the injection is sometimes necessary to sclerose all the prominent veins of the legs.

Exposure and ligation of a vein may be carried out in the groin near the junction of the long saphenous with the femoral vein or in the popliteal fossa near the junction of the short saphenous with the popliteal vein.

Stripping is a method of removing the affected vein. It is exposed and ligated at the groin and again lower down the leg. A Babcock's or Myer's stripper is threaded along the vein and pulled through. The end of the stripper is shaped so that it strips the vein through the subcutaneous tissues.

After operation pressure bandages are applied from the toes to the top of the leg to control bleeding. On return to bed the leg is elevated. The following day the patient is allowed out of bed and encouraged to walk about a little. He should sit with the legs supported horizontally on a stool and not hanging down. These measures help to prevent swelling of the leg and soon the collateral circulation takes over the work of the vein removed. The patient may go home, returning after 10 days for removal of the stitches.

9
Investigations

If a patient is to receive the best possible treatment, whether medical or surgical, careful investigation is necessary to diagnose the abnormality, assess the severity of the condition, determine the effect of treatment and discover any side-effects.

Much can be learnt by the doctor from the appearance of the patient, the history of the condition, percussion to assess the size of the heart, auscultation to hear the sounds in the heart and lungs and palpation to detect the site of the apex and any 'thrills' (through the chest wall these feel rather like a cat purring, and are caused by the blood flowing over calcified valves). A good nurse can assist by reporting any dyspnoea and cyanosis, whether they appear at rest or during exercise, and any orthopnoea, oedema or excessive tiredness.

However, more sophisticated techniques are now available to provide the scientific evidence necessary to complement the doctor's clinical expertise and experience. It is important that the nurse should know enough about these to be able to reassure the patient and to help in performing the investigations when necessary.

Postero-anterior chest X-ray

This shows the size and shape of the heart, any increased vascularization of the lungs and calcification of the valves or aorta, and may show the outline of any vessels whose position or size is abnormal, e.g. the dilatation of an aortic aneurysm. It also shows the widened mediastinal shadow caused by a collection of blood, for example when cardiac tamponade occurs.

As far as possible all metal or other X-ray opaque objects should be removed from the area being X-rayed.

Barium swallow and screening

During screening the movement of the heart, lungs and major vessels can be seen on the fluoroscopic screen. This may be combined with barium swallow and oblique X-rays taken to show the deflection of the oesophagus round a selectively enlarged left atrium as it bulges out at the back of the heart. It is not necessary to starve the patient before this.

Cardiac catheterization (Fig. 92)

A thin hollow tube is passed via a peripheral vein, usually the antecubital vein in the arm, into the right side of the heart. A

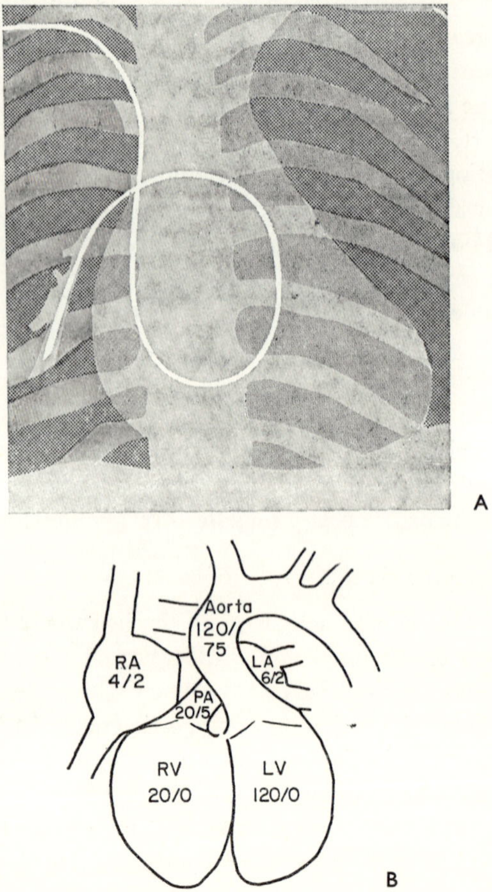

FIG **92. Cardiac catheterization.**
A, A diagrammatic representation of a radiograph, showing the catheter in position. B, Normal pressures in each chamber of the heart and in the great vessels.

sharp stilette may be passed through it and a transeptal puncture performed to reach the left side of the heart, or the catheter may be passed in retrograde fashion up to the aorta via the femoral artery. Manipulation of the catheter is guided by X-ray, the procedure being viewed on an image intensifier. The pressures and oxygen saturations are measured in each chamber of the heart, the pulmonary artery, and the 'wedge pressure' is measured with the catheter tip 'wedged' in the most distal pulmonary vessel it can reach.

The procedure must be explained beforehand to the patient, who can be assured that passage of the catheter through the vessels will not cause any sensation.

Cardiac catheterization via a vein. A premedication is usually given to reduce anxiety and the procedure is performed with full aseptic precautions, usually under local anaesthetic. The proximal end of the catheter is attached via a series of taps to electronic equipment which produces an oscilloscope display and a permanent paper tracing of the pressures recorded. Samples of blood are drawn from the various sites into heparinized syringes and sent to

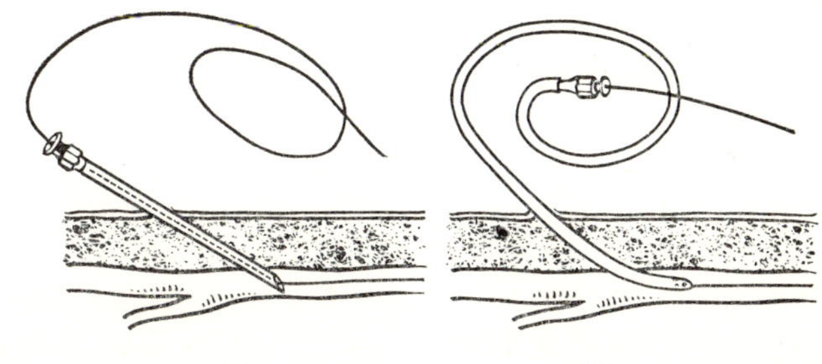

FIG **93. Percutaneous catheterization by the Seldinger technique.**

the laboratory for estimation of the oxygen content. The difference between the pressure before and after a valve is known as the gradient; a high gradient indicates obstruction to flow through the valve. When the catheter is withdrawn the incision is sutured and a firm dressing put on.

Cardiac catheterization via an artery. The catheter is usually passed via the femoral artery. It may be introduced percutaneously, i.e. a small incision is made, a Seldinger needle is inserted pointing towards the heart, a thin guide wire is passed through it for a few centimetres and the catheter is threaded over it and passed up the artery to the heart so that pressures and oxygen saturations can be measured as in venous catheterization (Fig. 93). When the catheter is withdrawn firm pressure must be maintained over the site for at least 5 min to prevent haematoma formation. In fat or very young patients it may be necessary to make a small incision in the artery to facilitate introduction of the catheter. A general anaesthetic may be necessary.

The role of the nurse

The responsibilities of the nurse in cardiac catheterization are:

1. To make sure that the patient has received sufficient explanation of what is to be done and is prepared for it. For example, it may be necessary to prepare for general anaesthetic or to shave the area where incision is to be made.

2. To make sure that any equipment provided is complete and sterile. (A technician may be responsible for sterilizing some of the equipment.)

3. To assist the doctor in performing the procedure when necessary.

4. To provide reassurance by voice and touch for the patient who is lying on a hard X-ray table and may find the darkness and strange sounds and procedures quite alarming.

5. To help to observe the patient's condition, including the electrocardiogram pattern, which is usually displayed on an oscilloscope where the doctor can also see it.

Oxygen and resuscitation equipment should be readily available whenever cardiac catheterization is performed, and the nurse must be prepared to assist in resuscitation if necessary. Serious cardiac dysrhythmias may be provoked, particularly in the more ill patients.

Most patients do not suffer ill effects from catheterization, but it is often wise to keep them in bed until the following day. The nurse must be alert for cardiac dysrhythmias or hypotension, particularly in patients with severe valve disease, congenital abnormalities or pulmonary hypertension. The catheterization sites must be observed for signs of bleeding.

Angiocardiogram

This may be obtained during cardiac catheterization. A catheter with multiple side holes is passed up into the heart and the proximal end attached to a pressurized injection device loaded with radio-opaque fluid (1 ml/kg patient's body weight). The fluid is then injected as a single bolus, and its passage through the heart and blood vessels recorded by a series of X-rays taken in rapid sequence, or as a cine X-ray (cine angiogram). These demonstrate any abnormal connection between the right and left sides of the heart, or the great vessels, the function of the valves, and the size, shape, patency and position of the great vessels.

The patient may feel hot and possibly nauseated when the injection is made, but he should be reassured that this will soon pass.

Aortogram

This may be performed by passing a catheter up the aorta as described for left heart catheterization, injecting radio-opaque fluid and recording its flow by a rapid series of X-rays. A catheter with an angled tip may be manipulated to allow injection of fluid into a specific artery, to provide, for example, renal or coronary angiograms. The cerebral vessels may be demonstrated by 'arch aortograms' (with the catheter tip in the aortic arch) or by an injection directly into the carotid artery.

Translumbar aortogram

This is performed under general anaesthetic, with the patient lying prone on the X-ray table. The skin is cleaned and 30 ml of radio-opaque fluid are injected through a needle which has been passed below the twelfth rib anteriorly and medially into the aorta. The size, shape and patency of the lower aorta and lower limb arteries are demonstrated on the X-rays taken after this.

Venogram

This may be taken to show venous obstruction, e.g. deep

vein thrombosis. Radio-opaque fluid is injected into a vein distal to the area being investigated, and X-rays are taken to record its flow.

Electrocardiograph

This is a tracing on special graph paper strips, and is obtained by recording the electrical changes in the heart muscle as each part is stimulated to contract and then relaxes. It can demonstrate heart rhythm and rate, block in the conduction system and myocardial ischaemia or disproportionate increase in the size and work of the various heart chambers (strain).

For detailed information on electrocardiography the reader is

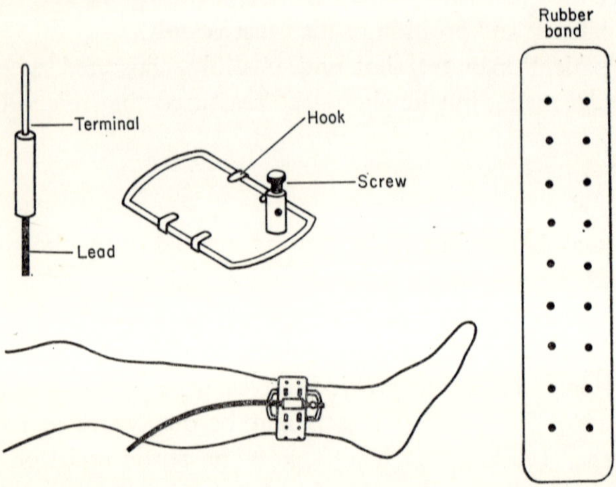

FIG 94. Limb electrodes are flat metal plates with a socket on the top side into which the lead terminal of the patient cable is connected.

advised to consult a textbook entirely devoted to this complicated subject. The method of recording a 12-lead ECG is best learnt by watching an experienced technician. However, it is necessary for the nurse to know a few basis facts in order to use monitoring equipment and read simple rhythm strips. The 12-lead ECG consists of 3 standard leads, 3 augmented or modified leads and 6 V leads when the exploring electrode is applied to various specified areas of the chest wall. These are recorded by applying metal electrodes to the skin, with electrode jelly to increase contact, and connecting them to the appropriate wires (usually labelled). The standard leads are:

Lead I	Right arm and left arm	(positive electrode)
Lead II	Right arm and left leg	(positive electrode)
Lead III	Left arm and left leg	(positive electrode)

An 'earth' electrode is usually attached to the right leg to carry away currents from other sources than the heart. A normal ECG may have its biggest deflection upwards or downwards, depending on which lead is recorded. When the current flows towards the positive electrode a deflection upwards is shown, when it flows away from the positive electrode a deflection downwards occurs. Resting muscle is said to be polarized; when stimulated to contract it becomes depolarized and subsequently, in the recovery period, it is repolarized. Put simply, depolarization occurs from left to right across the ventricular septum, then outwards through the ventricular walls. Depolarization of the left ventricle wall causes a greater deflection because the muscle is thicker. Therefore a standard Lead II would normally show deflections as follows:

A small one up, P (atrial depolarization and contraction)
A small one down, Q (depolarization across the ventricular septum)
A larger one up, R (depolarization outwards through the left ventricle)
A small one down, S
A small one up, T (period of recovery or repolarization).

The P wave represents atrial stimulation and contraction (depolarization), the QRS represents ventricular stimulation and contraction, and the T ventricular relaxation (repolarization). The P–R interval represents the time between atrial and ventricular contraction, i.e. the time taken for the impulse to cross the atrio-ventricular node.

It will be seen that if the left ventricle wall is facing the left shoulder (same as the left arm) and the right ventricle faces the

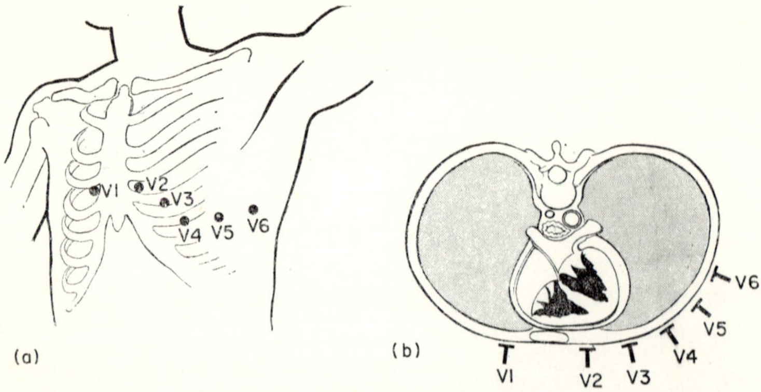

Fig **95.** *Above,* **The position of precordial, chest or V electrodes.** *Right,* **Placement of electrodes.**
1, Standard lead I. Positive pole to left arm. 2, Standard lead II. Positive pole to left leg. 3, Standard lead III. Positive pole to left leg.

left leg, then in Lead III the greatest deflection will be downwards, i.e. 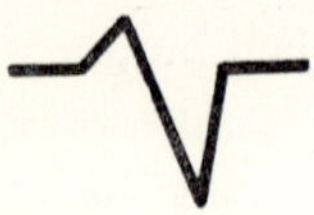 instead of 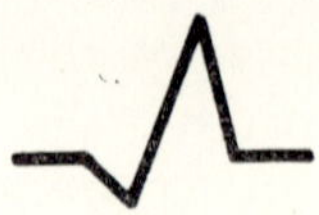

Further information on ECG patterns is in Chapters 4 and 6.

Blood volume

This may be measured by various dilution techniques. One is to inject intravenously a given quantity of albumen labelled with a radio-active substance such as iodine 131. A stabilization period of about 15 minutes is allowed and blood samples are then withdrawn. By measuring the radio-activity of the samples the degree of dilution can be calculated and the blood volume assessed.

Phonocardiogram

For many years doctors have used heart sounds as a guide to the condition of the heart, its valves and the major vessels. However, the sounds may be quite difficult to hear and analyse, particularly if the heart rate is rapid. It is now possible to produce on an oscilloscope or paper a tracing of the heart sounds by placing a small microphone over the heart and recording the sounds through it. This is called a phonocardiogram.

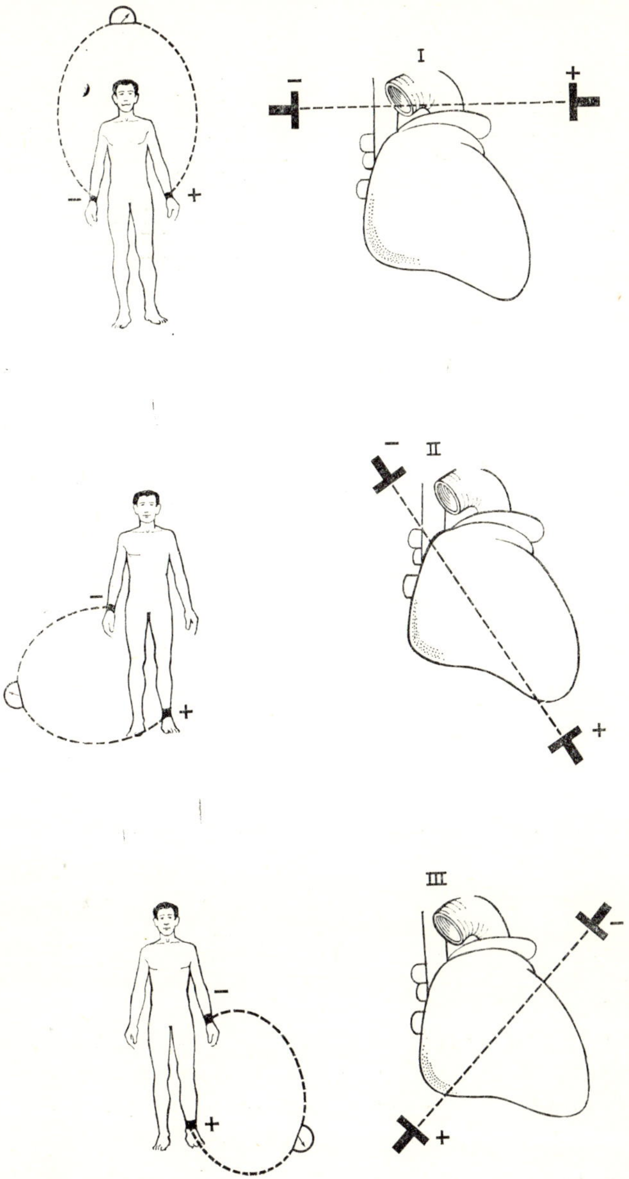
I
II
III

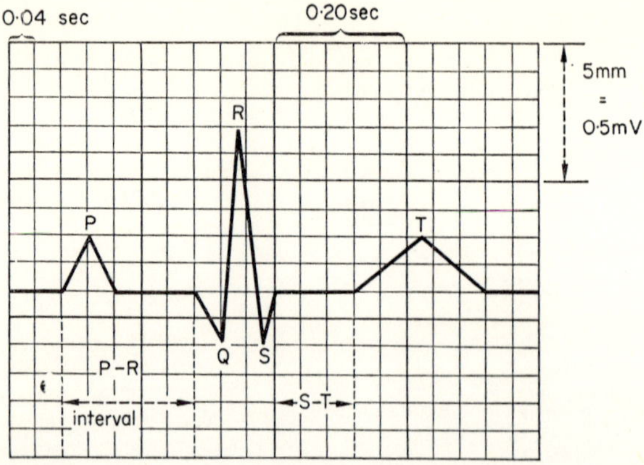

FIG **96. ECG graph paper and a standard lead 2 ECG.**

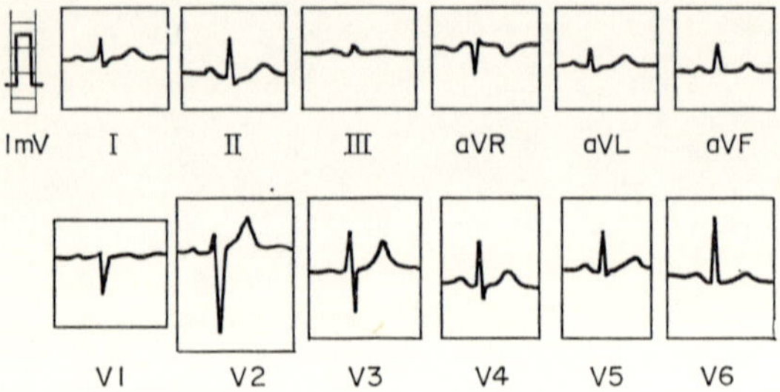

FIG **97. A normal 12 lead electrocardiogram.**

Respiratory function tests

These test the capacity and efficiency of the lungs from the mechanical point of view. (To test the efficiency of gas diffusion it is necessary to estimate blood gas, or perform other more sophisticated tests.) Only the investigations most commonly used in relation to cardiovascular disease are described here.

Vital capacity. This is the greatest amount of air which can be expired after maximal inspiration.

Forced expiratory volume (FEV_1). This is the proportion of the vital capacity volume which can be expired in one second. It is expressed as a percentage, and is normally 80–85%. It is reduced when expiration is impeded, e.g. by bronchospasm.

Maximum breathing capacity or maximum ventilatory volume (MBC or MVV). This is the amount of air which can be inspired and expired with maximum effort in one minute.

These three tests involve expiring air into a machine via a mouthpiece. With modern equipment all three results can be obtained from one maximal inspiration and expiration into the machine.

Prothrombin time and prothrombin index

These tests are of particular importance when anticoagulant therapy is in progress, since such drugs as warfarin and phenindione increase the prothrombin time and lower the prothrombin index. Dosage of such drugs is usually controlled by estimating the prothrombin index at regular intervals and adjusting the drug dosage to maintain the desired level.

Normal prothrombin time is 15–20 seconds at 37° C (Fullerton method). The prothrombin index is obtained by comparing the prothrombin time of the patient with that of a normal control taken at the same time. The formula is:

$$\frac{\text{Normal prothrombin} \times 100}{\text{Patient's prothrombin time}}$$

and the result is expressed as a percentage.

Prothrombin is formed in the liver, using vitamin K. The prothrombin time may be increased when there is liver damage, for example, if cardiac failure over a prolonged period has resulted in an enlarged and engorged liver.

Prothrombin is one of the factors concerned in blood coagulation. Therefore if the prothrombin time is much increased and the prothrombin index is below 30%, severe haemorrhage can occur.

Platelet count

This is performed to determine the number of platelets /mm^3. The normal is 250 000 – 600 000. Reduction in the number of platelets may increase the likelihood of bleeding. After cardiopulmonary bypass the platelet count is usually reduced, though less so with the use of modern bypass machines.

Erythrocyte sedimentation rate

This test demonstrates the rate at which the red cells sink to the bottom of a column of blood, leaving clear plasma at the top. It is often not of great diagnostic value since the sedimentation rate is increased by menstruation, pregnancy and a number of other factors which may not be significant. However, serial estimations may be used to indicate progress in a disease such as acute rheumatism.

The normal rate is up to 13 mm/ hour for women and children and 2–6 mm/ hour for men.

Other blood tests

Normal results and containers which may be used are shown in Table 2.

Table 2. Laboratory tests commonly performed

Test	*Type of container*	*Amount required (ml)*
Absolute count (Hb, PCV)	Sequestrene bottle	2·5
Agglutinins (cold and warm)	W.R. tube	4
Alkali reserve	Heparin bottle	5
Bilirubin	W.R. tube	3
Bleeding time	Capillary	–
Blood gases (pH, $P\text{CO}_2$, $P\text{O}_2$)	Special syringe	5
Blood grouping	W.R. tube	4
Calcium	W.R. tube	3
Chlorides	Heparin bottle	3
Cholesterol	W.R. tube	3
Clotting time, kaolin–cephalin	Prothrombin bottle	2
Creatinine	Sterile Universal Container for blood	15
Cross-matching	W.R. tube	4
Electrolytes (Na, K, Cl, urea)	Heparin bottle	8

Table 2. *continued*

Test	*Type of container*	*Amount required (ml)*
Erythrocyte sedimentation rate (ESR)	Sequestrene bottle	2·5
Fibrinogen	Prothrombin bottle	2
Full blood count (Hb, WCC film)	Sequestrene bottle or capillary	2·5
Grouping and cross-matching	W.R. tube	4
Heparin assay	Prothrombin bottle	2
Lactic dehydrogenase (LDH)	W.R. tube	3
Latex agglutination tests for rheumatoid, LE and thyroid antibodies	W.R. tube	4
Liver function tests	Sterile Universal Container for blood	10
Magnesium	Heparin bottle	5
Platelet count	Capillary	–
Proteins (A/G ratio, electrophoresis)	W.R. tube	3
Prothrombin index	Prothrombin bottle	2
Sugar	Fluoride bottle	2
Transaminases (SGOT and SGPT)	Sterile Universal Container for blood	5
Urea	Heparin bottle	3
Uric acid	W.R. tube	3
Wasserman reaction (WR)	W.R. tube	4
White cell count (WCC)	Sequestrene bottle or capillary	2·5

For more detail regarding serum enzymes and electrolytes see Chapter 10.

10

Chemistry and haemodynamics in cardiac conditions

Body fluids

Although Hamlet bewails his 'too, too solid flesh', he did not, presumably, realize more than 60% of the weight of the body is fluid. In an adult weighing 70 kg (11 stone) there are some 45 litres of water. It is not found as pure water, but rather as a solution containing salts, digested foodstuffs, metabolites, gases and as a vehicle for the transport of proteins and blood cells. The water and its contents are referred to as body fluids.

The body fluid is distributed throughout the body but can be differentiated according to where it is found, thus:

Intracellular fluid (ICF)	30 litres, actually inside the tissue cells.
Extracellular fluid (ECF)	15 litres, outside the cells. This can be further differentiated into:
Interstitial or tissue fluid	12 litres, in the spaces between the cells.
Intravascular fluid	3 litres, being circulated round the body in the blood vessels as blood plasma.

Thus the fluid can be thought of as being in 'compartments' (Fig. 98). The contents of each compartment are kept fairly constant; however, there is a continual passage of fluid from one compartment to another.

Before discussing the disturbances which may take place in body fluids in cardiovascular conditions, it would be well to consider the contents in the average healthy person.

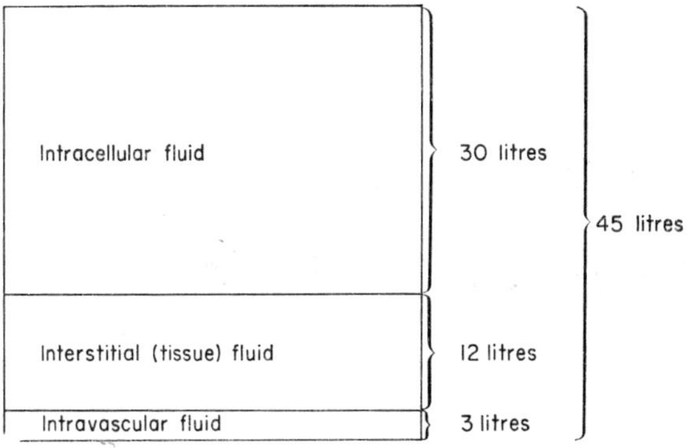

FIG 98. The representation of the body fluids in 'compartments'.

Water

As has been stated, in the average adult of 70 kg there are some 45 litres of water. Water is of utmost importance to life and it would be safe to say that each physiological process takes place in the presence of water. Reference has been made to its power as a solvent. It also has the power to take up heat and, by circulating round the body, it distributes heat from the deep structures to the surface of the body. In the process of sweating water is exuded to the surface of the body, from which it takes heat to cause evaporation. Thus water can be seen to be of importance in the regulation of body temperature. Waste products such as urea and excess substances such as salts are eliminated by the kidney only if they are dissolved in water. Exchange of gases in the alveoli of the lungs takes place across a moist membrane. The water in this moisture evaporates and is breathed out as water vapour.

The water content of the body remains fairly constant in health, but as some is continually being lost, the same amount must be put back in some way or other. The average adult loses the following amounts each day:

In sweat	500 ml
In expired air	500 ml
In faeces	100 ml
In urine	1400 ml
Total	2500 ml

If the water content is to remain the same, and the individual loses 2500 ml in the day, it will be seen that he must take in 2500 ml as food or drink. With the same individual, the amounts put out and the amounts required to be taken in vary from day to day, but a balance is kept between the one and the other. This is maintained by the antidiuretic hormone from the posterior pituitary gland, which affects the reabsorption of water in the uriniferous tubule of the kidney.

Electrolytes

Water is rarely found alone in the body but rather as a solution of salts and other substances as we have seen. While the term 'dissolved salts' is used frequently, it would be more accurate to refer to them as 'dissolved electrolytes'.

The smallest part of a chemical element is the atom. Each atom consists of a nucleus carrying positive electrical charges, the number of which depends upon the element concerned. The nucleus is surrounded by a group of electrons, each of which carries a negative electrical charge, the number of negatively charged electrons being the same as the number of positive electrical charges on the nucleus, thus keeping the atom in a state of electrical neutrality.

In certain circumstances two (or more) atoms may combine to form a molecule, but in doing so one atom may lose one (or more) of its electrons to the other atom. In this way one atom has gained an electron and is now carrying additional negative electrical charge, whereas the other has lost an electron and now carries an extra positive charge on its nucleus. For example, an atom of sodium combined with an atom of chlorine to form a molecule of sodium chloride; in so doing an electron leaves the sodium and joins the chlorine, leaving the sodium with an extra positive charge on its nucleus, and the chlorine (now chloride) with an extra negative charge on its electrons. In the dry state they remain in close association with each other as sodium chloride and balance each other in electrical neutrality. Neither of them is in its original atomic state, each having lost or gained an electron. Each is now referred to as an ion.

When a salt such as sodium chloride is dissolved in water the sodium and chloride ions dissociate. Although they are now separate they can soon reform the association. If an electrical current is passed through the solution, the sodium ion is attracted to the negative pole (and is referred to as a cation), while the chloride ion is attracted to the positive pole (and is referred to as an anion). Both anion and cation are referred to as electrolytes.

The following electrolytes are found in body fluids:

Cations	*Anions*
Sodium	Chloride
Potassium	Bicarbonate
Magnesium	Protein
Calcium	Phosphate

Proteins in body fluids usually carry a negative electrical charge. Glucose and urea do not carry charges and are not electrolytes.

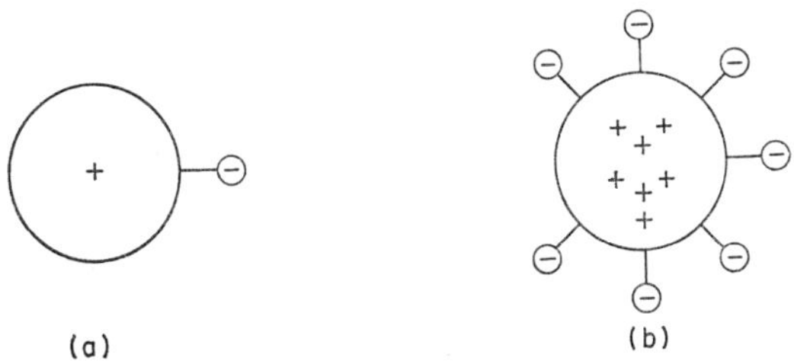

FIG **99. Electrical balance of atoms.**
A, Sodium, 1 positive (nucleus) and 1 negative (electron). B, Chlorine, 7 positive (nucleus) and 7 negative (electrons). The electrons represent the number in the outer circle.

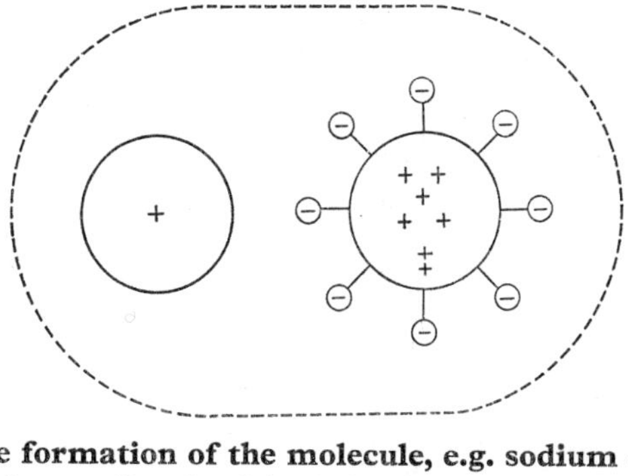

FIG **100. The formation of the molecule, e.g. sodium chloride.**
The electron from sodium has joined chlorine. Each is now an ion and is no longer an atom.

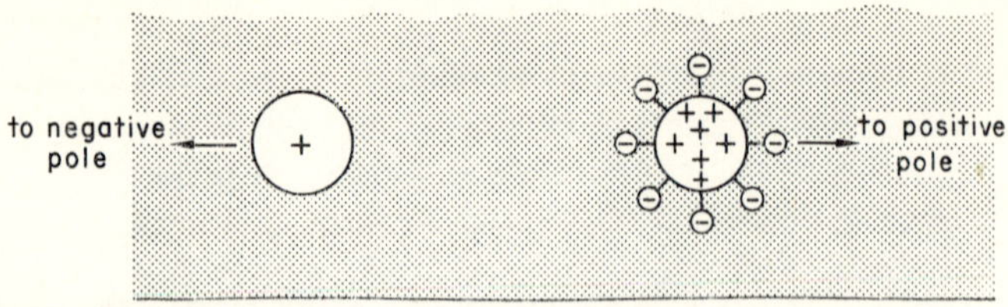

FIG **101. The dissociation of ions in solution in water.**
Sodium (Na^+) is attracted to the negative pole and chloride (Cl^-) to the positive pole.

The concentration of electrolytes in body fluids is measured as the number of milliequivalents in each litre of fluid (mEq/litre).

In solution the various electrolytes differ in their activity. Whereas a sodium ion carries one positive charge on its nucleus, a calcium ion carries two. Thus it will be seen that the sodium ion can combine with one bicarbonate ion, but since the calcium carries two charges, it will combine with two bicarbonate ions and can be thought of as being twice as active as sodium. An electrolyte is measured according to its power of chemical activity rather than according to its weight.

In a solution at electrical balance (neutrality), the total number of charges on the anions equals the total number of charges on the cations. Chemical analysis would show that the number of mEq of the one is the same as the number of mEq of the other. A sample of plasma from a healthy person might reveal the following electrolyte content:

Cations			*Anions*		
Sodium	(Na^+)	140	Chloride	(Cl^-)	103
Potassium	(K^+)	5	Bicarbonate	(HCO_3^-)	25
Calcium	(Ca^+)	5	Phosphate	(HPO_4^-)	2
Magnesium	(Mg^+)	2	Sulphate	(HSO_4^-)	1
			Organic acids		5
			Proteins		16
Total mEq		152	Total mEq		152

The composition of extracellular fluid differs considerably from that of the intracellular fluid. In the extracellular fluids there is only a slight difference between the electrolyte content of the plasma and that of the tissue fluid. The electrolyte concentration of the principal constituents in each is shown below, expressed in mEq/litre.

	Plasma	*Tissue fluid*	*Intracellular fluid*
Sodium	136–146	146	5–10
Potassium	3·5–4·5	3·5–4·5	145–150
Calcium	4·5–5·5	3	1–2
Chloride	95–105	110–115	1
Bicarbonate	25–32	25–32	15–25
Protein	16	1	65

It will be seen that the concentration of sodium is higher in the plasma and tissue fluid than it is in the intracellular fluid, whereas the concentration of potassium is the reverse. It is helpful to think of the potassium as the prisoner inside the cell, for the cell membrane seems to play an active part in keeping the potassium inside the cell. Sodium enters the cell but is very quickly pumped out if the potassium level is normal. If the cell is damaged the potassium may pass out into the tissue. Also, if there is a deficiency of sodium in the tissue fluid, so leaving a large proportion of negatively charged ions, the potassium will pass out of the cell in order to neutralize the electrical state of the fluid. This may lead to an unusually high amount of potassium in the tissue (extravascular) fluid; the salts there pass into the plasma and will later be eliminated by the kidney. Chloride and bicarbonate seem to have easy entry and exit from the cells.

Disturbances in water and electrolyte content of body fluid

Water depletion usually occurs when patients are not drinking enough water and more is being lost than is taken in. There is thirst; the urinary output is low and the specific gravity rises. For a time water from the cells helps to maintain the volume of extracellular fluid and the blood pressure remains normal. Pyrexia may develop, which will worsen the condition, and the patient becomes delirious.

The patient is given salt-free fluids. If he can drink, he is given water until his thirst is quenched, but if he cannot drink he may be given an intravenous infusion of 5% glucose in water. The output of urine is measured and compared with the daily intake, and with the disappearance of clinical symptoms the condition may have been rectified.

Although dehydration may be due to water depletion alone, it usually occurs in association with electrolyte deficiency, e.g. sodium as well as water.

Water intoxication or overhydration occurs when the intake of water exceeds the output. Healthy persons can drink large quantities of water without any harm to themselves the excess water being eliminated by the kidneys, the urine being pale, of low specific gravity and in large volume. However, if the function of the kidneys is impaired the water will collect in the body. Oedema is not common but may be noticeable round the eyes. There may be a gain in weight. The lungs may be affected, causing 'bubbly' respirations. The functioning of the cerebrum may be disordered, causing dizziness, headache, nausea and mental confusion. The serum sodium concentration may be reduced.

The intake of water by the patient is restricted sometimes for several days, during which the excess water will be eliminated as urine and evaporated as sweat. The amount of fluid taken in and put out will be measured, and the daily totals compared. An intravenous injection of 100 ml of 5% saline may be given.

Sodium

Sodium has the power of attracting water and because of this plays a considerable part in maintaining the volume of the extracellular fluid. This volume is important because the blood volume, the heart's output and thus the whole circulation depend upon it. Sodium also has some action in maintaining the conductivity of the nerve impulses and in the contraction of muscle.

In the average diet there is an adequate supply of sodium for daily requirements. A small amount is lost in sweat. The larger part of sodium lost from the body is in the urine; the kidneys regulate the amount of sodium in the plasma, their action being governed by the amount of the hormone aldosterone produced by the suprarenal cortex. When the blood volume is reduced, more aldosterone is secreted, causing a tendency for the blood volume to be increased.

Sodium depletion may occur as a result of insufficient intake in the diet, but as the kidneys can conserve sodium even if little is taken in, there may be sufficient to maintain a normal sodium balance. As sweat contains sodium, excess sweating may add to a mild degree of sodium depletion or add to a tendency to depletion from other causes. Because of the close association between sodium and water, sodium depletion is usually accompanied by water depletion; this condition is known as dehydration and occurs when the kidneys fail to conserve sodium, either because the kidneys are diseased or because the suprarenal gland produces insufficient hormone to control the loss, as occurs in Addison's disease. It may also occur as a result of diuretic drugs. Much sodium is lost when there is diarrhoea and vomiting, as a result of continued aspiration of the gastric contents. As sodium is the main cation in the extra-cellular fluid, a depletion in content may lead to the movement of potassium out of the cell in an attempt to maintain electrical balance. Depletion of sodium and its accompanying water leads to a fall in volume of extracellular fluid. The skin loses its elasticity and becomes dry and wrinkled. The tongue may become dry, but the patient may not complain of thirst. The eyes are sunken. There is a fall in blood pressure and a rise in pulse rate. The patient complains of nausea, vomiting, loss of energy and muscular cramps. He becomes apathetic and mentally confused. The urine becomes scanty in quantity and dark in colour; renal failure may occur. Severe depletion of sodium may cause disturbance in the acid-base balance and in potassium and magnesium metabolism.

The treatment of this extracellular dehydration is to restore the volume of the circulating fluid either orally or by the intravenous infusion of 0·9% normal saline. The return of the blood pressure and pulse rate to normal and the disappearance of the clinical features indicate an improvement of the condition. The doctor will further control the amount of saline infusion to be given by the estimation of the amount of sodium in the plasma (average Na^+ being 136–147 mEq/litre). It is important to avoid giving too much sodium, and observations should be made on the neck veins for any signs of increased venous pressure, such as swelling or pulsation, and for pulmonary congestion, such as sounds of 'bubbly' breathing.

Excess sodium usually brings about an increase of water in the extracellular fluid, and generalized oedema results. Sodium and water retention may be due to renal failure. It may also be due to the administration of corticosteroids. After trauma the hormone aldosterone is secreted and can cause retention of sodium by the kidney (see also congestive heart failure, p. 21). Finally, retention may occur as the result of overinfusion of saline.

The first part of treatment is to restrict the intake of sodium and water. A diet completely free of sodium is both unpalatable and difficult to obtain; however, restriction of added salt is possible, as is also the giving of salt-free butter and bread made without salt. It should also be remembered that baking powder contains sodium bicarbonate, so bread and pastry made with it should be avoided. Diuretics can be given as the doctor prescribes; with some diruetics it may not be necessary to restrict water and sodium to any severe degree.

Potassium

Potassium is found largely in the cells, which seem able to store it, and without it the cells themselves would not function properly. It has some action in maintaining the conduction of nerve impulses and in muscular contraction. A diet containing fruit, meat and tea contains a rich supply of potassium.

Potassium depletion occurs after injury to the tissues, when potassium leaves the cells, increases in the extracellular fluid and is lost via the kidney. It also occurs in starvation and wasting disease, when there has been continued gastric aspiration, and in conditions of the gastro-intestinal tract when there is vomiting and diarrhoea. It may also occur when a patient has been having intravenous fluids for a long time without addition of potassium, and also when there is increased loss in the urine due to the action of some diuretics such as the thiazide group. It also occurs in acidosis due to hypoxia. The patient becomes apathetic, drowsy and eventually mentally confused. Muscular movements may become weak, e.g. drooping of the eyelids may be one of the first things which a nurse may notice to cause her to be suspicious. Abdominal distension, retention of urine and even paralytic ileus may occur; there may be thirst and polyuria and the blood pressure may fall. The patient may appear flushed; his pulse may be slow. Cardiac dysrhythmias may develop, usually with ventricular extrasystoles, leading to cardiac arrest. Lack of potassium increases the tendency to intoxication by digitalis.

When the depletion has been recognized it can be treated by giving the patient fruit and fruit juices, this is a common and safe procedure. He can be given potassium chloride orally, usually in a slow release form otherwise it may irritate the gastro-intestinal tract. Some patients find it nauseating, and prefer an effervescent form of potassium containing potassium bicarbonate and potassium tartrate. When potassium cannot be taken by mouth, it may be given intravenously, e.g. 2 g of potassium chloride in 500 ml of normal saline or 5% glucose slowly over 2–3 hours. The uptake of potassium by the tissue cells is facilitated when there is a high level of carbohydrate metabolism taking place in the cell, so soluble insulin may be given at the same time as the glucose, in the ratio of 1 unit soluble insulin to every 2·5 g of glucose.

There must be a repeated analysis of the blood to estimate the content of potassium. It is wise to give potassium prophylactically when the patient is having drugs which are known to increase the urinary loss of potassium, as this combination is sometimes prescribed.

Excess potassium occurs when the kidneys fail to excrete it from the plasma, and it may occur when too much has been given as medical treatment. It also occurs when sodium is not being retained as in Addisonian crises. The effects of excess are not easily distinguished from deficiency of potassium, with the patient being lethargic, possibly mentally confused and with muscular weakness in both conditions. In potassium excess there may be paralysis of the respiratory muscles. The pulse becomes slow and irregular, and cardiac arrest may ensue.

The intake of potassium is restricted by withholding fruits and proteins. Any acidosis and any water sodium depletion are corrected. In order to prevent absorption of potassium from the intestinal tract, exchange resins may be given by mouth. Sometimes 20 units of soluble insulin may be given by injection, at the same time as 25–50 g of intravenous glucose, as a result of which there may be depletion of potassium in the plasma. 10 ml of 10% calcium gluconate may be given intravenously. If these efforts are insufficient, dialysis may be necessary.

Magnesium and calcium

Magnesium, like potassium, is usually found inside the cells of the tissues, and the metabolism of potassium seems closely linked with that of magnesium. The action of magnesium seems to be closely linked with that of calcium also. When potassium is lost from the body, it seems that magnesium is also lost. Consequently, if only potassium is returned to the body, there remains a depletion of magnesium. Thus, if a patient is being treated for potassium depletion and he does not make much progress, the doctor may order magnesium to be given, probably as magnesium hydroxide by mouth or as 2–4 ml 50% magnesium sulphate by intramuscular injection.

Spasm of skeletal muscle occurs in tetany when there is *depletion of calcium*, calcium being necessary for relaxation of muscle. If the tetanic spasms of tetany are not diminished when calcium has been given, the spasms may be due to the depletion of magnesium.

The most frequent causes of *magnesium depletion* is prolonged vomiting or diarrhoea, malnutrition, the malabsorption syndrome, loss of intestinal contents from fistula etc., and when fluid and electrolytes have been given as treatment but no additional magnesium. The patient has tremors and there may be involuntary jerky movements. Depression and mental confusion may occur, with hallucinations and aggressive behaviour. The serum concentration of magnesium should not be less than 1·5 mEq/litre.

Excess magnesium occurs in renal failure and when too much magnesium has been given as part of treatment. When the concentration in the plasma exceeds 5·0 mEq/litre, the symptoms of hypotension and weakness occur and eventually coma. Tendon reflexes are diminished and lost; respiration may be depressed. When there is a very high serum concentration cardiac arrest occurs.

Effects of electrolytes (ions) on the heart

The action of various electrolytes on the heart has been studied in mammals, and similar effects on the human heart have been noted as a result of clinical investigations and following electrolyte therapy.

If the animal heart is perfused with isotonic sodium chloride, the beating ceases to be regular and eventually stops altogether.

When calcium ions are added to the fluid, the heart beats for a time, but then stops in systole (contraction).

If potassium is added to the fluid, the beats continue for a time but the heart stops in diastole (relaxation).

If sodium chloride, calcium and potassium are all added to the fluid perfusing the heart, the heart continues to beat regularly and indefinitely. Solutions such as Ringer's lactate and Darrow's contain all these ions.

From the point of view of the nurse, the action of the electrolytes on the heart should be remembered when any fluid containing them is being administered, especially if it is being given intravenously. Any clinical features associated with excess (or depletion) should be looked for, the patient's general condition kept under constant review and observations made in particular on the pulse, blood pressure and muscle tone.

Acid–neutral–alkali (or base)

Water itself dissociates into ions only very slightly, forming hydrogen ions (H^+) carrying the positive charge, and hydroxyl ions (^-OH) carrying the negative charge. The number of hydrogen ions equals the number of hydroxyl ions; thus water is in a state of electrolyte neutrality (or balance).

A chemical may be added to water and if, on dissociation, the fluid is found to have more hydrogen ions than water alone, then that fluid is said to be an acid. Conversely, if the fluid contains less hydrogen ions than water, it is said to be an alkali or base.

There are various methods of testing whether a fluid is an acid or alkali. Most nurses are familiar with the use of litmus paper when testing urine, acid turning the litmus red while alkali turns it blue. Some acids are stronger than others; for example, hydrochloric acid is much stronger than acetic acid. To assess the strength of an acid, colour reagents are sometimes used, but in laboratories, other more accurate methods are available. The strength of an acid or alkali is often expressed using the term pH, and it is as well to understand what this, and the number that accompanies it, means.

Pure water does not easily dissociate into ions; so few hydrogen ions are produced that in order to make one gramme of them, 10 million litres of water would be required. As a logarithm this is written as 10^7, ten to the power of seven. An acid contains more hydrogen ions than water, consequently less than 10 million litres would be required to produce one gram of hydrogen ions, e.g. the amount required might only be 1 million litres—the logarithm of 1 million being written as 10^6. On the other hand, an alkali contains fewer hydrogen ions than water, and thus more would be required to produce one gram, e.g. the amount might be 100 million litres. The logarithm of 100 million is written as 10^8.

If pH is used to represent hydrogen ion content followed by the logarithm of the number of litres required to produce one gram of hydrogen ions, then pH 6 would indicate that the fluid is an acid of that strength, or pH 8 that the fluid is alkali. Water would be pH 7—it will be remembered that water is neutral and neither acid or alkali. The total range of pH is from pH 1, a very strong acid, to pH 14, a very strong alkali.

Blood plasma is at a pH 7·4, i.e. slightly on the alkali side of neutral. It varies only slightly in health, between pH 7·35 and pH 7·45 and life cannot exist for long outside the range of pH 7·1 to pH 7·8. Any great change in the pH level of the plasma would disrupt the action of enzymes and the condition of protein.

As a result of metabolism the cells produce sulphates, urates and phosphates, all of which are acid substances, and also carbon dioxide, some of which is converted into carbonic acid. Thus the tendency of the plasma is to become less and less alkaline—or nearer and nearer to acid—but there are several built-in mechanisms whereby the body maintains its pH 7·4 and eliminates the acid substances: the sulphates, urates and phosphates are excreted by the kidneys, and the carbon dioxide by the lungs.

If carbon dioxide is bubbled through water, some of it will be dissolved in the water, but some of it will react with the water to form carbonic acid. The carbonic acid dissociates to form ions of hydrogen and bicarbonate (HCO_3). Carbonic acid (H_2CO_3) is a weak acid which is volatile in the sense that it soon breaks up into water and carbon dioxide, the latter quickly dispersing into the atmosphere.

When hydrochloric acid is added to water, the water becomes a strong acid, dissociating into hydrogen and chloride ions. If sodium bicarbonate is dissolved in water the resultant solution dissociates into sodium and bicarbonate ions. If hydrochloric acid is added to the sodium bicarbonate, it produces the neutral salt sodium chloride and the weak acid carbonic acid which, being volatile, soon disperses into the atmosphere leaving water behind. The sodium ion linked with the chloride ion to form sodium chloride, while the hydrogen ion linked with bicarbonate to form carbonic acid. In the presence of bicarbonate, a strong acid is turned into a weak acid.

A similar reaction takes place when the sulphuric acid produced by the cells meets the sodium bicarbonate dissolved in the plasma, with the production of sodium sulphate and carbonic acid. The sulphate can be removed by the kidneys, the carbon dioxide of the carbonic acid by the lungs. The sodium, too, and the hydrogen ions can be removed by the kidneys. By converting the strong acid into the weak acid which is easily eliminated, the bicarbonate has protected the body from the adverse effects of the strong acid, and in this sense is said to have acted as a 'buffer' against it. A buffer has been described as a chemical substance which, when present in a solution, permits little or no change to occur in that solution when acid or alkali is added.

In its role as a chemical buffer, bicarbonate in the plasma protects against the acid products of metabolism, and in this sense is sometimes referred to as the 'alkali reserve'.

Other buffers are the plasma proteins which form proteinases and also the haemoglobin in the erythrocytes.

Carbon dioxide and bicarbonate

The tissue cells produce carbon dioxide as a product of metabolism. This diffuses through the tissue fluid and the capillary wall to the plasma, and then into the erythrocytes. In the erythrocytes an enzyme called carbonic anhydrase quickly combines the carbon dioxide with water to form carbonic acid. This dissociates into the ions of hydrogen and bicarbonate. The hydrogen links with, and is buffered by the haemoglobin which is losing its oxygen. The bicarbonate ion links with the potassium ion in the cell to balance the electrical charges. The bicarbonate ion moves out of the erythrocyte into the plasma, but, as will be remembered, the potassium remains inside the cell, leaving a tendency for an imbalanced electrolyte charge. To maintain the electrolyte balance inside the erythrocyte, chloride ions, which had been linked with the sodium ions in the plasma, move into the erythrocyte. The bicarbonate links with the sodium ion in the plasma, and there is thus a balanced ionized solution of potassium chloride in the erythrocyte and sodium bicarbonate in the plasma. This movement of the chloride ion into the erythrocyte is often referred to as the 'chloride shift'.

When the blood reaches the lungs, the changes take place in the reverse order. The bicarbonate ions move into the erythrocyte and the chloride ions move out into the plasma. In all this the chloride ions have been taking quite a passive, though necessary, part. The haemoglobin takes on oxygen and releases the hydrogen ion to do so. The hydrogen ion links with the bicarbonate to form carbonic acid. The carbonic anhydrase breaks up the carbonic acid into water and carbon dioxide. The carbon dioxide diffuses out of the erythrocyte into the plasma, and then into the alveoli for elimination from the body.

Thus it will be seen that bicarbonate plays an important part in the transport of carbon dioxide, as well as acting as a chemical buffer.

Under normal circumstances, with the plasma at a pH 7, the amount of bicarbonate ions in the plasma is between 21 and 30 mEq/litre. It is sometimes referred to as 'standard bicarbonate' and sometimes as 'alkali reserve'.

Acid-base balance and imbalance

The blood plasma is usually at a pH 7·4. As a result of the intake and the metabolism of foodstuffs, acid and alkali (base) substances, not necessarily in equal amounts, enter the bloodstream and are likely to upset the slight alkalinity of the plasma. It will be realized that the addition of acid (or base) to the plasma must be balanced by an equal addition of base (or acid as the case may be), if the pH 7·4 is to remain constant; or the additional acid or base ions must be removed from the plasma. In the body one can distinguish three mechanisms which take part in this acid–base balance:

1. As a result of metabolism, the tissues form large amounts of carbon dioxide and, to a lesser extent, acetoacetic, sulphuric and other acids. The first mechanism of the body to maintain the acid–base balance and the subsequent pH 7·4 is that the acids are taken on by the buffer systems of the body, of which mention has already been made. These are limited in the extent to which they can continue to be effective and can be thought of as a temporary measure.

2. The carbon dioxide which may be dissolved in the blood plasma or, as carbonic acid or as bicarbonate, will be carried to the lungs for elimination. This will be referred to again in conjunction with its importance in cardiovascular conditions.

3. Eventually the acids and bases produced by the metabolic processes, other than carbonic acid, will be eliminated by the kidneys. This renal process is somewhat complicated, involving the formation of carbonic acid in the renal tubules and the subsequent elimination or retention of electrolytes as the body requires. The process involves the use of a considerable amount of water, so that in cases of dehydration, there is always the possibility of acid–base disturbance being an additional difficulty.

Thus it can be seen that both the lungs and the kidneys are instrumental in maintaining the normal acid–base balance, and between them there is a degree of compensation, as will be seen later.

In cardiovascular disorders, the state of the acid–base balance can be estimated by analysis of the plasma, and is assessed by the relationship of (*a*) the actual pH, i.e. hydrogen ion content, (*b*) the partial pressure of carbon dioxide ($P\text{CO}_2$) which gives an indication of the quantity of carbon dioxide solution in the plasma and (*c*) the amount of bicarbonate in the plasma. When the amount of plasma bicarbonate is known, the amount which must be added or subtracted in order to restore it to the normal or standard bicarbonate can be assessed; this is known as 'base excess'. Under normal circumstances, the proportion of carbonic acid to bicarbonate in the plasma is in the ratio of 1:20.

Under normal circumstances, the buffers, the lungs and the kidneys maintain a constant pH 7·4, but in certain conditions may be unable to do so, as a result of which acid or alkali may collect in the blood.

Acidaemia and acidosis mean that there is an excess of acid substances (hydrogen ions) in the plasma, with a lowering of the pH. It can be considered as being of respiratory or metabolic origin.

Respiratory acidosis occurs when carbon dioxide is not being eliminated by the lungs and is accumulating in the body. This may happen when the patient is not breathing satisfactorily (hypoventilation) or when the eliminating process in the lungs is interfered with, as in pulmonary infection with bronchospasm. The patient becomes flushed and pink and if, in addition, there is anoxia he will become cyanosed. He becomes restless and confused, sweats and eventually may become comatose. The pulse rate rises and so does the blood pressure. Treatment is aimed at the cause. Any infection should be dealt with, secretions should be removed and bronchospasm relieved. Artificial ventilation may be required.

Metabolic acidosis occurs when the tissues are producing additional acids and when the kidneys are unable to remove acids in excess of requirements for the normal pH 7·4. Insufficient supply of oxygen to the tissue causes incomplete metabolism and the release of lactic and other acids. In diabetes mellitus ketone bodies are released in abnormally large amounts and at a rate too great for their oxidation. In renal failure, the kidneys may not be able to make carbonic acid and bicarbonate and so the release of hydrogen ions is interfered with. The tendency to compensate by the bicarbonate acting as a buffer to these acids brings about a reduction in the plasma bicarbonate. Direct loss of bicarbonate can occur in severe diarrhoea and when drugs such as acetazolamide are used. The increase of hydrogen ions in the blood stimulates the respiratory centre and respirations may become rapid and deep. The patient is restless and often confused. When there is an associated loss of water and other salts, as in diabetic ketosis, there may also be a fall in blood pressure with a rise in pulse rate. Treatment usually includes the administration of sodium bicarbonate intravenously, e.g. 100 ml of 8·4% sodium bicarbonate intravenously in the course of 15 minutes, repeated according to the results obtained on analysis of the blood content.

Alkalaemia and alkalosis mean that there is an accumulation of base (alkali) in the blood or a reduction in the acid (hydrogen ion) content, with a rise in the pH. It too can be considered as being of respiratory or metabolic origin.

Respiratory alkalosis occurs as a result of hyperventilation, which may be of emotional onset, as in the overbreathing of hysteria. It may be caused by a lesion of the central nervous system; it also tends to occur when a patient is having mechanically assisted ventilation. As a result of the overbreathing, excess amounts of carbon dioxide are removed from the plasma; the amount of bicarbonate may remain within normal limits, but the pH rises. The patient may complain of tinglings and numbness; he may develop tetany. Treatment is aimed at increasing the carbon dioxide tension of the alveolar air and thus of the plasma passing around the alveoli. When the onset is from emotional causes, the patient needs reassurance and is encouraged to try to be calm. Rebreathing into a paper bag helps. Occasionally sedation may also be required. If the patient is attached to a mechanical respirator, this will require the appropriate adjustments to be made.

Metabolic alkalosis may occur as a result of prolonged vomiting and continued gastric aspiration due to the loss of hydrochloric acid and of potassium, with resultant electrolyte imbalance. It may also occur as a result of the ingestion of large amounts of sodium bicarbonate and after rapid large blood transfusions. Respiration is diminished due to the raised pH failing to stimulate the respiratory centre; there may even be periods of apnoea in severe cases. Tetany may develop.

Treatment is aimed at restoring the body fluids to normal where depletion has occurred; this is associated with attempts to rectify the electrolyte balance. The intravenous administration of a solution containing sodium chloride, potassium chloride and ammonium chloride has been used in this connection.

An indication of the changes in the blood chemistry can be obtained from the following table which shows what happens when acidosis or alkalosis of respiratory or metabolic origin occur:

Condition	pH	*Standard bicarbonate*	P_{CO_2}
Respiratory acidosis	Down	Normal	Up
Metabolic acidosis	Down	Down	Normal
Respiratory alkalosis	Up	Normal	Down
Metabolic alkalosis	Up	Up	Normal

However it must be remembered that a metabolic acidosis will develop a compensatory respiratory alkalosis and vice versa. Several factors may be present in the same patient.

Chemistry of respiration

The need for oxygen

In order to live and perform work the tissues require energy, which they obtain from the oxidation of carbon and hydrogen in the food. The whole process by which they achieve this is termed metabolism. It is a complex process taking place as a series of changes, the end result of which is the liberation of energy and the production of carbon dioxide (CO_2) and water (H_2O) as waste products. The carbon dioxide is carried by the blood to the lungs where it is eliminated into the air. The water adds to the water content of the body, any excess being eliminated by the kidneys as urine. If the oxygen supply is insufficient, the cells are at first inactive and later die. The oxygen which originates in the outside (room) air, is breathed into the alveoli, passes into the blood in the capillaries surrounding the alveoli and is carried round the body to the tissue capillaries, where it passes out into the tissue fluid and then to the tissue cells. The ways in which these changes take place are worth consideration, as there is the possibility of interference at various stages.

Pressure or tension of gases

The molecules of a gas are continually moving at a high speed. If in a confined space they strike against the walls of the container: the more gas in the space the greater will be the total force with which the molecules are striking the walls; this is referred to as the pressure of the gas.

If a gas of high pressure is brought into contact with the same gas at a low pressure, molecules from the higher will move into the space occupied by the lower until the pressure of both is equal. This process is referred to as diffusion.

When there is a mixture of gases, each individual gas behaves as if it were the only one present, exerting its own pressure. The sum of pressures exerted by all the gases would be the total pressure of the mixture. The individual gas would exert only a part of the total pressure, hence the term 'partial pressure' when referring to the gases of respiration. At sea level, dry room air is at a total pressure (known as barometric pressure) of 760 mm Hg. The following table shows the approximate partial pressures of the component gases:

Gas	*Percentage in air*	*Partial pressure*
Oxygen	20·93%	160 mm Hg
Carbon dioxide	0·03%	Negligible
Nitrogen	79·04%	600 mm Hg
	100%	760 mm Hg

Gases in solution

When in contact with a water, the molecules of gas exert pressure on the surface of it and pass inside, i.e. are dissolved in it. The pressure of the gas molecule in the water will be the same as that in the air above it. Air is a mixture of gases; each of the component gases becomes dissolved in the water and each gas will exert its own partial pressure. The term sometimes used to indicate the partial pressure exerted by a gas is its tension and is expressed as P, e.g. Po_2 will express the partial pressure of oxygen.

The carriage of oxygen and carbon dioxide

The air in the alveoli of the lungs is separated from the blood by two thin layers of cells, through which diffusion of gases takes place. Oxygen passes from the alveoli into the blood and carbon dioxide from the blood into the alveoli, the extent and rate of the diffusion being determined by the differences in the partial pressures of those gases in the alveolar air and the blood. The composition and partial pressure of the alveolar air is as follows:

Gas	*Percentage in air*	*Partial pressure*	
Oxygen	14%	PO_2	100 mm Hg
Carbon dioxide	6%	PCO_2	40 mm Hg
Nitrogen	80%	PN_2	573 mm Hg
Water vapour	Saturated	PH_2O	47 mm Hg
	100%		760 mm Hg

It will be noticed that the proportion of oxygen and carbon dioxide in the alveolar air differs from that in atmospheric air or room air. This is because, after quietly breathing out, the respiratory tract and the lungs themselves still contain a quantity of air containing carbon dioxide. This is known as the 'dead space'. When the individual breathes in, the dead space air mixes with the additional room air, altering the proportion of the contents as indicated.

Replenishing the alveolar air with room air is most important, otherwise there would be insufficient partial pressure of oxygen, and that of carbon dioxide would increase beyond permitted limits. This can occur when there is insufficient intake of room air, as in obstruction of the respiratory tract, or when breathing is so shallow that the amount required to dilute the residual alveolar air is insufficient. Deep breathing, on the other hand, will increase the intake of room air and dilute the residual alveolar air, increasing the partial pressure of oxygen and lowering that of carbon dioxide. Thus, carbon dioxide will leave the blood and oxygen will enter more easily. The amount of blood circulating through the lungs must be sufficient to bring the carbon dioxide for elimination and to take away the oxygen required for metabolism. This is interfered with in pulmonary hypertension, when changes take place in the blood vessels. When areas of the lungs are collapsed or when there are secretions present in the alveoli, the quantity of air may be insufficient to supply the oxygen requirements and take away the carbon dioxide eliminated.

As the blood leaves the alveoli, the oxygen in it is at a partial pressure of 100 mm Hg, the same as that of alveolar air. When it reaches the tissues it is still at the same partial pressure. Only a thin layer of cells separates the blood in the tissue capillaries from the tissue fluid. The partial pressure of oxygen in the tissue fluid is low—40 mm Hg—because the tissues have been using it in the process of metabolism. Because of the difference in partial pressures, oxygen diffuses out of the blood and into the tissue fluid,

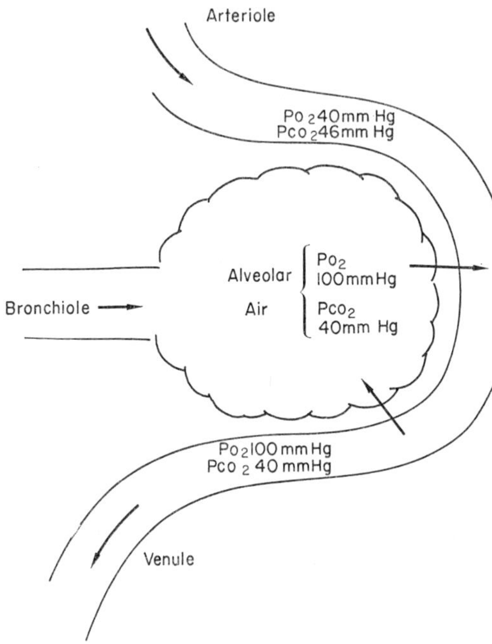

FIG **102. Gas exchange in the alveoli.**

until the pressure in the blood has fallen to 40 mm Hg, i.e. the same as that of the tissue fluid. With oxygen at a partial pressure of 40 mm Hg the blood returns along the veins to the heart and then to the lungs, where it comes into contact with the alveoli, in which the air is at the partial pressure of 100 mm Hg. Diffusion of oxygen again takes place until the two partial pressures are equal. The uptake of oxygen by the blood can be facilitated if the oxygen pressure in the alveoli is increased, as for example, by the administration of oxygen.

Diffusion of carbon dioxide takes place along similar lines but in the reverse direction. The partial pressure of carbon dioxide in the alveolar air is 40 mm Hg and this is the pressure in the blood when it reaches the tissues. The partial pressure of carbon dioxide in the tissue fluid is 46 mm Hg, so diffusion takes place into the blood until equilibrium is reached. Blood returns via the veins and the heart to the lungs, where it comes into contact with alveolar air, in which the partial pressure of carbon dioxide is 40 mm Hg. Carbon dioxide diffuses out of the blood into the air until equilibrium is reached.

The partial pressure (tension) of the gases in blood can be estimated in the laboratory. Blood is taken from an artery using a heparinized syringe, but care must be taken that the blood is not exposed to air, as this would alter the partial pressures.

The quantity of oxygen carried by the blood depends upon the ability of oxygen to combine with haemoglobin. When haemoglobin has associated or combined with oxygen it is referred to as oxyhaemoglobin and is bright red in colour. Dissociation of the oxygen from the oxyhaemoglobin leaves reduced haemoglobin which is darker in colour.

When haemoglobin has combined with all the oxygen it is able to combine with, it is said to be saturated. When oxygen is at a partial pressure of 100 mm Hg, as is found in alveoli air, the amount taken up is almost at the maximum, and the oxyhaemoglobin is in the region of 95–97% saturation capacity.

In a person who has the average amount of 15 g of haemoglobin in 100 ml of blood, there would be some 19 ml of oxygen in the 100 ml of blood leaving the lungs and passing along the arteries to the tissues.

In venous blood returning from the tissues to the lungs, the oxygen is at a partial pressure of 40 mm Hg but there would be 14 ml of oxygen in every 100 ml of the blood. That is, it would be still holding oxygen to 70% of its saturation capacity. Although the oxygen tension in the blood and in the tissue fluid was equalized, there is still, as it were, a reserve of oxygen associated with the haemoglobin after the blood has left the tissues. Should the tissues be more active, using up more oxygen and producing a rise in the carbon dioxide (carbonic acid) content and/or a rise in temperature of the tissue fluid, a greater amount of oxygen will dissociate from the oxyhaemoglobin and this dissociation will also be more rapid.

However, once the partial pressure of the oxygen is below 50 mm Hg there is a rapid fall in the quantity or percentage of saturation capacity. A graph showing the changes in the relationship between the oxygen capacity (saturation) and the partial pressure in the blood is called the 'oxygen dissociation curve'.

It is often a matter of surprise that the blood contains more

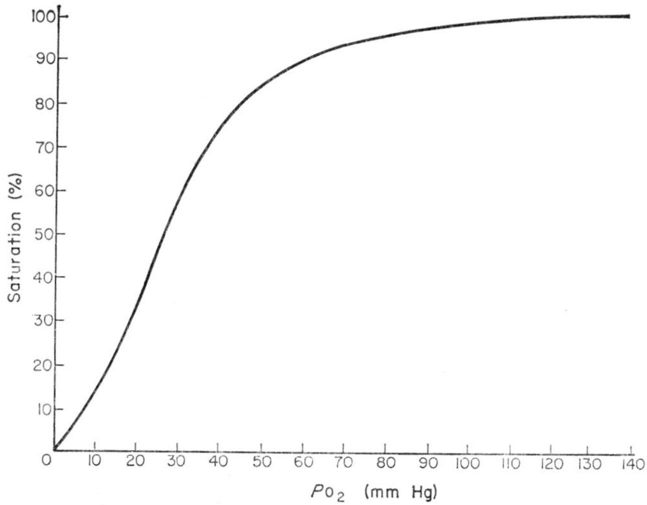

FIG **103. Oxyhaemoglobin dissociation curve at 38° C, pH 7·4.**

carbon dioxide than it does oxygen. Leaving the lungs the blood contains 19 ml of oxygen but 40 ml of carbon dioxide in every 100 ml of blood. Leaving the tissues on its return to the lungs, the figures are 14 ml oxygen and 52 ml carbon dioxide. The reason for this is that carbon dioxide is more than a waste product; much of it is converted into carbonic acid and into bicarbonate, thus participating in the acid–base balance of the blood.

Breathing—the stimulus

The action of breathing takes place on the reception by the appropriate muscles of nerve impulses from the respiratory centre situated in the medulla oblongata. The respiratory centre is influenced by several factors, but the most important are the pH (hydrogen ion content) of the blood and the level of carbon dioxide of the blood. Should there be a rise in the carbon dioxide content or of the hydrogen ion content (pH) it is stimulated and breathing takes place, the effect of which is that more room air will enter the alveoli, the carbon dioxide content of the alveolar air will be decreased and carbon dioxide will leave the blood until an equilibrium between its partial pressures in the air and in the blood has been formed. On the other hand, if the carbon dioxide content of the blood is diminished there will be less stimulus to the respiratory centre and breathing will also be diminished until the carbon dioxide content of the blood reaches its usual level. It should be noted that if the respiratory centre is subjected to a high level of carbon dioxide for a long period, it becomes insensitive to the carbon dioxide and breathing will not be stimulated by it. A slight reduction in oxygen content of the blood (hypoxia) will then stimulate chemoreceptors situated in the carotid bodies to send impulses to the respiratory centre which will, in its turn, send out impulses resulting in breathing. However, if the shortage of oxygen is severe, the respiratory centre itself will become depressed by the shortage, so that impulses from the chemoreceptors will have no effect. This is why, in chronic respiratory failure, when the respiratory centre becomes insensitive to the prolonged high carbon dioxide level, respiration is stimulated by the slight hypoxia, so that if a high concentration of oxygen is administered it will remove the hypoxia and thus the stimulus to respiration, resulting in hypoventilation and even apnoea. To avoid this, calculated regulated amounts of oxygen between 20 and 30% can be given using a Venturi mask, so that carbon dioxide can be allowed to escape and a slight level of oxygen lack maintained at the same time.

Cholesterol

This is a steroid, that is a physiological compound based on a hydrocarbon structure, found in most tissues as free cholesterol or combined with fatty acids. It seems to be mainly formed in the liver, but it is also taken in when eating eggs, animal fats (saturated fats), liver, kidney and brain. It is excreted in bile. Cholesterol plays some part in the formation of the cell membrane, where it is found in conjunction with other lipids (fatty substances), and it is a precursor of bile salts and acids, oestrogens, corticosteroids and the ergosterol in the skin from which vitamin D is made.

Usually there are 100- 250 mg/100 ml of blood, but the amount seems to be determined by the amount of animal (saturated) fat in the diet—the higher the intake of animal fat, the higher the amount of cholesterol and lipids in the blood (hyperlipidaemia).

Atherosclerosis is characterized by the deposition of large amounts of cholesterol in the walls of the arteries. Patients with atherosclerosis and coronary artery disease sometimes have high levels of cholesterol in the blood, and these conditions are common among those whose diet includes a high amount of animal fat. Those whose diet contains a small amount of animal (saturated) fat but more vegetable and fish oils (non-saturated fats) seem to have normal cholesterol levels and few seem to suffer from coronary artery disease. It is not always agreed that there is any connection between a diet high in animal fat, high cholesterol levels and coronary artery disease. Attempts have been made to lower the level of cholesterol in the blood by dietary means and by drugs such as clofibrate.

Plasma proteins

In the average person the total plasma proteins are 6–8 g/100 ml of blood. Analysis shows the following differentiations:

Albumin	3·5–5·5 g
Globulin	1·5–3·0 g
Fibrinogen	0·2–0·4 g

Collectively the plasma proteins act as a reserve supply of protein readily available for transformation into the other tissue proteins in times of starvation. They exert an osmotic pressure of 25 mm Hg necessary for the formation and reabsorption of tissue fluid; in this albumin seems to play the greater part. They are capable of buffering both acids and alkalis. They increase the viscosity of the blood, thus necessitating that an adequate blood pressure is maintained. They act as a transport media for bilirubin, certain hormones and antibodies, globulin playing the greater part in the latter. Fibrinogen is necessary for the clotting of blood.

Albumin, the smallest of the plasma proteins, is made in the liver. Globulin, of which there are three fractions, namely α, β and γ, is probably made in the reticulo-endothelial system and lymphatic tissue.

The ratio of albumin to globulin is important and under usual circumstances is 1·7:1. The ratio is reversed in liver diseases due to the reduction of albumin formation by that organ.

A fall in total plasma, proteins, especially albumin, will lower the osmotic pressure of the plasma, leading to the diffusion of fluid from the plasma into the tissue spaces, resulting in oedema, and in a low blood pressure.

Should the membrane of the glomeruli of the kidney be damaged, albumin, being the smallest protein, will easily pass into Bowman's capsule and thence into the uriniferous tubule, and appear in the urine. Similarly, if the capillaries of the tissues are damaged or injured, albumin leaks into the surrounding tissue space causing localized oedema of inflammatory response. Perhaps it is because of this that there is a reduction of the albumin in the plasma protein after injury.

Laboratory tests can be made to estimate the quantity of plasma proteins and also the albumin/globulin ratio.

Transaminase

The transaminases are enzymes by means of which changes take place in the amino acids.

The body proteins are built up from some 20 amino acids. It is essential that 10 of these be taken in the diet, hence they are called 'essential amino acids', and from these, after changes in their structure, the remaining amino acids (non-essential) can be formed. The tissues are continually deteriorating and being broken down into amino acids, some of which may be used again to form other amino acids or other proteins, but some of them will be further broken down and will be converted in the liver into urea for excretion by the kidney (see below). Excess amino acids are not stored in the body, but are broken down and eliminated as urea.

For these changes in amino acids to take place, the enzymes transaminases are necessary. Those which are commonly met with in cardiovascular work are *serum glutamic oxaloacetic transaminase* (SGOT), of which under normal circumstances there are some 5–30 Karmen units in 100 ml of blood, and *serum glutamic pyruvic transaminase* (SGPT), of which there are up to 25 Karmen units.

As some protein is always being broken down, some transaminase is always present in the blood. However, if large amounts of tissue (and therefore of its proteins) are being broken down, the amount of transaminase needed will increase, and thus the amount in the blood will be raised. While this occurs in damage to liver, pancreas, kidney and skeletal muscle, it is particularly noticeable when metabolically active tissue such as the myocardium is breaking down.

When a patient suffers a myocardial infarction, the levels of serum transaminase will be estimated at the onset, and during the course of the condition. From the first to the fourth day following the infarction the SGOT and the SGPT are elevated.

Lactic dehydrogenase (LDH), normally 100–400 units, is also elevated following myocardial infarction, but for longer periods. This is an enzyme which brings about oxidation of lactic acid, not by the addition of oxygen, but by the loss of hydrogen, a process which is necessary when the supply of oxygen is depleted, as in infarction.

Urea

In the deamination of amino acids, the amino (NH_2) part is separated from the acid (COOH) part. The acid part is oxidized to produce heat and energy, leaving water and carbon dioxide as waste products. The amino part is converted into ammonia (NH_3). In the liver the ammonia is converted into urea ($CO(NH_2)_2$), which is taken by the blood to the kidney for elimination.

Under normal circumstances it is eliminated by the kidney, which maintains the usual amount of from 20 to 40 mg/100 ml of blood.

For about a week after injury (including surgery), there is increased breakdown of body proteins, but provided its function is not impaired the kidney can eliminate the increased amount of urea formed, keeping the urea level in the blood within normal limits.

The elimination of urea by the kidney depends upon the rate of filtration in the glomeruli, and will be adequate providing that more than 30% of the normal glomerular filtration rate is present—that is, roughly, if more than a half of one kidney is working normally—below which the urea cannot be eliminated and the amount in the blood will rise.

Interference with glomerular filtration occurs if there is insufficient blood flowing through the kidney, as happens when the blood pressure is low or when there is narrowing or constriction of the blood vessels to and in the kidney. The functioning of the glomeruli themselves may be impaired as a result of hypoxia due to insufficiency of oxygenated blood or to renal disease such as nephritis.

Estimation of the amount of urea in the blood is made in the laboratory and the result will give an indication of the functioning of the kidney. A more accurate indication will be obtained if an estimation is also made of the amount of urea in the urine, as well as the measurement of the amount of urine passed as compared with the fluid intake during the previous 24 hours.

Bleeding and clotting

Bleeding or haemorrhage occurs when blood escapes from the blood vessels, and if it continues will result in exsanguination and death. Clotting or coagulation is a process which takes place in the plasma and is one of the ways in which the body prevents the loss of blood.

When the escape of blood is small, as in a pin-prick, a cluster of platelets will stick together near the point at which the blood is escaping; they will release serotonin, which causes vasoconstriction and reduces the bleeding, and may together form a plug preventing blood leaving the capillary. After such a pin-prick it takes 2–6 min for the bleeding to stop: this is referred to as the bleeding time.

Larger amounts of blood form a clot, which is a network of fibrin fibres entrapping the blood cells, the fibrin network gradually shrinking and squeezing out the fluid, which is now called serum.

Blood in a glass dish takes less than 10 minutes to form a clot; this is termed clotting time.

Clotting of blood is a complex process, much of which is still not completely understood (Fig. 104). The following is the theory at present accepted. When tissue is damaged or blood shed, the tissue cells and the blood platelets release thromboplastin (thrombokinase). The formation of thromboplastin is itself a complicated

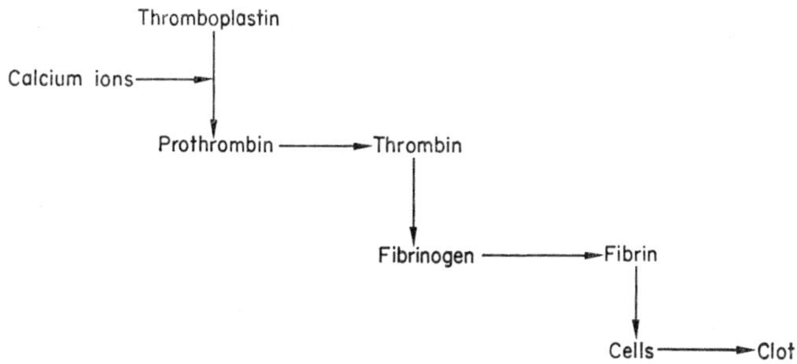

FIG 104. The mechanism of the clot formation.
Thromboplastin, released by the platelets in the presence of calcium ions, acts upon prothrombin, converting it into thrombin. The thrombin in turn acts upon fibrinogen, converting it into fibrin, which entraps cells in the blood, causing a clot.

process. The thromboplastin in the presence of calcium ions converts prothrombin (already in the plasma, having been formed in the liver) into thrombin. The thrombin acts upon the soluble protein fibrinogen converting it into strands of fibrin. The fibrin strands form a net which, as it shrinks, traps the blood cells forming a red jelly-like mass called the clot. The clot sticks to the tissues and prevents any further loss of blood. The fluid squeezed out is called serum and is the same as plasma except that the fibrinogen has been removed.

The blood in the circulation does not clot, partly because it is moving along the vessels with a smooth lining and partly because of the presence of heparin in the plasma which prevents the formation of thrombin and of fibrin.

If the walls of the vessels are damaged or roughened, platelets may gather at the roughened site, release thromboplastin and eventually form a clot. The clot in the vessels is referred to as a thrombus, and the thrombus formation as thrombosis. The clot may become dislodged and travel in the blood stream as an embolus, and eventually it may block an artery causing infarction (as in coronary thrombosis and myocardial infarction).

In some people there is a defect in the formation of thromboplastin, giving rise to disorders such as haemophilia and Christmas disease. They are apt to sustain severe haemorrhage from even a small cut and it is hazardous for them to undergo surgery. Clotting can be prevented by the administration of anticoagulants such as heparin. It is given intravenously; the doctor orders the dose to be given, e.g. 10 000 units, initially and this is followed by smaller amounts at intervals of 4–5 hours. Should it be necessary an injection of protamine sulphate may be given to neutralize the effects.

Anticoagulants such as dicoumarol, phenindione and warfarin may be given orally. They act by preventing the formation of prothrombin in the liver. The dose ordered by the doctor depends on the prothrombin time or prothrombin content in the blood. Vitamin K, necessary for the formation of prothrombin, is absorbed from the small intestine in the presence of bile salts. To counteract the effects of oral anticoagulants, phytomenadione or Vitamin K may be given.

When anticoagulants are being given, observations should be made for signs of bleeding from the kidney (haematuria), into the skin (purpura) and from internal organs.

When blood is taken for transfusion purposes, a preparation containing citrate is added, which combines with the calcium ions so that thromboplastin is unable to act upon prothrombin and coagulation is prevented.

Clotting can be speeded up by the addition of thromboplastin or thrombin. These are sometimes used on bleeding surfaces, as are other substances such as fibrin foam and oxidized cellulose.

Fibrinolysin is an enzyme which dissolves fibrin. Plasmin is a fibrinolysin which dissolves the fibrin fibres in blood clots. Plasminogen is its precursor found in the plasma, and can be activated by streptokinase from streptococcal infection and by urokinase from urine, to form plasmin. Purified streptokinase has been given to stimulate the formation of plasmin and thus prevent clotting and to dissolve clot which has formed in a blood vessel, thus allowing the circulation of blood through it.

On the other hand, an increased production of plasmin may, by preventing clot formation, result in further bleeding. When the tendency to bleed is due to increased plasmin, aminocaproic acid may be administered orally or by intravenous infusion. This will inhibit the formation of plasmin, prevent the breakdown of fibrin and thus indirectly assist clotting.

The cardiac cycle

The term cardiac cycle (Fig. 105) is used to denote the series of events which happen in the heart from one point in a heart beat to the same point in the next. For convenience one can follow these events from the moment of cessation of systole and commencement of diastole of the ventricles.

At this point the ventricles are in the contracted (i.e. smaller) state, having ejected most, if not all, of the blood they contained into the great vessels. The pressure of the blood in the aorta and pulmonary artery closes the semilunar valves (aortic and pulmonary), preventing the blood from flowing back into the ventricles.

Blood from the superior and inferior venae cavae on the right and from the four pulmonary veins on the left pours into the atria, through the atrioventricular valves (tricuspid and mitral) and into the ventricles. As the blood enters the ventricles the walls are stretched to the full position. Eddies in the current of blood flow lift up the atrioventricular valves almost to the closed position. Both the atria and the ventricles are now filled with blood.

The sinu-atrial node or pacemaker causes the adjacent cardiac muscle fibres to contract. The impulse spreads over both atria and the contraction which follows presses the blood through the atrioventricular valves into the ventricles. Both atria contract simultaneously, the whole contraction, atrial systole, taking 0·1 second to complete.

The impulse causing the wave of contraction stops at the ring of fibrous tissue which separates the walls of the atria from the walls of the ventricles. The atrioventricular node, situated in the wall of the atria, picks up the stimulus and transmits it down the atrioventricular bundle of His. This modified cardiac muscle runs down the septum between the ventricles, giving off branches to both ventricles.

During the period of atrial systole, the ventricles are relaxed, but as the stimulus passing down the atrioventricular bundles of

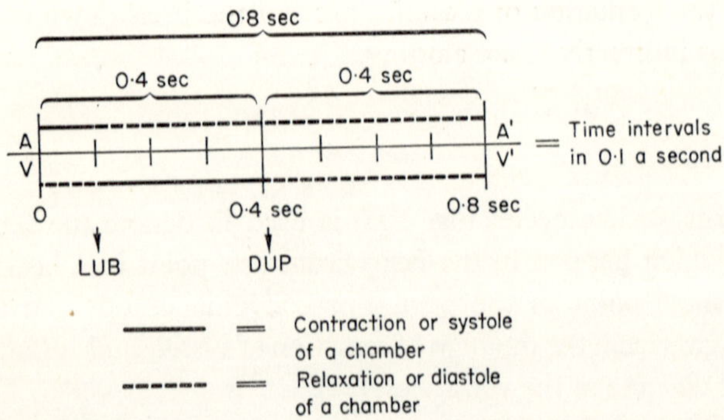

FIG 105. The sequence of events in the cardiac cycle.
A-A[1], The contraction and relaxation of the atrium. V-V[1], The contraction and relaxation of the ventricle. The cycle occupies 0·8 sec, of which 0·4 sec are occupied by the contraction of both atria and ventricles, and the remaining 0·4 sec by relaxation of all chambers of the heart. Note that 0·8 sec is the time of 1 beat if the pulse rate is 72/min.

His reaches them, they contract simultaneously. The rise in pressure closes the atrioventricular valves. The ventricles continue to contract, increasing the pressure of the blood inside until it is greater than that of the blood in the aorta (about 80 mm Hg) and in the pulmonary artery (about 15 mm Hg). The pressure in the left ventricle will probably reach a height of 120 mm Hg, while that of the right ventricle will probably reach a height of 25 mm Hg. The semilunar valves are then forced open and the blood in the ventricles ejected. Having completed the contraction the ventricles relax, the pressure inside falling to about 0 mm Hg.

The walls of the aorta and pulmonary arteries contain a considerable amount of elastic tissue which stretches as the blood is forced out of the ventricle into the vessel, thus allowing it to accommodate the sudden increase of content. The elastic tissue then recoils, pressing on the blood. This increased pressure pushes the blood.

The ventricles have relaxed and no more blood is being ejected, so the blood in the vessels tends to rush back into the ventricle. However, the aortic and pulmonary valves close, thus preventing the blood from re-entering the ventricles. Both ventricles contract together (ventricular systole), taking 0·3 sec to do so.

By now the blood is already flowing through the atria into the ventricles, thus commencing another cardiac cycle.

The heart beats, that is the cardiac cycle takes place, about 70 times in 1 min in the healthy adult, so that each beat (or cycle) takes 0·8 sec to complete. The atrial systole occupies 0·1 sec, the ventricular systole occupies 0·3 sec, thus the remaining 0·4 sec is for the period of diastole or relaxation. When the heart beats faster than 70 times/min, each beat (cycle) occupies the same 0·4 sec, but the period of diastole or relaxation is reduced.

Cardiac output

The function of the heart is to maintain a constant flow of blood throughout the body. The blood circulates from the heart, round the body, back to the heart, through the heart to the lungs, back to the heart, through the heart and out to the body once again. Thus it will be realized that the amount of blood pumped out of the heart can only equal the amount of blood which has entered. If more blood returns to the heart, the heart must also put out more, and if less returns there is less to pump out.

In health and at rest the heart beats about 70 times/min; this is referred to as the heart rate. At each beat, each ventricle ejects 70 ml of blood; this is referred to as the stroke volume. Thus it will be seen that in the space of one minute, 70 beats ejecting 70 ml of blood will mean that the heart has put out, from each ventricle, 4900 ml of blood. This is referred to as the cardiac output. The formula for calculating the cardiac output is:

Heart Rate × Stroke Volume = Cardiac Output.

Heart rate

In the first place the rate at which the heart beats is determined by the inherent rhythmicity of the sinu-atrial node (or pacemaker), from which the cardiac muscle fibres conduct the wave of contraction which spreads to the whole of both atria.

The sinu-atrial node is influenced by several factors:

1. The cardiac centre in the medulla oblongata, from which the nerve impulses via the vagus nerve slow down the heart rate (vagal inhibition), and also from which nerve impulses via the sympathetic nerves increase the heart rate (sympathetic stimulation). The cardiac centre itself is influenced by:

   a. The higher centres of the brain, e.g. emotional stress which usually causes an increased rate.
   b. The baroreceptors, e.g. a fall in blood pressure is followed by a rise in heart rate.
   c. Oxygen lack and carbon dioxide excess, both of which cause a rise in heart rate.

2. Sensory nerves associated with pain, e.g. a fair amount of pain increases the heart rate, but severe pain may slow it down.

3. The temperature of the blood entering the right atrium, e.g. a rise in temperature causes an increase in heart rate, whereas a subnormal temperature tends to slow it down.

4. The presence in the blood of hormones such as (*a*) adrenaline and noradrenaline from the adrenal gland and (*b*) thyroxin from the thyroid gland, both of which increase the heart rate.

Stroke volume

The amount of blood ejected from each ventricle when it contracts is referred to as the stroke volume and, if the individual is resting, it is usually 70 ml. Contraction of the ventricle does not necessarily mean its complete emptying.

The stroke volume depends very much upon the amount of blood returning to the heart. If the amount entering the ventricle is large, the walls of the ventricle will be distended and the muscle fibres lengthened. This is followed by a more forceful contraction and thus the ejection of more blood; for example, in a young man taking exercise, it can be as much as 200 ml. This is the essence of the law of the heart, formulated by the physiologist Starling (1914), that 'the energy of contraction is proportional to the initial length of the cardiac muscle fibres.'

Sympathetic stimulation also causes a stronger contraction, leading to more complete emptying of the ventricle.

On the other hand, if less blood returns to the heart, there is less to pump out, and the contraction is less forceful. This is often seen after severe haemorrhage, when the pulse can be felt to be weak and thready. If the stroke volume is low, the blood pressure in the arteries will most probably be low, the baroreceptors will affect the cardiac centre, and there will be rise in the rate at which the heart beats, as part of the compensatory mechanism to maintain an adequate arterial pressure.

Blood flow and velocity in the vessels

From the heart the blood is ejected at each ventricular systole, so that its flow along the great arteries is somewhat intermittent and, if such an artery is severed, the blood escapes in spurts. In the capillaries, where changes take place between the blood and the tissue fluid, the flow is in a steady and continuous stream.

In the aorta, the blood flows rapidly at a speed of 0·4 m/sec. In a capillary, the rate of flow is 0·5 mm/sec. In the veins it gradually speeds up until the rate at which it enters the heart will be the same as that at which it leaves it, it being remembered that the amount of blood leaving the heart is the same as that entering.

In order to understand the reason for this considerable change in both speed and manner of flow, one might compare it with water flowing from a river entering a lake, passing through the lake and out by a river at the far end (Fig. 106). The water in the river entering will be the same in amount as that leaving the lake. The water in the river entering will be doing so at quite a rapid rate. As it enters the lake, it meets the water already there, and begins to slow down. The rate at which the water flows across the lake will depend upon the size of the lake: if it is wide the flow will be slow, whereas if it is narrow the flow will be somewhat quicker. As it reaches the far end of the lake, the water is pushed by the water flowing from behind it and, as the width of the lake gets smaller, the speed gradually increases until it is flowing out of the lake as fast as the water is doing in the river entering.

In the circulation the artery is like the river entering, the vein is like the river leaving. The capillaries are like the lake, indeed sometimes they are referred to as the 'capillary lake', except that whereas the water in the lake flows freely, the blood is flowing through millions of small tubes, i.e. capillaries. A cross-section of the aorta shows its diameter to be about 3 cm. As the blood flows into the branches and out into the capillary lake, the passage is

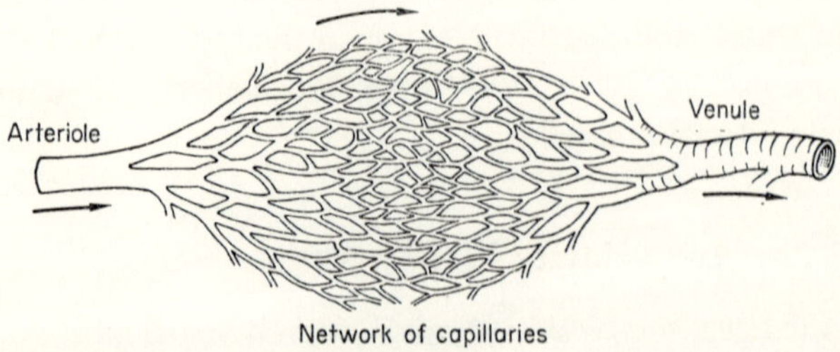

FIG **106. The effect of a 'capillary lake' on the velocity of blood flow.**
The area of cross-section of the capillaries is greater than that of the arteriole.

broader, the flow is reduced in speed. Under normal circumstances the body regulates the flow at 0·5 mm/sec in the capillaries. However, if for any reason the vessels become dilated, or too many vessels become dilated, the total width of the capillary lake would be broader and the flow would be even further slowed down, until the blood might tend to 'stagnate' and not be returned to the heart. After leaving the capillaries the blood passes via the small veins into the larger ones, but the total cross-section of these vessels gets narrower, so that the flow gets quicker.

Blood pressure in the vessels

The importance of an adequate arterial blood pressure and the means by which the body maintains it are discussed under hypertension (p. 179). The objective of this section is to compare the pressure of blood at various points in the circulation.

Blood is ejected by the left ventricle into the aorta at a pressure of 120 mm Hg. By their elasticity the large arteries adjust to accommodate to the input of blood and they recoil, pushing the blood forwards; after this the pressure has usually fallen to 80 mm

Hg before the heart beats once more. Thus in the arteries the mean pressure is 100 mm Hg.

As blood flows from one larger artery to many small arteries it gradually slows down in speed and also drops slightly in pressure. By the time it has reached the arterioles, the branching of the vessels is greatly increased and the pressure of the blood in them is greatly decreased until, by the time the blood reaches the capillaries, the pressure is 32 mm Hg. At the proximal end of the

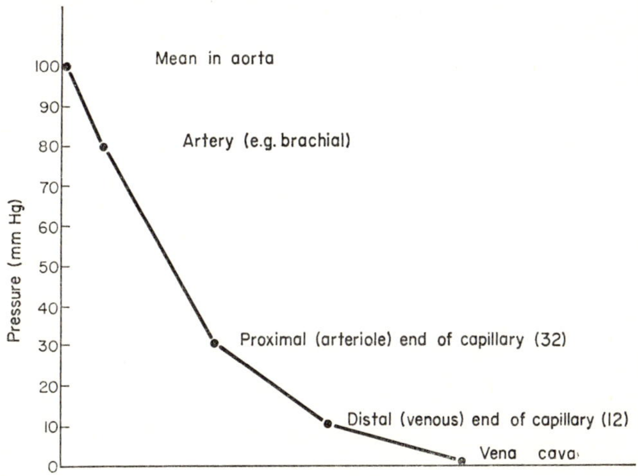

FIG **107. Pressure in the systemic vessels.**

capillary this pressure of 32 mm Hg, known as the hydrostatic pressure, is sufficient to force fluid out through the capillary wall into the tissue spaces, thus forming tissue fluid. The blood passes along the capillary in a steady flow until, at the distal end, the pressure is reduced to 12 mm Hg. When the osmotic pressure (25 mm Hg) exerted by the plasma proteins exceeds the falling hydrostatic pressure of the blood in the capillary, part of the tissue fluid is attracted back into the blood stream, the rest remaining as tissue fluid or returning via the lymphatics. The blood thus leaves the capillaries at a pressure of 12 mm Hg. After leaving the capillaries the blood flows along the veins into the large veins. It flows more quickly but the pressure is even lower. In the veins the pressure is measured in centimetres (cm) of water (H_2O), and not

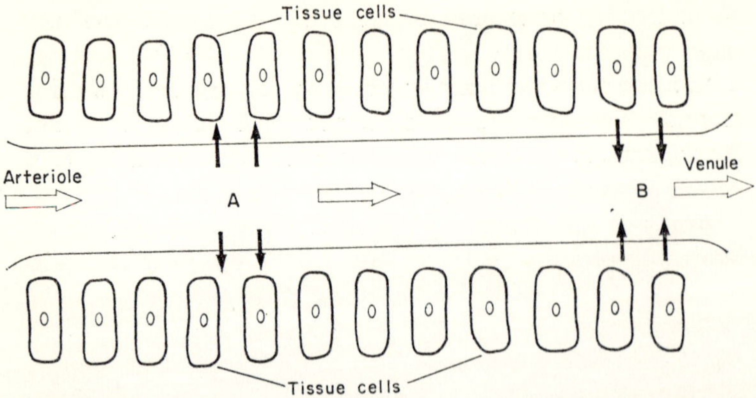

FIG 108. The changes in pressure as blood passes along the capillary, and the formation of tissue fluid and its return to the blood stream.
At point A the blood pressure is 32 mm Hg and the osmotic pressure 25 mm Hg, therefore fluid is forced out. At point B the blood pressure is 12 mm Hg and the osmotic pressure 25 mm Hg, therefore fluid is attracted in.

of mercury (Hg). The pressure in the peripheral veins may be from 6 to 10 cm H_2O, this pressure falling as the blood passes into the larger and more central veins, until at the entrance to the right atrium it may be as low as 0·5 cm H_2O. This small pressure is sufficient to stimulate the heart into contracting and ejecting the usual stroke volume. In practice the central venous pressure is usually measured by passing a cannula 60 cm (24 in) long through one of the peripheral veins of the arm as far as the subclavian vein or even the superior vena cava. As with arterial blood pressure, for clinical purposes it is not so much the exact pressure which matters, but rather whether it is rising or falling and how this fits in is associated with the clinical condition of the patient.

Observations can be made on the jugular vein in the neck. Gravity draws the blood to the lower (cardiac) end of the vein, the upper part remaining emptied and collapsed. When the individual is lying at rest and at an angle of 45°, the lower end can be seen to be distended usually for not more than 2–3 cm above the sternal angle, if the blood cannot enter the right atrium, distension of the vein can be seen at higher levels. The vein may also be seen to pulsate at each contraction of the atrium.

As indicated, the pressure at which the blood enters the right atrium, although low, is sufficient to stimulate the heart into contracting, a high venous pressure is caused by the heart failing to pump the blood forwards. If this condition continues over a long period of time, the heart may become dependent on this abnormally high venous pressure to stimulate it into contraction.

When such a patient has an open heart operation, it may be necessary to maintain the venous pressure at an abnormally high level until it regains the ability to be stimulated by a normal pressure.

If the right side of the heart is unable to pump the blood from the venae cavae forward into the pulmonary artery, the blood will collect in the veins and eventually back into the capillaries. This interferes with the flow of blood out of the capillaries, and also causes an increase in the pressure at the distal (venous) end. When this rise in pressure is greater than the osmotic pressure of the plasma proteins (25 mm Hg), water will not be attracted back into the capillary, but will remain in the tissue spaces, causing oedema.

The venous return

Blood is pumped by the heart along the arteries and arterioles. The walls of the latter determine the blood pressure by their state of constriction or dilatation. However, at any one time, about two-thirds of the blood in the general circulation is in the veins.

Veins have a similar structure to the arteries except that the tunica media is much smaller; thus the walls of the veins are comparatively thin and the vessel easily collapses if empty or can easily distend when filled. The muscle layer is under the influence of the sympathetic nervous system, which maintains a degree of muscular tone thus preventing the distension of the veins. Distension of the veins would lead to a pooling of blood in them thus reducing the amount in the circulation, and with less blood returning to the heart there would be smaller stroke volume and lower cardiac output.

Several mechanisms are known to take part in ensuring the return of venous blood to the heart (Fig. 109):

1. *Valves* are found in the walls of the veins in the lower limbs

which permit the blood to flow in the direction of the heart only.

2. Nearby *skeletal muscles*, alternately contracting and relaxing as in exercise or movement such as walking, squeeze on the veins, compressing the thin walls and forcing the blood to move. Because

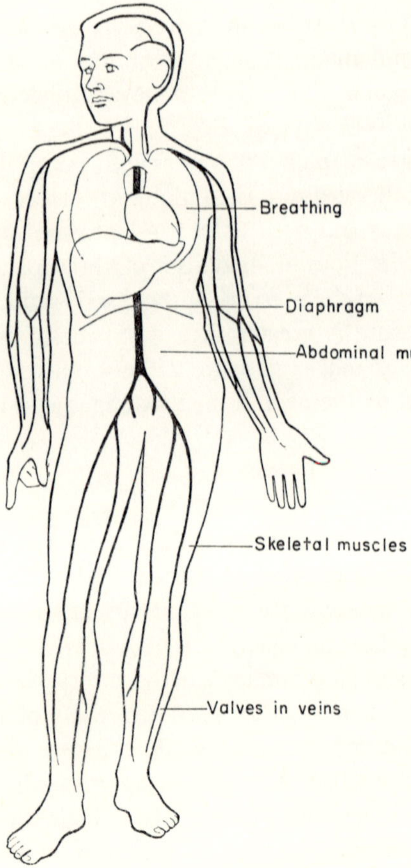

FIG **109. Factors affecting the venous return.**

of the valves it can move in the direction of the heart only. The mechanism is sometimes referred to as the 'muscle pump'.

3. *Muscles of the abdominal wall*, by supporting the abdomen, also cause pressure on the veins of the abdomen, preventing their distension with blood when in the upright position, e.g. standing.

4. *Breathing* brings about changes of pressure in the thorax. The intrathoracic pressure is always a little below atmospheric pressure, but fluctuates between −2·5 mm Hg on expiration and −6 mm Hg on inspiration. This intrathoracic 'negative' pressure acts as a suction pump pulling the blood up the abdominal veins and into the thorax where very quickly it is poured into the right atrium.

During inspiration the diaphragm contracts and presses downwards on to the abdominal cavity, increasing the intra-abdominal pressure. The pressure on the abdominal veins forces the blood upwards, as the valves in the veins of the lower limb prevent it from flowing downwards.

Thus breathing has both a force and a suction effect in pumping the venous blood back to the heart.

Pulmonary pressures

At systole, the right ventricle ejects blood into the pulmonary artery at a pressure of 25 mm Hg, a much lower pressure than that of the left ventricle, which is 120 mm Hg. The stroke volume of both ventricles is the same, 70 ml.

The pressure of the blood in the pulmonary artery is 25 mm Hg at systole, falling to 8 mm Hg in diastole. It falls a little on inspiration and rises a little on expiration. The walls of the aterioles are thin and easily distended, offering little resistance to the blood flow, in contradistinction to those of the systemic circulation. The blood flows at the same rate as in the aorta, 0·4 m/sec, a total of 5 litres/min while at rest, rising to 30 litres/min on exercise.

The arterioles are supplied with sympathetic nerve fibres, but the extent of vasoconstriction is less than in the systemic circulation.

The pressure in the pulmonary capillaries is 10 mm Hg, compared to 32 mm Hg in the systemic capillaries. It is measured by passing a thin catheter through the right side of the heart and along the pulmonary artery until it is 'wedged' and occludes one of the pulmonary arterioles.

Although the pressure is less than that of the capillaries in the systemic circulation, it is adequate, because there is little space between the tissues in the lungs, and no tissue fluid is formed.

The pressure of the blood in the pulmonary veins is about 5 mm water, depending upon the pressure and flow throughout the left atrium.

When the left side of the heart is unable to transfer blood from the pulmonary veins to the aorta, the excess blood may collect in the left atrium, and also in the pulmonary veins, making it difficult

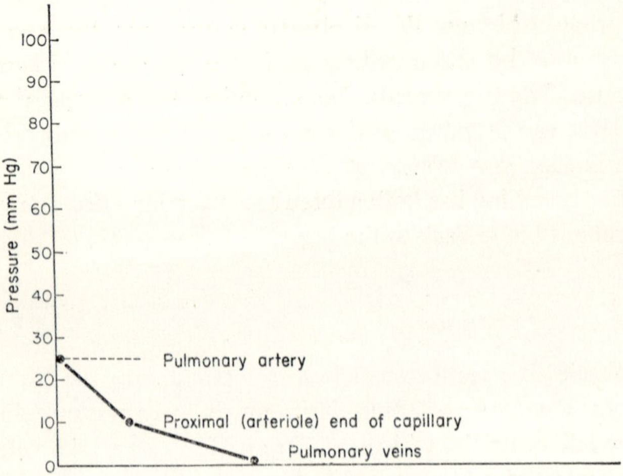

FIG **110. Pressure in the pulmonary vessels.**
Compare with Fig. 107.

for blood to leave the capillaries. The pressure in the capillaries may rise and when it reaches 30 mm Hg tissue fluid forms. As there is little space between the tissues, the fluid passes into the alveoli causing pulmonary oedema. It is this which causes the breathlessness of cardiac asthma.

The right ventricle contracts even more forcefully, raising the pressure in the pulmonary artery and aterioles. As their walls are thin, they distend and this distension presses on the alveoli decreasing even further the quantity of air in them. The lungs, being filled with blood, become less compliant than usual, so that they inflate and deflate less easily when breathing.

There is considerable impairment in the exchange of air between the lungs and the atmosphere; this condition is known as pulmonary hypertension. If pulmonary hypertension persists for a number of years, changes in the arterioles cause narrowing and increased resistance to the flow of blood with consequent rise in pressure. It is as though by doing so it protects against a raised capillary pressure and the formation of pulmonary oedema.

Effects of gravity

When a person is lying down the normal systolic pressure is 120 mm Hg in the aorta and in the arteries of the head and in the legs. When he stands up, gravity pulls the blood away from the head and into the legs. However, compensating mechanisms are brought into action. There is an increase in the tone of the muscle of the walls of the veins with subsequent constriction pushing the blood back to the heart and preventing pooling in the legs. The abdominal muscles contract to support the abdominal organs and at the same time press on the abdominal veins. Some blood does remain in the lower part of the body, thus reducing the stroke volume, yet the cardiac output is only slightly diminished as there is a rise in pulse rate.

If he stands up slowly his body has time to make the necessary adjustments, but if he stands up suddenly there may be a temporary reduction in cardiac output and possible fainting. This may also occur in a patient who has been lying in bed for some time and whose veins have lost their muscle tone and power to contract. It may also occur in patients who are having some hypotensive drugs which, by blocking the sympathetic nervous stimuli, bring about a paralysis of the veins of the muscle of the vein walls, so that they are unable to constrict, and become distended with blood.

In the healthy adult, standing in the erect position, the pressure in the aorta is 120 mm Hg, but in the arteries of the head it is only about 90 mm Hg, while in the legs it is as much as 200 mm Hg.

11
Drugs

The body is a whole composed of several parts or organs, each of which has its own special part to play in the functioning of the body as a whole. In the majority of cases the organ will also exert an influence directly or indirectly on other organs.

When a drug is introduced into the body its action will be directly upon some tissue or organ, but it may also act indirectly upon others. For example, in congestive cardiac failure, digitalis strengthens the heart beat and improves the circulation of blood to the kidney, which, having a better blood supply, functions better.

A drug may be given for an intended effect upon one organ or tissue, but it may also have effects upon others which were not intended; these are sometimes referred to as side-effects. For example, guanethadine, given for its action on peripheral blood vessels and to lower the blood pressure, may also have the side-effect of diarrhoea and nasal stuffiness. It may happen that the intended effects are off-set by the side-effects, especially with new drugs. As further investigations and trials are made upon the drug in the laboratory, it may be possible to isolate the active principle from these parts which caused the side-effects and, by removing the latter, enhance the intended effect of the drug. Sometimes the drug molecules may be slightly altered so that the modified drug has fewer or no side-effects.

The newly discovered drug may be in a near original or crude state, requiring the administration of large amounts in order to obtain the intended effects. Later, as the drug undergoes further analysis, modification and testing, it may be possible to produce it in a more refined, purified state, so that a much smaller dose will be required. For example, the average dose of digitalis folium is from 60 to 120 mg, whereas that of its glycoside digoxin is 0·25 mg.

Thus it will be understood that when a new drug has been produced and established in use, there may follow other drugs related to the original, with slightly different overall effects, stronger intended effect or less side-effects. The recent modification may also be given in lower doses, hence the importance of noting the dosage of each drug, whether or not it is related to another.

The nurse who is caring for a patient suffering from cardiovascular disorder will encounter many drugs. Some will be from different sources and given for different reasons, but others may be related to an earlier drug. Some, such as adrenaline, may be given for an intended effect upon the heart and blood vessels, while others may be given for their effect upon another organ which will in turn affect the diseased organ. Diazepam (Valium) may be given for its effect upon the patient's nervous system; it is a tranquillizer which keeps the patient in a calm state of mind and thus eliminates the possibility of the emotions sending sympathetic stimuli to the heart.

In this chapter it is proposed to give details of drugs which are commonly used for their more or less direct effect upon the circulation—the heart, blood vessels and kidney. Should the reader require details of drugs not found in this chapter, reference should be made to books dealing purely with pharmacology.

Drugs affecting the heart

Those decreasing the heart rate

Digitalis and its derivatives

Digitalis, obtained from the leaf of the foxglove, has been used in the treatment of heart conditions since 1785, when William Withering first introduced it for the relief of dropsy. It can still be given in the form of digitalis folium, 60–120 mg, but more frequently it is one of the glycosides which is ordered.

Digitoxin is a glycoside obtained from *Digitalis purpurea*. It is completely absorbed from the intestinal tract when given by mouth. The dose is usually 0·1 mg. It is slow to act when given orally or intravenously, but its action lasts up to 18 days.

Digoxin is a glycoside obtained from *Digitalis lanata*. It may not be completely absorbed from the intestinal tract. However, it is quick to act, its action lasting up to 5 days. It is given orally in doses of 0·25 mg, and can be given intramuscularly or intravenously. If given intravenously, careful observation is necessary as cardiac dysrythmias may be provoked.

Lanatoside C is another glycoside obtained from *Digitalis lanata*. Its action is quick and brief and it is soon eliminated from the body. Hence it is of use in emergency; furthermore, it is less likely to accumulate in the body.

Digitalis is used mainly in chronic congestive cardiac failure. It exerts a direct effect on fatigued heart muscle, allowing better usage of available energy and resulting in a more powerful and more effective contraction. In turn the cardiac output is increased, venous pressure reduced, dyspnoea relieved and oedema cleared. The circulation is improved, the increased supply to the kidney enabling it to function better with resultant diuresis. The enlarged heart is reduced in size. The heart beats more slowly so that it rests better and longer during diastole; there is more time for the ventricle to fill, the muscle fibres are stretched more and, as Starling's law determines, this leads to a more forceful contraction. The exact reason for the slowing is not completely known — it may be because of better emptying or because the digitalis stimulates the vagus nerve, whose action is to inhibit the heart rate, because it antagonizes (blocks) the action of the sympathetic nerves on the pacemaker or because it inhibits the conduction of impulses along the bundle of His to the ventricles.

It is common practice for the doctor to order a loading dose of digitalis, and when there is sufficient in the body for full effect, a smaller dose to maintain that level in the body, e.g. 0·5 mg digoxin by mouth or by injection if required urgently, followed by a maintenance dose of 0·25 mg two or three times a day. Digitoxin being more potent and longer-acting, the maintenance dose may be 0·1 mg once weekly.

Unfortunately digitalis is excreted slowly and may easily accumulate in the body, producing toxic effects. The early signs are nausea and loss of appetite; later vomiting and diarrhoea may occur. The pulse rate becomes very slow (bradycardia) and in many hospitals the nurse is advised to count the pulse rate before giving digitalis. If it is below 60–70/min, it may be worth while to check the apex beat as this may be higher, and report these to the doctor before administering the dose. Elderly patients may not tolerate digitalis well, and become irrational and confused. Other toxic signs are coupled beats, extrasystoles and tachycardia; this indicates that the muscles of the ventricles have an increased sensitivity to stimuli, which may lead to ventricular fibrillation resulting in cardiac arrest.

Low serum potassium, as caused by diuretic which leads to potassium loss, increases the effect of digitalis on the heart muscle, increased sensitivity and extra systole taking place. Should this occur, potassium is given.

Ouabain

Ouabain is the active principle of *Strophanthus*, its action being similar to that of digitalis. It may be given orally in doses of 1 mg twice daily. It is excreted more rapidly than digitalis, and does not accumulate in the body. Sometimes 0·2 mg is given intravenously for rapid short-lived effect when the ventricular rate is over 100.

Quinidine

Quinidine, of use in atrial fibrillation of recent onset, e.g. thyrotoxicosis, acts on the myocardium, mainly of the atrium. It reduces the excitability of the atrium, thus decreasing both the initiation of contractions and the conduction of the impulses across the atria; the resting period between atrial contractions is lengthened and normal rhythm restored.

Ventricular fibrillation may occur; to prevent this a course of digitalis is sometimes given first. There may be side-effects of tinnitus, low blood pressure, nausea and vomiting. A test dose of 200 mg is often given. The patient is kept in bed for 12 hours. If no adverse reactions are noted, the drug is given in doses of 300 mg 5 to 6 times a day for 7–10 days. When normal rhythm has been restored the dose is reduced to a maintenance dose of 300 mg twice daily. When possible, the patient's heart beat should be monitored by an oscilloscope of ECG.

Sometimes clots of blood may have formed in the atria and when normal rhythm has been restored these may become dislodged and enter the circulation to form emboli. It is for this reason that some doctors, when ordering quinidine for the control of atrial fibrillation, also order anticoagulants. Because of the possible danger of quinidine, electrical cardioversion is now frequently used in order to re-establish normal cardiac rhythm.

Procainamide

Procainamide (Pronestyl), a derivative of the local anaesthetic procaine, has action similar to quinidine. It is used mainly to restore normal rhythm in patients with ventricular dysrhythmias, especially as may occur suddenly as a result of cardiac catheterization or cardiac surgery. It is given orally in tablets of 0·25–1·0 g every 4–6 hours, or it may be given intravenously in doses not exceeding 20–50 mg/min until a total of 1 g has been given. The cardiac rhythm may suddenly return to normal but, as ventricular fibrillation may occur, followed by cardiac collapse, it is advisable to monitor the heart beat by oscilloscope or ECG. When intravenous injections are being given, the blood pressure should be taken at frequent intervals as procainamide is a vasodilator and may cause lowering of the blood pressure.

Lignocaine

Lignocaine, chemically related to procainamide, is sometimes used in acute cardiac dysrhythmias. An initial dose of 50–100 mg is given intravenously, followed by 1–5 mg/min as a solution of 500 mg lignocaine in 500 ml 5% dextrose solution. It is of shorter duration than procainamide. A look-out should be kept for side-effects such as drowsiness, twitchings or respiratory arrest. Heparin (500 units) is sometimes added to the infusion as there is a tendency for thrombophlebitis to occur.

Lignocaine is used during cardiac catheterization and cardiac surgery. It may also be used after myocardial infarction to control serious cardiac dysrhythmias.

It is often used as a local anaesthetic in conjunction with adrenaline. In view of the effects of adrenaline on the heart, it will be realized that it is necessary to ensure that the lignocaine being given in cardiac conditions does not contain adrenaline.

Those increasing the heart rate

Adrenaline

Adrenaline, 0·2–0·5 ml of 1 in 1000 solution, or 5–10 ml of 1 in

10 000 solution, is given by injection—hypodermic, intravenous and on occasion directly into the heart muscle. It affects the β-receptors, increasing the concentration of adenosine triphosphate (ATP) and creating phosphate in the muscle fibres. The metabolic process is increased, more energy is released and the muscle contracts. There is an increase in rate as well as in force of the contraction, the increased cardiac output bringing about a rise in blood pressure. Vasoconstriction of the peripheral blood vessels also brings about a rise in blood pressure. Muscles of the bronchioles relax, thus facilitating entry of air into the alveoli. Arterioles of skeletal muscle relax. Dextrose is released from the liver. There may also be tremors, feelings of anxiety and palpitations. Toxic doses may produce ventricular fibrillation.

Isoprenaline

Isoprenaline (Saventrine, Suscardia) is a bronchodilator, for which purpose it may be given sublingually in tablets of 10–20 mg. It may also be incorporated in spray aerosols. It stimulates the rate at which the heart beats, acting on the β-receptors, and is inotropic (increases the contractility of the heart muscle), any rise in blood pressure resulting from the increased cardiac output. Its effect on the arterioles is vasodilatation, and thus may bring about a fall in blood pressure. It is given in doses of 2–8 mg in 500 ml 5% dextrose solution by intravenous infusion, the rate of flow being carefully adjusted to maintain that ordered by the doctor. The slightest increase in rate of infusion may lead to tachycardia. Should there be any hypoxia of the myocardium, ventricular irritability may lead to fatal dysrhythmia.

Beta-blocking agents

Propranolol

Propranolol (Inderal), blocks the effect on the β-receptors in the myocardium of sympathetic (adrenergic) stimulation, of adrenaline and of noradrenaline. Consequently, in response to physical and emotional stress, there is no increase in either the heart rate or the force of contraction, and no increase in oxygen requirements. For this purpose it is given orally in doses of 5–30 mg every 6 hours, or even higher quantities up to 240 mg/day, for patients with myocardial ischaemia, e.g. to reduce the severity and frequency of anginal attacks. The decrease in cardiac rate decreases the cardiac output and thus the arterial blood pressure; hypotension may result. In smaller, controlled dosage it is used for the treatment of hypertension. It is also used to abolish ventricular dysrhythmias occurring during anaesthesia and in digitalis intoxication. In emergency it can be given slowly by intravenous injection in doses up to 5 mg. It sometimes causes dizziness, nausea, vomiting, an erythematous rash and hypoglycaemia in diabetes mellitus treated with insulin and oral agents. By inhibiting the relaxation of bronchial muscle, it may cause bronchospasm, especially in asthmatics. In those with an already damaged heart it may precipitate heart failure. Adverse effects can be treated by the administration of 1 mg atropine intravenously.

Practolol

Practolol (Eraldin), oxprenolol (Trasicor) and alprenolol (Aptin) are similar to propranolol but produce fewer side-effects. They are regarded as cardioselective in action, in that they block the β-1-receptors in the myocardium, without blocking the β-2-receptors in the bronchioles, and thus do not induce bronchoconstriction. Orally in doses of 50–100 mg 2 or 3 times daily they are useful in preventing attacks of angina. Intravenously in doses of 5–25 mg they are effective in the management of ventricular dysrhythmias. They appear to be less successful than propranolol as hypotensive agents.

Drugs acting on blood vessels

A description of the blood vessels is given in Chapter 8, to which the reader's attention is drawn, as an appreciation of the physiological principles assists in a better understanding of those drugs used for their action on blood vessels and of the subsequent possible side-effects.

Vasoconstrictors

Vasoconstrictors cause contraction of the muscle fibres in the walls of the arterioles with consequent narrowing of the vessel. Generalized vasoconstriction results in a raised peripheral resistance and a rise in blood pressure. It is with this intention that these drugs are usually prescribed.

Noradrenaline (*Levophed*) is a powerful but short-acting constrictor of all blood vessels, and consequently after its administration there is a rapid rise in blood pressure. Usually it is given slowly by intravenous infusion, 2–4 ml being diluted in 500 ml normal saline. It appears to have little or no direct effect on the heart. If allowed to leak into the tissues, the vasoconstriction of the superficial blood vessels may lead to necrosis of the surrounding area. During the administration, the blood pressure is taken at frequent intervals, so that the infusion can be adjusted to maintain the desired level.

Metaraminol (*Aramine*) is a powerful general vasoconstrictor, its effects being maintained for longer periods than those of noradrenaline. It is given by hypodermic or intramuscular injection of doses of 2–10 mg, or slowly by intravenous infusion, 15–100 mg being diluted in 500 ml normal saline or 5% glucose. It has been given to raise the blood pressure in conditions such as myocardial infarction, haemorrhage and traumatic and surgical shock, but it is now less used because vasoconstriction of the renal arteries diminishes the blood supply to the kidney and may interfere with diuresis. It has mild but quite transient effects upon the central nervous system, improving breathing and lightening consciousness.

Mephentermine (*Mephine*) and *methoxamine* (*Vasoxine*) have a similar effect to metaraminol.

Vasodilators

Vasodilators can be considered according to their site of action or, alternatively, according to the purpose for which they are given.

Ganglion blocking agents, as their names suggest, act at the synapses in the ganglia, blocking the transmission from the pre- to the postganglionic fibres by preventing the release or the usage of acetylcholine. Both sympathetic and parasympathetic ganglia are affected, so that in addition to the inhibition of sympathetic adrenergic fibres with consequent dilatation of the blood vessels and lowering of the blood pressure, there is also inhibition of the parasympathetic cholinergic fibres with a consequent dryness of the mouth, blurring of vision and reduction of peristalsis. Such drugs include hexamethonium compounds, mecamylamine (Inversine) and pempidine (Perolysen).

Adrenergic blocking agents prevent the release or the usage of noradrenaline and adrenaline at the junction of the adrenergic postganglionic fibre with the muscle of the blood vessel. Vasoconstriction is inhibited and a corresponding vasodilatation occurs. The activity of the parasympathetic nerves is not affected; indeed it may become dominant when the counteracting effect of the adrenergic nerves has been removed. Such drugs are guanethidine (Ismelin) and its derivatives, bretylium (Darenthin) and methyldopa (Aldomet).

α-Blocking agents prevent the α-receptor cells in the muscle of the blood vessels from being acted upon by noradrenaline and adrenaline. Vasoconstriction is inhibited and vasodilatation occurs. Such a drug is phenoxybenzamine (Dibenyline).

Vasodilators used in myocardial ischaemia

Angina pectoris occurs when the work demanded of the heart is increased, as in sudden physical exertion and emotional excitement, but the amount of oxygen required is less than that being supplied by the blood, usually because of narrowing of the coronary arteries. The ischaemic myocardium causes an acute gripping pain in the front of the chest, the patient stops his activity until the work demanded of the heart is lessened to the point where the oxygen requirements are being met. Dilatation of the coronary arteries increases the supply of blood and oxygen to the myocardium. Some parts of the coronary artery may dilate, but some sclerosed parts may not be able to do so. Vasodilating drugs bring about a degree of dilatation of the coronary arteries, and also of the arterioles and veins of the periphery. There follows a pooling of blood in these vessels, especially the veins; consequently less blood returns to the heart and with a diminished venous return the work required of the heart is also decreased.

Nitrites and nitrates are the oldest group of vasodilators used to relieve or prevent angina pectoris; they appear to have considerable effect on the coronary arteries. They act directly on the smooth muscle in the walls of the blood vessels. Other arteries are also dilated, so the patient may become flushed and complain of a throbbing headache. There may be hypotension as explained above, the patient may feel giddy and faint.

Amyl nitrite, 0·12–0·3 ml, is contained in a glass ampoule. When the patient has an attack of angina the ampoule is crushed and the fluid released. It is soaked by the absorbent material in which the ampoule is wrapped, where it evaporates, and the vapour inhaled by the patient. Its action is rapid, but soon passes off. The vapour is recognizable to bystanders. Nowadays this method of relieving the attack is not often used.

Glyceryl trinitrate. A tablet of 0·5–1 mg is crushed between the teeth and the fragments are held under the tongue where they dissolve and are absorbed through the mucous membrane. It takes effect in 2–4 min and the effect lasts 15–20 min. Some patients develop a tolerance to it. When a patient is about to take some more than usual physical effort, such as climbing the stairs, he is advised to take the tablet at the outset, thus preventing a possible attack.

Pentaerythrityl tetranitrate (*Peritrate*) has an action which is slower in onset than glyceryl nitrate but which lasts up to 5 hours; consequently it is readily considered as a prophylactic measure. Tablets containing 10–30 mg are taken before food, in the morning and during the day. Patients are less likely to develop tolerance.

Sorbide nitrate (*Cedocard*, *Vascardin*), 10 mg dissolved in the mouth, has an effect within 10–15 minutes and which lasts up to 4 hours.

Prenylamine (*Synadrin*), 60 mg 3 times daily, is effective as a long-term prophylactic agent. It has a slight hypotensive action, so that if hypotensive drugs are being given, the dosage may need appropriate adjustment.

Propranolol (*practolol and alprenolol*) (see p. 266), the β-blocking agent, by preventing an increase in heart rate and cardiac activity and thus also an increase in the oxygen requirements resulting from exertion, are of value in angina pectoris.

Peripheral vasodilators

In general, these are given in conditions caused by an insufficiency of blood to some part of the periphery, such as those giving rise to intermittent claudication, e.g. Buerger's disease, Raynaud's phenomenon, chilblains, arteriosclerosis and Menière's disease of the ear. When administered the skin may become flushed and warm and there may be a throbbing headache. Lowering the blood pressure may cause giddiness and fainting; there may be palpitations and nervous unrest. They tend to permit an increase of gastric juice, and may exacerbate any peptic ulcer present.

Alcohol, among other effects, produces a measure of peripheral vasodilatation as for example the feeling of warmth and flushing of the skin after a tot of whisky has been drunk on a cold day. It is sometimes recommended along with other vasodilator drugs.

Nicotinic acid tends to cause a moderate vasodilatation as well as to promote the oxidation process in the tissue. It is sometimes given in doses of 25–250 mg. *Inositol nicotinate*, a derivative, is given in doses of 200 mg 3 times daily. It is often given for the treatment of Menière's disease.

Tolazoline (*Priscol*), 25–50 mg orally 3 times in the day or 10–20 mg by intramuscular or intravenous injection, is one of the oldest vasodilators. An α-blocking agent, its action is of short duration and it can be used to relieve vasospasm as occurs in Raynaud's phenomenon. Other drugs having a similar action include:

Isoxsuprine (*Dilavase*) 10–20 mg 3 times daily.
Cyclandelate (*Cyclospasmol*) 400 mg 3 times daily.
Buphenine (*Perdilatal*) 6–12 mg 3 times daily.
Thymoxamine (*Opilon*) 40 mg 4 times daily or 5 mg/ml by injection.

Phenoxybenzamine (*Dibenyline*) is an α-blocking agent having an action of longer duration than tolazoline. It antagonizes the vasoconstrictive power of noradrenaline, but does not interfere with the stimulation of heart muscle, nor with bronchodilatation. Orally in doses of 10–20 mg it has been used in the treatment of chilblains, but its absorption in the intestinal tract is irregular. It has been used as an intra-arterial injection, 0·5–1 mg in 1 ml, when acute ischaemia of a limb occurs. As an intravenous infusion it is sometimes used when circulatory failure is accompanied by intense vasoconstriction. 50 mg are dissolved in 500 ml normal saline or

5% glucose. The infusion is given slowly and takes at least an hour. A rapid fall in blood pressure may occur unless the circulating blood volume is maintained by the infusion of extra fluid. In particular this may occur if phenoxybenzamine is administered too rapidly. Care should be taken to avoid injection into the tissue; intramuscular injection is not recommended. Skin reactions may occur; it is wise to avoid contamination of the skin by the drug. It has also been used in hypertensive conditions such as may be due to phaeochromocytoma (see phentolamine, p. 273).

Hypotensive agents

Hypertension is described in Chapter 8; the object of this section is to consider some of the drugs which are used specifically for the reduction of high blood pressure. Although their site of action may differ, the effect of these drugs is usually one of generalized vasodilatation.

The doctor usually prescribes a dosage to be taken and then observes the effects over a period of time. The dosage is increased or decreased as necessary, according to its effect upon the blood pressure and according to the general effect upon the patient. The process of stabilization can take place at home or the patient may be admitted to hospital. During stabilization, the blood pressure is taken with the patient lying down and also when he is standing up. In health, as the individual stands up, there is a fall in blood pressure of about 10 mm Hg, the reflex vasoconstriction compensating for the fall. When drugs which inhibit vasoconstriction are given, the reflex is abolished, compensation does not take place and there is a resultant fall in blood pressure, sometimes of 30 mm Hg. This is postural hypotension. If this is too low for the patient, he may experience dizziness and actually faint. The dosage ordered is adjusted until the patient's blood pressure is no longer too low when he is standing.

Reserpine, from the *Rauwolfia* plant, is a mild hypotensive, depressing in some way the higher sympathetic centres of the brain. It also appears to reduce the noradrenaline usually present in the muscle of the arteriole. It has a mild sedative effect which may lead to drowsiness and depression, and it has been reported as producing suicidal tendencies in susceptible patients. Other side-effects include feelings of fatigue, agitation, diarrhoea, nasal congestion and bradycardia. It is given in doses of 0·25 mg orally 3 times a day for a week, and then a maintenance dose adjusted to suit the individual patient.

Ganglion blocking agents block transmission of impulses of the autonomic nerves at the synapses from the pre- to the postganglionic fibres. The effect on the adrenergic sympathetic nerves leads to vasodilatation and fall in blood pressure, but as the parasympathetic cholinergic nerves are also affected, there follow the side-effects of dry mouth, constipation and blurred vision.

They are used less frequently these days, the tendency being to use those drugs having a more selective action. Hexamethonium and similar compounds were first used as ganglion blocking agents; those at present in use include:

Pentolinium (*Ansolysen*), 10–20 mg orally.
Pempidine (*Perolysen*), 10–80 mg orally.
Mecamylamine (*Inversine*), 5–60 mg orally.

Adrenergic blocking agents act on the postganglionic adrenergic nerve fibres, interfering with the formation or release of noradrenaline or release of adrenaline, or with their usage after release. Vasoconstriction is inhibited and a fall in blood pressure takes place. The action of the parasympathetic cholinergic nerves is unaffected and even unopposed, so that side-affects such as diarrhoea, nasal stuffiness, muscular weakness, frequency of micturition, bradycardia and exacerbation of peptic ulcer may occur. The patient is advised to avoid sudden change of position, standing for long periods, to take care of himself in warm weather and to avoid emotional excitement. When he feels faint he is advised to lie down until the feeling passes off, and then to sit for a time before standing.

Guanethidine (*Ismelin*) and its derivatives are adrenergic blocking agents. Initial doses are 10 mg daily, being gradually increased to 30–60 mg daily. The effect of guanethidine lasts 24 hours, so it need be given only once daily, preferably in the morning.

Bethanidine (*Bethanid*, *Esbatal*) is more quickly absorbed and excreted than guanethidine, so the dose of 10 mg is given twice daily. Since its action is rapid, lasting about 12 hours, it is used for prompt and easy stabilization, and is advantageous when surgery is necessary and treatment for hypertension suspended as part of the preparation. Side-effects are milder and of lower incidence than of guanethidine.

Debrisoquine (*Declinax*), related to guanethidine, is also given twice daily in doses of 10 mg initially gradually increasing to 30–80 mg. There is a low incidence of side-effects. It appears to have a better response in women than in men. It can be used when the patient is in heart failure.

Guanoxan (*Envacar*) is given in daily doses of 10 mg increasing to 50 mg daily.

Methyldopa (*Aldomet*) interferes with the synthesis of noradrenaline from its precursor dopamine by inhibiting the enzyme responsible for it. The interference with production and availability of noradrenaline leads to a reduction of high blood pressure both when lying down as well as when standing up. It is given in doses of 250 mg 3 times daily and increased until a total of 1–1·5 g is being given. Although side-effects of drowsiness, fatigue, dry mouth and even pyrexia may occur, they do not appear very frequently.

Phentolamine (*Rogitine*) is an α-blocking agent which has been used in arteriospasm, vasospasm and diabetic arteriosclerosis for its vasodilatory properties. It neutralizes the vasoconstrictor effort of adrenaline and is of use when high blood pressure is caused by excessive amounts of adrenaline and noradrenaline released in phaeochromocytoma. Phaeochromocytomas arise in the chromaffin tissue in the adrenal gland or in other parts. They usually secrete noradrenaline and adrenaline in excessive amounts. As a diagnostic means of distinguishing between hypertension due to phaeochromocytoma and essential hypertension, an injection of phentolamine will bring about an immediate fall of pressure if due to phaeochromocytoma, but there is no significant change if it is essential hypertension.

Propranolol (*Inderal*) has already been mentioned. It is sometimes used as a hypotensive agent.

Thiazides (diuretics) also have a hypotensive effect. The administration of such a diuretic at the same time as other hypotensive drugs will result in potentiation of the hypotensive drug. There is therefore the possibility of giving a thiazide diuretic with a smaller amount of hypotensive agent. Thiazide diuretics may cause a rise on the level of serum uric acid (normal 2·0–5·0 mg/100 ml blood). While this may produce no symptoms, it may precipitate an attack of gout. Some manufacturers are now making tablets containing both substances. An example is Ismelin–Navidrex, which contains guanethidine 10 mg cyclopenthiazide 0·15 mg and potassium chloride 400 mg.

Promazine (Sparine) and chlorpromazine (Largactil), often used for their anti-emetic and/or tranquillizing effect, may also cause paralysis of vasomotor control with resultant hypotension.

Anticoagulants

The process of bleeding and blood clotting is described in Chapter 10. The following drugs are at present in frequent use.

Heparin

The dose is 5000–10 000 units intravenously. Some heparin is normally found in the blood, having been formed in the liver. Given therapeutically it inhibits the conversion of prothrombin into thrombin and neutralizes the action of any thrombin present. It has a quick action, but the action passes off quickly, lasting only a few hours and thus requiring repeated administration. It does not dissolve clots, but prevents any further clotting from taking place; for this reason it is sometimes ordered in forms of thrombosis. Should prolonged administration be necessary, the daily dose is estimated on the clotting time. However, it is usually given only for a 36–48-hour period. An oral anticoagulant is given at the same time as the initial dose of heparin; this becomes effective after 36–48 hours, after which the heparin is discontinued.

Coumarin group

These have a delayed action, but the action is prolonged. They inhibit the formation of prothrombin by the liver, and the dose is estimated according to the level of prothrombin in the blood.

Phenindione (Dindevan). Initial dose 200–300 mg orally; maintenance dose 25–100 mg daily.

Warfarin sodium. Initial dose 30–50 mg by intramuscular or intravenous injection. Maintenance dose 3–10 mg orally each day. Smaller doses, e.g. 5–10 mg, may be given after valve replacement. Warfarin is excreted slowly so that one dose daily is adequate.

Ancrod (Arvin)

Ancrod (Arvin), an enzyme in the venom from a Malayan pit viper, has anticoagalant properties. Trials have been carried out using it intravenously to ascertain its usability in dissolving established thrombosis but it is not fibrinolytic. Once it is administered its action is prolonged, investigations being made frequently on the clotting mechanisms of the blood. For the first 24 hours, it is given by intravenous infusion, but afterwards by twice daily intravenous injection in doses of 2 units/kg body weight. A tendency to develop a resistance to ancrod has been reported, especially when it was given by the intramuscular route.

Modifying factors

The effectiveness of oral anticoagulants is reduced when barbiturates, chloral hydrate, steroids or griseofulvin are being given at the same time. On the other hand, their effectiveness is increased when salicylates and phenylbutazone, chlorpromazine and related drugs, quinidine, clofibrate and anabolics are being given, and also if the amount of vitamin K in the intestines is reduced as a result of the administration of liquid paraffin, sulphonamides, chlorampenicol, tetracyclines and neomycin.

Observations

When anticoagulants are being given, observations should be made for signs of bleeding from the kidney (haematuria), into the skin (purpura), from the nose (epistaxis) and from internal organs (haematemesis, melaena).

Antidotes

An antidote may be required. *Protamine sulphate* will neutralize heparin. It is given intravenously, and 1 g protamine sulphate will neutralize 100 units heparin. *Vitamin K* causes a rise in the prothrombin level in the blood and reverses the action of anticoagulants given orally. The forms used are: (*a*) *phytomenadione* 5–50 mg intravenously or 2·5–10 mg orally; (*b*) *acetomenaphthone* 5–20 mg orally or intramuscularly; and (*c*) *menaphthone sodium bisulphate* 1–2 mg by hypodermic or intramuscular injection.

Fibrinolytics and thrombolytics

Fibrin fibres are continually being made in the blood, but clots do not form because the fibres are dissolved by the action of the plasmin. Should a clot form, it will gradually be dissolved by the action of the plasmin. Plasmin is formed from plasminogen by the action of streptokinase. This dissolving of clots is called fibrinolysis or thrombolysis.

Streptokinase (*Kabikinase*)

Streptokinase is administered directly into the blood vessel following pulmonary embolism or venous and arterial thrombosis of not more than 24 hours duration. To avoid any hypersensitive reaction, 100 mg hydrocortisone or 25 mg prednisolone are given before the streptokinase and repeated 6-hourly for 2 days. Tests of bleeding time, clotting time and prothrombin times may be taken. The streptokinase is dissolved in 150 ml of 5% glucose solution or normal saline, and 1200 000 units are given over a period of 30 minutes. It may be continued by continuous drip infusion of 100 000 units/hour for up to 3 days.

Streptokinase may cause severe bleeding from needle punctures and operating sites; it is not usually given for at least 3 days after operation. When given in deep vein thrombosis there is always the possibility that, as the clot breaks up, parts may enter the circulation, leading to pulmonary embolism. The nurse must continually observe the patient for such bleeding and for signs of other embolism.

Aminocaproic acid (*Epsikapron*)

When fibrinolysis leads to haemorrhage, aminocaproic acid may be given as an antidote. It may be given orally or intravenously, the dosage being 0·1 g aminocaproic acid/kg body weight. It may be repeated four-hourly or as frequently as ordered. For intravenous infusion it may be mixed with 5% glucose solution or isotonic saline.

Reducing the cholesterol level

Clofibrate (Atromid S)

The precise action of clofibrate is not known, but when given to those with a high cholesterol level in the blood it reduces the amount of cholesterol and triglycerides. Since a high incidence of thrombosis occurs in those with a high cholesterol level, clofibrate is regarded as an antithrombotic agent. The dosage is usually reckoned on a basis of 1·5–2 g/kg body weight.

Cholestyramine

This is a resin which binds bile acid and salts in the intestines, thus preventing their re-absorption, with a consequent reduction in the cholesterol level of the blood. It is given orally, the dose being 16–32 g daily.

Fenfluramine (Ponderax)

This is a drug given in the treatment of obesity. It is referred to as a glycoliptic agent and is of use when an imbalance exists between glucose and fat metabolism in the tissues. It causes muscles to take up glucose, thus reducing the amount available for conversion into fat; it also tends to inhibit the synthesis of fat from glucose. It also decreases the appetite, so that loss in weight occurs without stimulation of the central nervous system. The dose is 20 mg 2 or 3 times daily. Side-effects include diarrhoea, giddiness and mild sedation. It increases the activity of hypotensive and sedative drugs.

The xanthine group

These originate from tea, coffee and cocoa, the active principles being theobromine and theophylline. They stimulate the heart muscle and increase cardiac output. They have a stimulating effect on the cerebrum producing wakefulness. Mild diuresis also follows administration as they decrease the re-absorption of sodium and water in the kidney. The usual reason for giving these drugs is that they stimulate breathing and dilate the bronchioles.

Theophylline

It may be given alone in a dose of 60–200 mg orally, but it is also found in preparations containing other drugs.

Aminophylline

The dose is 100–500 mg orally, intramuscularly or slowly intravenously. 500 mg suppositiories are also available. It consists of theophylline and ethylene diamine. It is frequently used to assist breathing in acute left ventricular failure (cardiac asthma) and pulmonary oedema.

Diuretics

An accumulation of fluid occurs gradually as a result of heart failure, presenting as oedema of the lungs and of the dependent parts of the periphery. This in turn embarrasses the heart's action and makes the heart failure even worse. If excretion of the fluid by the kidney can be increased, the accumulation in the body is decreased, the embarrassment to the heart removed and the heart can function even though it may be limited. The formation of the urine by the kidney can be considered under two processes:

1. Filtration under pressure in the Malpighian body (Fig. 111) whereby the blood under pressure enters the glomerulus and much of the fluid part is filtered through the walls into Bowman's capsule.
2. Selective reabsorption of substances required by the body as the filtrate passes along the uriniferous tubule. About 75% of the dissolved salts and accompanying water are absorbed in the proximal tubule. Absorption in the distal convoluted tubule varies according to the body's needs at the time—sodium, potassium, chloride and bicarbonate and the accompanying water (Fig. 112).

The absorption of sodium takes place as a result of the action of carbonic anhydrase, as a result of the cells lining the tubules actively selecting it and as a result of the influence of the hormone aldosterone from the adrenal cortex. When sodium is absorbed, water is also absorbed.

When the blood supply to the kidney is poor, little filtration occurs, so any means of improving the circulation to the kidney will result in an improvement in kidney function and diuresis.

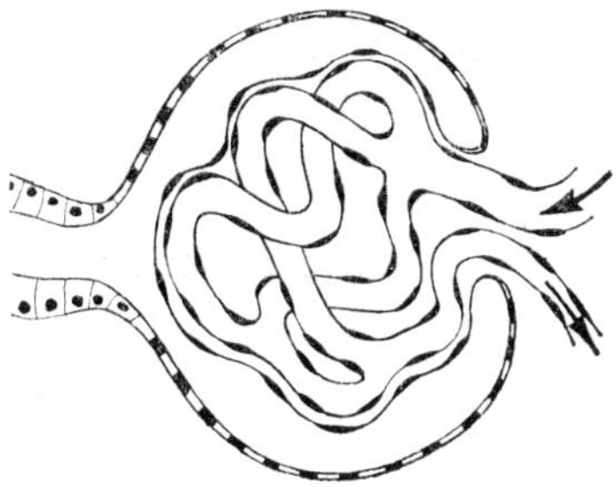

FIG 111. The Malpighian body (renal corpuscle), showing the glomerulus and Bowman's capsule.

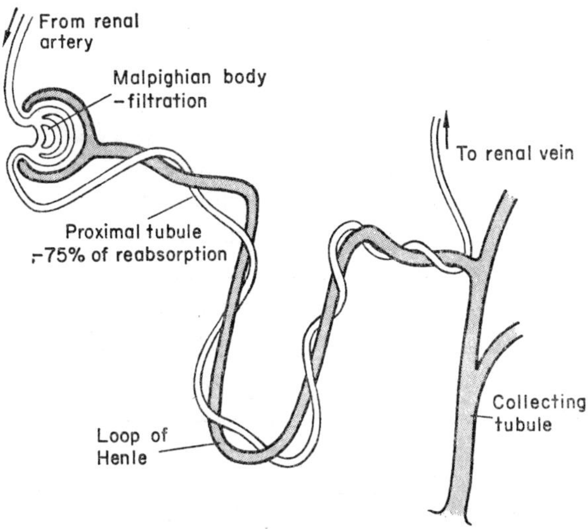

FIG 112. The site of filtration and reabsorption in the nephron.

When a patient with congestive heart failure rests, blood is diverted from the muscles and allowed to go to the kidney, thus increasing the blood supply and the urinary output. Drugs which stimulate the heart, such as digitalis, increase the cardiac output and by increasing the blood supply to the kidney they help diuresis.

Interference with the absorption of sodium will also result in less water being absorbed; the sodium and the water will pass along the tubule and out in the urine. Drugs such as the mercurial *mersalyl* diminish the selective action of the cells of the tubule in absorbing sodium. It is given by intramuscular injection as early as possible in the morning. It is now used much less frequently, its place having been taken by new oral diuretics.

Drugs such as *thiazides* inhibit the action of carbonic anhydrase in the cells of the walls of the tubules, and prevent the absorption of sodium, bicarbonate, chloride and potassium ions. The loss of potassium may lead to hypokalaemic alkalosis. Depletion of potassium causes weakness of muscles and dysrhythmia of the heart. If the patient is also having digitalis, the heart is even more sensitive to the digitalis, and cardiac irregularities occur, which may prove fatal.

Potassium supplements may be given by mouth to counteract the depletion. Sometimes they are incorporated in the same tablet as the thiazide.

Some doctors prefer the thiazide to be given on alternate days only, so that the body has a chance to replenish its potassium stores.

Chlorothiazide (*Saluric*), 1–2 g on alternate days, was the first of this group of diuretics. It is poorly absorbed in the intestines. Since then modifications in the molecule have been made to make it more stable and more soluble. The side-effects of these drugs are a tendency to purpura and agranulocytosis; it may aggravate diabetes mellitus in susceptible patients. Other thiazides are *hydrochlorothiazide* (*Esidrex*, *HydroSaluric*), 25–100 mg on alternate days and *bendrofluazide* (*Centyl*, *NeoNaclex*), 2·5–10 mg on alternate days.

Frusemide (*Lasix*) is a more powerful diuretic than the thiazides, giving a speedy diuresis, its effect being completed in 6 hours. The dose is 40–80 mg orally spread throughout the day, on alternate days; 20 mg repeated as necessary intravenously. It is a carbonic anhydrase inhibitor. Massive diuresis may occur and it may cause potassium and sodium depletion, sudden hypotension and circulatory collapse.

Ethacrynic acid (*Edecrin*) is another powerful diuretic with a speedy rapid onset. The dose is 50–100 mg orally, increasing on subsequent days. It is recommended that it be taken with food. It may also be given intravenously to produce very rapid diuresis.

Triamterene (*Dytac*) decreases the reabsorption of sodium but not of potassium. It is not as potent as the thiazides, but is sometimes used to supplement their usage. The dose is 50–100 mg twice daily.

Spironolactone (*Aldactone*) is sometimes used when other diuretics do not completely remove the oedema. It is usually given at the same time as other diuretics. The dose is 25 mg 6-hourly, by mouth. Spironolactone antagonizes the action of aldosterone and this inhibits the absorption of sodium. There is often a large diuresis, at first, but as this decreases the doctor may discontinue the administration. It tends to retain potassium rather than cause its loss, so that when it is being used, potassium supplements may be withdrawn.

Clopamide (*Brinaldix*) causes a marked diuresis of water and excretion of sodium, but when compared with other diuretics the loss of potassium is small. The dosage is 20–60 mg daily given orally.

Amiloride (*Midamore*) is a drug which helps the body to conserve potassium when diuretic therapy is likely to cause potassium depletion. It allows the loss of water and sodium, but blocks the loss of potassium. Given in conjunction with a prescribed diuretic, it removes the need for potassium supplements. It is given orally in doses of 5–10 mg daily. During vigorous diuretic therapy, amiloride may cause hyperkalaemia, therefore the patient should be carefully observed for its occurrence. Other possible side-effects include skin rash, pruritus, mental confusion and visual disturbances.

12

Ward organization

Good organization, communication and interpersonal relationships are important in any ward or unit. These become even more vital where cardiac patients are cared for, since for them recovery, palliation of their condition or even survival often depend on good teamwork by a number of people.

As in any ward, so in the cardiac ward, the Sister or her deputy tends to be the key figure. She can do much to set the tone of the ward and provide the calm, efficient, yet friendly atmosphere which is so necessary to the cardiac patient, and which allows other staff to do their work well. It is her task to try to coordinate the activities of nursing and medical staff, physiotherapists, technicians, domestic and other ancillary staff, patients and relatives, to provide the maximum benefit and minimum harm and inconvenience to the patient. For example, if the patient is to benefit fully from physiotherapy, he must not be tired already because he has had a bed-bath and full examination by a doctor immediately before treatment. It is usually quite possible to arrange periods of rest and activity alternately. It is to the Sister that nursing staff look for clinical expertise, advice, support and encouragement, the medical staff for information and execution of the treatment ordered and the patients and relatives for reassurance, information and further explanation of what is happening. Many people are still so anxious and overawed when spoken to by medical staff that they fail to comprehend what is said and will turn to nursing staff for clarification.

All this becomes even more important when, because of the nature of cardiac disease, the situation is potentially an anxious one for all concerned. Medical and nursing staff are mutually dependent in providing good patient care. Nursing staff need from the doctors clear medical orders and adequate explanation; medical staff need from nurses help in examining the patient, observations relating to the patient and intelligent execution of treatment. There must be mutual confidence and understanding, and cooperation for the patient's benefit. Willing and cooperative domestic staff are an essential part of the team. Their work and that of other staff must be arranged so that all runs smoothly. It is clearly undesirable for floor cleaning to take place with a noisy vacuum cleaner while doctors are trying to listen to heart sounds or patients are having a rest period.

All personnel must be trained to tell senior nursing staff if they are asked by patients to bring in food or other things which may be harmful. It is not unknown for a patient who is receiving oxygen therapy to acquire cigarettes and matches from relatives or untrained staff, or for those needing a restricted diet to ask for salty or other unsuitable foods.

Emergency call systems

In any cardiac ward there are usually a number of patients who may need urgent assistance, and it is imperative that help and effective treatment should be readily available. Emergency call systems must therefore be easy to use, always effective, and known to all staff. Two systems are needed:

1. An *internal system* to call help from within the ward or unit. This may be a light, bell or buzzer, workable from all areas where there may be patients, including bathrooms.

2. An *external system* to call help from outside the ward or unit. Some systems connect the wards with the cardiac outpatient department, theatre and other areas where there are likely to be staff attached to the cardiac unit. These may be helpful, but may not be effective at night or week-ends, when such areas may be unoccupied. Probably the best system is a telephone number used only for absolute emergencies. The operator, on receiving the call, then informs other specified personnel, such as an anaesthetist, physician, cardiac surgeon and possibly cardiac technicians. This may be done by the hospital call system, e.g. 'bleeps', or by a 'cardiac call' or coded call over the loudspeaker, so that everyone relevant goes to the location specified. If the emergency trolley is not within the ward then there should be a definite arrangement for someone to bring it when the call goes out.

Ethics of performing life-saving measures

People have a right to die in peace and dignity. Extreme measures to maintain life can only be justified if it is thought that resuscitation can lead to some worthwhile period of life as a person, not just a 'biological preparation'.

If there is to be a real chance of successful resuscitation circulation and respiration:

1. *Must not* be stopped for more than 3 minutes before being restored.

2. *Must not* have failed as the end result of a progressive pathological process, unless there is a chance that the condition can be relieved. For example, if a patient with known valvular disease has a cardiac arrest, it is just possible that resuscitation could be followed by an emergency valvotomy or valve replacement.

Resuscitation at the expense of the care or peace of mind of other patients (especially where there is lack of privacy or staff) can only be justified by a real possibility of success.

Usually medical staff will give guidance as to who is to be resuscitated. It is no more unethical for a doctor to say that a patient is not suitable for resuscitation than to say that a patient's disease is inoperable. He may well feel that it is unnecessary and unkind to restore 'life' to someone whose cardiac function has finally failed after deteriorating over a period of years. To resuscitate the patient in these circumstances is merely to put him through the suffering of dying twice without compensatory benefit. Age is not an infallible guide in deciding whether to resuscitate, but there are circumstances when one might do this for a patient of 17 years but not of 75 years. The capacity of the human body to recover completely from severe physical stress decreases with increasing age. If there is any doubt resuscitation should be attempted; it is too late to start 10 minutes later. Any nurse dealing with cardiac patients must be able to think clearly about the ethics of resuscitation if she is to have peace of mind, and be able to support junior staff, patients and relatives when necessary.

In-service training and education

The knowledge of investigation and treatment of cardiac disease has increased considerably over the last twenty years, and the work is still developing. It needs continuous interest and effort on the part of all staff to keep up-to-date with changes.

Formal education and in-service training play a part in the development of good cardiac nurses, especially in coronary or intensive therapy units or postoperative care wards where the nurse has much to learn about specialized techniques and equipment. Just as important, however, is the frequent informal exchange of information between medical and nursing staff, or senior and less experienced nurses as they discuss their patients and the work of the ward. Because of their interest in people most nurses are much more likely to remember what happened when Mr Smith developed acute pulmonary oedema than they are to remember a list of signs, symptoms and treatment.

A good knowledge and understanding of cardiac work not only make it more interesting for the nurse, but are essential if she is to provide good care for the patient. A nurse who is interested in her patient's progress and understands the importance of fluid intake and output, heart rate or other such observations, is much more likely to record them faithfully and accurately. If she knows about possible complications and drug side-effects she is much more likely to notice them early.

Cardiovascular nursing demands good powers of observation, a high degree of technical competence and understanding, confidence in dealing with emergencies, and the ability to work well in a team. These can only be developed efficiently by deliberate training and education as well as experience, and then only if the nurse concerned is willing to make the necessary effort herself.

The nurse who is assuming duty for the first time in a cardiovascular unit will be prepared to give her best to the patients she meets. She will realize that there is much to know about the patients' conditions and the treatment each condition requires, and she will be eager to learn it. However, being in a new and unfamiliar setting she will undoubtedly feel somewhat apprehensive of what may be expected of her and of her present capabilities.

The nurses (and doctors) already working in the unit will assist her greatly if they remember what may be her feelings at the time. In assisting the newcomer to learn the principles and practice of cardiovascular nursing, the established members of staff assume the role of teacher. They may teach consciously by introducing her to new situations, demonstrating new procedures and explaining new conditions. They may teach unconsciously by caring for the patient and by maintaining interpersonal relationships at the highest possible level, for the newcomer, knowingly or unwittingly, will copy established staff.

Orientation to the unit, ward or department is always facilitated if the newcomer is shown the lay-out, and if the uses of various rooms are explained.

A knowledge of the scope of the unit will help to lessen confusion; these can be thought of as:

1. Why the patient is in the unit.
2. What will happen to him while he is there.
3. How long he is likely to remain.
4. Where he will go when he leaves.

The general routine of most hospital wards is similar, and that of a cardiovascular ward will soon be picked up. However, the work of the various departments may differ owing to their specialized nature, and consequently the routine may also differ. Early explanation will make for early familiarity with the different routine.

In some departments of a cardiovascular unit the equipment is specialized, expensive and, to the newcomer, somewhat bewildering. Gradually she will learn, but eventually she must know about each item of equipment:

1. What it is.
2. How it is used and when (under what circumstances).
3. Where it is kept and how it is stored.
4. After use, how it is cleaned or how it is disposed of.
5. How it is re-ordered.

While this knowledge is most important for the specialized equipment, the established staff must appreciate that the newcomer may need the same sort of information and instruction for what is often thought of as general equipment.

The location of the patient's case notes must be indicated, and what a set of notes consists of. Charts and records can sometimes be complicated, so careful guidance will be required on their maintenance and advice on their interpretation. As the nurse becomes more familiar with the unit and takes on wider responsibilities, she will learn the forms peculiar to the hospital for such clerical matters as re-ordering returns, submitting requisitions and admitting and discharging the patient.

The newcomer will be a member of a team whose sole objective is the care of the patient. This team, consisting of doctors, nurses, physiotherapists, technicians and others, will most probably be large, and may even be divided into smaller teams. The newcomer will need to know not only the name of each member of the team, large or small, but also her role and sphere of speciality. She will need to be informed of her own area of responsibility, which will increase as she gains experience.

The span of duty hours of each member of the team should be explained. Although nursing staff may be on duty throughout the 24 hours, some non-nursing personnel may not be, and it is important that they should be requested, and/or given facilities to perform their special duties during the time they are on duty.

Where more than one person is working to the same end, a system of communication is necessary to ensure a common purpose and to avoid duplication, omission and confusion. Good team work is assisted if members are informed of any special way they may, or must, communicate with:

1. Each other.
2. The doctor.
3. Teams on other spans of duty especially with regard to methods of reporting, both written and verbally.
4. Other wards and departments.

Although much may be predicted or at least anticipated when patients with cardiovascular conditions are being cared for, the unexpected does tend to occur and emergency situations arise.

The newcomer, at some time, will need to know:

1. What type of emergency is likely to occur.
2. How to recognize it has occurred.
3. The action she should take and which others may take.
4. The alarm call system so that more specialized assistance may be obtained with a minimum of delay.

The subject of cardiovascular disease covers a wide field, the nurses knowledge must be correspondingly wide and also deep. It cannot all be learned at once, and it may be that not all will be easily recalled. As there is much to learn, she will need guidance as to where to learn it. She will be advised as to which textbooks she herself should obtain. There should be a copy of prescribed textbooks in the unit. For reference it is advisable to have clinical, physiological and biochemical textbooks available, and current professional journals for information on recent changes. Written instructions for the use of equipment should be easily accessible, along with any nursing procedures and details of specialized nursing care.

The nurse newly entering the cardiovascular unit may be undertaking a special course, in which case a plan of formal instruction will most probably have been drawn up. In addition to this, for those who are gaining clinical experience, a doctor may give some instruction about the patients and their condition, the aims of treatment and what is expected of the nurses. In order that reference to particular patients may be facilitated, this instruction may be given within the unit, or in a room nearby. Such talks could be planned ahead or could be the result of some incident in the unit, an unusual condition, or because a nurse (or nurses) have asked for it. The nurse in charge may be instrumental in arranging it.

Perhaps more important will be caring for the patients alongside more experienced nurses who will pass on their knowledge and skill to the learner. For the experienced nurse who is teaching a newcomer, the following pointers may be helpful:

1. For a skill:
   (*a*) Explain why and how.
   (*b*) Show her how.
   (*c*) Allow her to practice under your supervision.

2. For observations:
   (*a*) Explain why the observation is made.
   (*b*) Show her what to observe, making sure she can observe it.
   (*c*) Allow her to observe, checking it yourself.
3. For clinical knowledge:
   (*a*) Tell her what you know.
   (*b*) Tell her what to find out.
   (*c*) Tell her where to find it.
   (*d*) Ask her what she has learned.

These guiding lines are indeed few. Good relationships between colleagues and working together as a team with the common desire to care for the patient are the basis on which nurses build their ability to learn from each other.

The coronary care unit

The majority of people who die from an acute heart attack do so during the first 72 hours. The coronary care unit is designed to provide the best possible staff, equipment and environment to care for these patients during the period of greatest risk, to prevent complications when possible and to detect and treat them early and effectively when they do occur. With such facilities the mortality and morbidity can be considerably reduced.

The patient's needs

Most of the patients admitted with coronary disease are conscious, anxious and very aware of their surroundings. They need constant observation and monitoring of cardiac rhythm, yet anxiety may be increased by the sight or sound of their own monitor or the apparatus and procedures associated with other patients. Anxiety may provoke cardiac dysrhythmias, and it is by no means unusual to see ventricular extrasystoles appearing on the oscilloscope of one patient who is watching that of another patient whose condition has suddenly deteriorated.

Good basic care is needed, but apart from this and some drug therapy the greatest needs are often observation, rest and reassurance rather than active treatment. However, emergency care may be needed at any time, and there must be staff, equipment and space available for this immediately.

The environment

To fulfil these needs in most well designed units the patients are nursed in single glassed-in cubicles (non-reflective glass) which are light and airy, allowing adequate space and visual contact with the world outside and with staff and the nurses' station. The unit should make an impression of peaceful, pleasant surroundings. The emergency call bell, monitoring and suction apparatus essential for each bed should be placed near the head of the bed so that they are convenient but not obtrusive. Lighting must be variable, so that it is adequate during treatment, but not disturbing to the patient during rest periods. Most patients prefer to be able to see the clock, so that they have some idea of the passage of time.

At the central station the monitor displaying the electrocardiograms of all patients in the unit is observed constantly by medical or nursing staff, so that appropriate action can be taken immediately when necessary. By selecting the 'recording' control an electrocardiography strip is recorded whenever new abnormal rhythms are seen, or at regular intervals. Much of the monitoring equipment now in use not only gives a visual or audible alarm signal (or both) when the heart rate passes the upper or lower limit set for each patient, but also records automatically the ECG rhythm from 15 sec before the alarm sounded. In some units a time clock is automatically started when the alarm sounds.

All requirements for cardiopulmonary resuscitation and the treatment of dangerous dysrhythmias must be immediately available, and it should be remembered that cardiac emergencies do not always occur singly. Some units have a small theatre attached, so that pacemaker catheters can be introduced under sterile conditions with X-ray screening without moving the patient far from the unit.

Privacy is necessary during resuscitation or other procedures so curtains or blinds at the communicating window are necessary.

The staff

It is essential that the coronary care unit should be staffed with enough well trained nursing staff to provide the necessary care and observation for each patient at all times, even when emergency procedures are in progress in one area of the unit. Good teamwork between all members of the unit staff, whatever their function, is vital. Some units have a doctor present at all times; all units must have medical staff readily available. Nevertheless nurses are certainly expected to undertake resuscitation when necessary and may be expected to perform procedures such as the intravenous administration of drugs or defibrillation. In such situations the nurse must be sure that:

1. She is trained and competent to perform the procedure.
2. It is in accordance with the policy of the nursing administration and the employing authority that she should do so.

Most of the nurses' time will be spent, not in dramatic situations, but in giving nursing care and observing and recording the various parameters which indicate the condition of the patient. This demands concentration and accuracy. Anyone engaged solely in watching the monitors must be relieved at least every 2 hours; it is not possible to maintain the same concentration for longer periods.

The nurse is not just a technician, but is important to the patient as a human being who can calm his fears, tell him what is going on and relieve his uneasiness. While performing other nursing tasks, she should establish a relationship which allows him to talk about his anxieties or other things, or remain quiet as he feels inclined. Even within the first few days, the patient may be worrying not only about his present condition, but about his future. Will he be able to support his family? Will he be a complete invalid? The doctor will usually explain the diagnosis, but it often falls to the nurse to help the patient understand it, to explain the importance of treatment ordered and the things to be avoided. Many of the patients with coronary disease are intelligent, active and positive in temperament and hold responsible positions in life. They therefore find it difficult to accept treatment or restrictions without understanding the need for them. Without proper support and teaching they may either disregard advice and treatment completely, or become depressed, anxious, overconcerned about themselves and irritable. This adds to the burden on both patient and family. The nurse can give the necessary psychological support and encouragement and, if the patient is not too ill, help him to lay the foundations for a positive but realistic attitude to his recovery and future life.

Some patients need a radio or light reading matter to stop them becoming bored and more anxious.

When the time for transfer out of the coronary care unit approaches the patient must be encouraged to look on this as a step forward, and given confidence that he will receive all the care and attention he needs after transfer, despite less numerous staff and lack of monitors. In some units monitoring equipment is discontinued for a period before transfer and the patient purposely given a little less attention than previously, so that the transition is not so abrupt. This is especially necessary for longer-term patients, who perhaps have needed treatment for persistent dysrhythmias.

The nurse in the coronary care unit needs to be calm, confident, cheerful and patient, willing and competent to assume the extra responsibilities associated with the work. She must be able to work well and conscientiously in the team when the unit is quiet and the work relatively routine, yet react immediately to work quickly and efficiently when the need arises. Her job satisfaction lies in knowing that she can 'cure sometimes, relieve often, and comfort always' these very ill patients, and that those who need readmission will return with confidence to the place where they have been so well cared for.

Visitors

Many patients want and need the support of their family or close friends during their illness. The family, too, need to see the patient and develop confidence in the staff. Nevertheless too much visiting is very tiring. Usually one or more short visits by a member of the family are allowed during each day. This helps the patient and the family, and allows staff to pass on any necessary information about the patient's progress. The family may make an important contribution to the patient's progress after discharge if they understand how to help and encourage him.

Continuity of nursing care

A recent tendency is to appoint a nurse who is responsible for continuity of care and psychological support of the patient and his family after he has been discharged from the unit. It is essential that she has experience of working in a coronary care unit. She visits the patient while he is in the unit to establish rapport with him, and by contact with the unit nursing staff learns of his condition and treatment. In conjunction with the medical social worker she makes any necessary arrangements circumstances may demand before the patient is discharged. When the patient has returned home, the nurse visits him and his family to answer any queries and to give advice about his condition, treatment and day-to-day activities. Such visits provide an opportunity for the patient and his family to ask those questions which they did not think to ask or did not dare to ask while he was in hospital.

Mobile coronary care units

> Overall mortality from an acute heart is in the region of 40% during the first 4 weeks. Of all deaths during this period at least 40% occur during the first hour, more than 50% within the first 2 hours, and 65% within the first 12 hours. A high proportion of deaths, therefore—60–70% according to several studies—occurs prior to hospitalisation.
>
> Report on Working Group EURO 5020 (2) of the World Health Organization

Mobile coronary care units are an attempt to save at least some of those who die before admission to hospital. In most cases the service consists of a physician specially trained in resuscitation, anaesthetic and electrocardiography techniques, a nurse trained in acute coronary care and an ambulance man to drive the specially equipped ambulance. The team must be able to be on the way to the patient within 3 minutes.

All the requirements for emergency diagnosis and treatment of acute coronary disease are taken to the patient, who is then transferred, as soon as any emergency treatment has been given, to a hospital coronary care unit. It is thus possible to watch for and treat any serious complications during transfer. Usually the doctor and nurse are part of the staff of the hospital unit, so there is continuity of care after admission.

As yet this service is available only in Belfast and Edinburgh in the United Kingdom, in parts of the U.S.S.R. and in a very few other places, thus there is insufficient evidence to show how much it could reduce the overall mortality from coronary disease in a community.

Principles of intensive therapy

The aim of the intensive therapy unit is to provide the best possible staff, equipment and facilities for patients whose good recovery or even survival depend on these things. Unfavourable signs and symptoms will then be observed early, and complications prevented or treated promptly and efficiently, so offering the best chance of success. All members of the staff, including domestic and para-medical staff, must work as a team for the benefit of the patient. Close cooperation and good communication between nursing and medical staff are particularly important and for this reason nurse–doctor relationships are usually relatively informal in these units.

Nursing in a cardiac intensive therapy unit can be very satisfying. It offers the nurse an opportunity to use many of her nursing, technical and personal skills in helping patients through the first difficult days after an operation or in acute cardiac illness.

Care of these patients can be divided into:

1. Observation.
2. Basic nursing and technical care.
3. Care of the patient as an individual.

Observation

Accurate observation and recording of such things as the patient's colour, general condition, arterial and venous pressure, heart rate and rhythm, respiration and fluid balance are essential. These records will indicate whether progress is satisfactory or not, and provide continuity as the patient passes from the care of one person to another. The nurse must learn to interpret them so that she can get help or take action herself when necessary. Many complications can be avoided if the warning signs are observed and prompt action is taken. Electronic monitors can assist but not replace observation by a good nurse.

Basic nursing and technical care

An ill patient needs to be kept clean and comfortable. However, the nurse must use all her skill to give the necessary care to skin, pressure areas, mouth and hair with the minimum disturbance to a very ill patient.

Many of these patients have in situ long arterial or venous cannulae, drainage tubes, pacemaker wires, a catheter and/or an endotracheal tube, each attached to some form of apparatus. It requires foresight and care to move such a patient without disconnecting or interrupting the function of these.

Many nurses are apprehensive when faced with respirators, oscilloscopes or other equipment. It is important that the intensive therapy nurse should learn not necessarily how these things work, but how to use them safely and efficiently as tools to give better care to the patient. This is not usually too difficult; after all even the sphygmomanometer was a strange tool for nurses a few years ago. However, the good nurse constantly uses her eyes and ears, and will notice a disconnected respirator tube or blood leaking back along the arterial line even when taking a blood pressure or talking to medical staff. All equipment must be kept clean and in good repair, and anything which might be needed in emergency must be instantly available. This means frequent and careful checking of equipment.

Accurate administration of drugs, intravenous fluids and other treatment ordered is important and the patient must be watched for side-effects. Adequate nutrition and fluids play an important part in recovery, and need to be given in as suitable and as attractive form as possible.

Cross-infection is always a hazard in the intensive therapy unit. Nursing staff must always be aware of this danger to the patients and must try to avoid it and set a good example to other staff in this respect.

Care of the patient as an individual

Each patient in the intensive therapy unit remains an individual with emotional, social and teaching needs. Pleasant-looking quiet surroundings, a view from the outside world, a clock and privacy when necessary are important to the conscious patient's well-being. These things, plus sufficient space to work efficiently, also reduce stress on the staff, which indirectly benefits the patient. Happy and confident staff who try to discover and fulfil all their patients' needs, to calm their fears and to provide encouragement, are more likely to have happy and confident patients. This makes physical care much easier.

The intensive therapy nurse aims to achieve all this while still allowing the patient adequate rest. She organizes her work calmly and efficiently, ever alert to see and deal with emergency situations. She must be able to realize that many of these patients are very ill, and mature enough to accept that not all of them will recover. The physical, mental and emotional demands on the intensive therapy nurse are considerable at times, but her reward is to see many ill people recover and to know that she has played a vital part in their recovery.

Intensive therapy is specialized work experienced by relatively few nurses. Those engaged in it must be prepared to interpret the work and purpose of the unit to others, and so clear up misunderstandings. It is inevitably expensive in terms of staff and equipment, but this is justified by the recovery of more very ill patients more quickly than can be achieved with ordinary ward resources.

Glossary

Haemodynamic state. The general state of the circulation. The haemodynamic state may be:

1. Adequate, when the pumping action of the heart produces a flow of blood which is sufficient to supply the needs of the tissues.
2. Poor, when the flow is insufficient to supply tissue needs.
3. Good, when there is a reserve which can be used, e.g. during exercise.

Changes in the haemodynamic state are reflected by changes in the arterial and venous pressures and the heart rate. In a patient who is haemodynamically unstable these are all abnormally variable.

Perfusion. The flow of blood (or other fluids) through an area, e.g. with good peripheral perfusion the peripheries (fingers, toes, ears etc.) are pink, warm, and have an obviously good circulation.

'*Peripheral shut-down*'. Inadequate flow through the periphera tissues due to vasoconstriction and/or poor cardiac output. The skin looks pale, and the extremities, including lips, ear-lobes, fingers and toes are cyanosed and cold. This is seen in the 'low cardiac output syndrome'.

Cyanosis. A bluish appearance of the skin or mucous membrane which occurs when there are at least 5 g of reduced haemoglobin/100 ml of blood passing through the area. This means that the lower the haemoglobin level in the blood, the greater must be the oxygen lack before cyanosis appears. Conversely, a polycythaemic patient (with abnormally high haemoglobin level) will become cyanosed more readily.

Central cyanosis results from an increased amount of reduced haemoglobin in the general circulation. This may be due to an inadequate oxygen intake, as may occur in respiratory insufficiency, or to blood from the systemic veins or right heart chambers passing via abnormal communications directly into the systemic arterial system, thus bypassing the lungs. Peripheral cyanosis occurs when blood flows so slowly through the peripheral tissues that a greater percentage of its oxygen is taken up, and the amount of reduced haemoglobin therefore increased. Increasing the circulation through an area, e.g. by rubbing the ear lobe, causes it to become pink for a short period.

Lung compliance. The 'stretchability' of the lungs, and the ease with which they can be expanded (not the elasticity, which is the degree to which they recoil after stretching). For example a patient with pulmonary oedema has poor lung compliance ('stiff lungs') and needs a higher artificial ventilation pressure to achieve a given tidal volume than would a patient with normal lung compliance.

Inotropic. A drug or other substance which produces an inotropic effect increases the contractility of the heart, i.e. the force with which it contracts.

Chronotropic. Something which increases the heart rate is said to be chronotropic.

Mole (mol). A term being used increasingly in chemistry. It expresses a standard number of specified particles, and is the same as the gramme molecular weight (molecular weight in grammes). In the case of an atom (or ion) of potassium, since the atomic weight (or ionic weight) is 39, a mole of potassium will be 39 grammes. A compound such as sodium chloride contains 1 atom of sodium (atomic weight 23) and 1 of chloride (atomic weight 35·5). Therefore the molecular weight of sodium chloride is $23 + 35{\cdot}5 = 58{\cdot}5$, and thus 1 mole of sodium chloride will be 58·5 grammes. The advantage of this scale of measurement is that it can be used for molecules which do not dissociate in water, e.g. glucose (molecular weight 180 g) as well as for electrolytes.

Since the amounts in biochemistry are small the term millimole (1/1000), abbreviated as mmol, is used.

Osmole (osmol). The standard unit of measure of osmotic pressure. Since osmotic pressure depends on the number of particles of solute, 1 mol of potassium exerts 1 osmol, and similarly 1 mol of glucose exerts 1 osmol. However, 1 mol of sodium chloride, by dissociation, present 1 mol of sodium and 1 mol of chloride ions, and thus exerts 2 osmol.

References and further reading

ANDREOLI, K. G. (1968) *Comprehensive Cardiac Care*. St Louis: Mosby.

BAILEY, R. E. (1971) *Pharmacology for Nurses*, 3rd ed. London: Baillière, Tindall & Cassell.

BAIN, W. H. & WATT, J. K. (1970) *Cardiovascular Surgery for Nurses*. London: Livingstone.

BRAIMBRIDGE, M. V. (1972) *Postoperative Cardiac Intensive Care*, 2nd ed. Oxford: Blackwell Scientific.

BUXTON HOPKIN, D. A. (1970) *Anaesthesia, Recovery and Intensive Care*. London: English Universities Press.

CHEST AND HEART ASSOCIATION (1970) *How to Stop Smoking*. London.

CHEST AND HEART ASSOCIATION (1970) *The Human Side of Heart Illness*. London.

CLARK, D. B. & BARNES, A. (1971) *Intensive Care for Nurses*. Oxford: Blackwell Scientific.

DAVIDSON, S. (1971) *Principles and Practice of Medicine*, 10th ed. Edinburgh: Livingstone.

DUNLOP, D., ALSTEAD, S. & MCGREGOR, A. G. (1971) *Textbook of Medical Treatment*, 12th ed. Edinburgh: Livingstone.

EDWARDS, F. R. (1966) *Foundations of Thoracic Surgery*. Edinburgh: Livingstone.

FAMILY WELFARE ASSOCIATION (1971) *Guide to the Social Services*. London.

GREEN, J. H. (1968) *An Introduction to Human Physiology*. London: Oxford University Press.

GREEN, J. H. (1969) *Basic Clinical Physiology*. London: Oxford University Press.

HOBKIRK, J. K. (1970) *Anaesthetics for Nurses*. London: Baillière, Tindall & Cassell.

HUBNER, P. (1971) *Nurses' Guide to Cardiac Monitoring*. London: Baillière, Tindall & Cassell.

JOHNSTON & WHILLIS (1972) *Gray's Anatomy, Descriptive and Applied*, 35th ed. London: Longmans.

JULIAN, D. G. (1970) *Cardiology*. London: Baillière, Tindall & Cassell.

MACLEOD, J. (1966) *Clinical Examination*, 2nd ed. Edinburgh: Livingstone.

MELZER, L. E., PINNEO, R. & KITCHELL, J. R. (1965) *A Manual of Intensive Coronary Care for Nurses*. Philadelphia: C. C. V. Fund, Presbyterian Hospital.

MEREDITH DAVIS, J. B. (1971) *Preventive Medicine, Community Health and the Social Services*. London: Baillière, Tindall & Cassell.

MOLLOY, A. & CHATER-JACK, H. S. M. (1970) *Heart Trouble in the Family*. London: Chest and Heart Association.

NURSING TIMES (1971) *How Drugs Act*. London.

PITORAK, E. F. (1969) *Nurses' Manual of Cardiac Surgery and Nursing Care*. New York: McGraw Hill.

RICHARDS, R. L. (1970) *Peripheral Arterial Disease*. Edinburgh: Livingstone.

ROBERTS, K. & EDWARDS, J. M. (1971) *Paediatric Intensive Care*. Oxford: Blackwell Scientific.

SCHAMROTH, L. (1971) *An Introduction to Electrocardiography*, 4th ed. Oxford: Blackwell Scientific.

SCHAMROTH, L. & SEGAL, F. (1960) *An Introduction to Congenital Heart Disease*. Oxford: Blackwell Scientific.

TROUNCE, J. R. (1970) *Guide to Drugs in Common Use*. Aylesbury: Medical and Technical Publishing.

WILKINSON, A. W. (1968) *Body Fluids in Surgery*, 3rd ed. Edinburgh: Livingstone.

WILLIAMS, H. (1970) *Learning to Live with Angina*. London: Chest and Heart Association.

WRIGHT, S. (1971) *Samson Wright's Applied Physiology*, 12th ed. London: Oxford University Press.

Up to date reading on this subject can also be found in the following publications:

Heart. A quarterly journal published by the British Heart Foundation.

Health. A quarterly journal published by Health Horizons.

On the State of the Public Health. Published annually by the Chief Medical Officer of the Ministry of Health.

Annual Report of the Department of Health and Social Services. Published annually by Her Majesty's Stationery Office.

Index